RADIOGRAPHIC IMAGING & EXPOSURE

FOURTH EDITION

TERRI L. FAUBER, EdD, RT(R)(M)

Associate Professor and Radiography Program Director
Department of Radiation Sciences
School of Allied Health Professions
Virginia Commonwealth University
Richmond, Virginia

with 205 illustrations

ELSEVIER
MOSBY

ELSEVIER
MOSBY

3251 Riverport Lane
St. Louis, Missouri 63043

RADIOGRAPHIC IMAGING & EXPOSURE, FOURTH EDITION   ISBN: 978-0-323-08322-5
Copyright © 2013, 2009, 2004, 2000 by Mosby, an imprint of Elsevier Inc.

Notices

Knowledge and best practice in this field are constantly changing. As new research and experience broaden our understanding, changes in research methods, professional practices, or medical treatment may become necessary.

Practitioners and researchers must always rely on their own experience and knowledge in evaluating and using any information, methods, compounds, or experiments described herein. In using such information or methods they should be mindful of their own safety and the safety of others, including parties for whom they have a professional responsibility.

With respect to any drug or pharmaceutical products identified, readers are advised to check the most current information provided (i) on procedures featured or (ii) by the manufacturer of each product to be administered, to verify the recommended dose or formula, the method and duration of adminis-tration, and contraindications. It is the responsibility of practitioners, relying on their own experience and knowledge of their patients, to make diagnoses, to determine dosages and the best treatment for each individual patient, and to take all appropriate safety precautions.

To the fullest extent of the law, neither the Publisher nor the authors, contributors, or editors, assume any liability for any injury and/or damage to persons or property as a matter of products liability, negligence or otherwise, or from any use or operation of any methods, products, instructions, or ideas contained in the material herein.

Library of Congress Cataloging-in-Publication Data

Fauber, Terri L.
  Radiographic imaging & exposure / Terri L. Fauber. -- 4th ed.
    p. ; cm.
  Radiographic imaging and exposure
  Includes index.
  ISBN 978-0-323-08322-5 (pbk. : alk. paper)
  I. Title. II. Title: Radiographic imaging and exposure.
  [DNLM: 1. Radiography. 2. Radiographic Image Enhancement. WN 200]
  616.07572--dc23   2011040614

Publisher: Jeanne Olson
Associate Developmental Editor: Anne Simon
Publishing Services Managers: Julie Eddy and Hemamalini Rajendrababu
Project Managers: Jan Waters and Srikumar Narayanan
Designer: Ashley Eberts

Printed in the United States of America

Last digit is the print number: 9 8 7 6 5 4 3 2 1

CONTRIBUTORS

James Johnston, PhD, RT(R)(CV)
Associate Professor
Director of Interdisciplinary Education
College of Health Sciences and Human Services
Midwestern State University
Wichita Falls, Texas

Kenneth A. Kraft, PhD, DABR
Associate Professor
Department of Radiology
School of Medicine
Virginia Commonwealth University
Richmond, Virginia

Elizabeth Meixner, MEd, RT(R)(MR)(CT)
Assistant Chair
Department of Radiation Sciences
School of Allied Health Professions
Virginia Commonwealth University
Richmond, Virginia

REVIEWERS

Caroline Burns, MS, RT(R)(M)
Assistant Professor, Industry Professional
St. John's University
Queens, New York

Deanna Butcher, MA, RT(R)
Program Director
St. Cloud Hospital
School of Diagnostic Imaging
St. Cloud, Minnesota

William J. Callaway, MA, RT(R)
Director, Associate Degree Radiography Program
Lincoln Land Community College
Springfield, Illinois

Marilyn H. Carter, BS, RT(R)
Program Coordinator, Radiologic Technology
    Program
Southeast Arkansas College
Pine Bluff, Arkansas

Carolyn L. Cianciosa, MSRT
Radiography Program Director
Niagara County Community College
Sanborn, New York

Mary Doucette, MS, RT(R)(M)(MR)(CT)(QM)
Program Director, Radiology Technology
Great Basin College
Elko, Nevada

Edward J. Goldschmidt, Jr., MS, DABMP, RSO
Radiation Safety Officer, Medical Physicist
Cooper University Hospital
Camden, New Jersey

Clyde R. Hembree, MBA, RT(R)
Program Director
School of Radiography
University of Tennessee Medical Center
Knoxville, Tennessee

Rebecca Keith, MS, RT(R)
Instructor
Northern Virginia Community College
Springfield, Virginia

Deborah Leighty, MEd, RT(R)(BD)
Clinical Coordinator
Hillsborough Community College
Tampa, Florida

Marilyn Maes, MS, RT(R)(MR)
Program Director
Gurnick Academy of Medical Arts
Concord, California

Karen Norris, BS, RT(R)
Interim Program Chair
Mercy College of Health Sciences
Des Moines, Iowa

Stacie (Maier) Smith, RT(R), MHA
Program Director
Holy Cross Hospital
School of Radiologic Technology
Silver Springs, Maryland

Andrew Woodward, MA, RT(R)(CT)(QM)
Assistant Professor
Department of Allied Health Sciences
Division of Radiologic Science
The University of North Carolina at Chapel Hill
Chapel Hill, North Carolina

PREFACE

Radiographic Imaging & Exposure takes a unique and more effective approach to teaching imaging and exposure by focusing on the practical fundamentals. With a topic such as radiographic imaging, it is impossible to depart from theoretic information entirely, and we do not want to do so. A concerted effort was made to present the most important and relevant information on radiographic imaging and exposure. This book highlights the practical application of theoretic information to make it more immediately useful to students and practicing radiographers alike. Our ultimate goal is to provide the knowledge to problem solve effectively to produce quality radiographic images consistently in the clinical environment.

WHO WILL BENEFIT FROM THIS BOOK?

Radiographic Imaging & Exposure provides a fundamental presentation of topics that are vital for students to master to be competent radiographers. Radiographers will also benefit from the practical approach to the topics of imaging and exposure presented here.

ORGANIZATION

Radiographic Imaging & Exposure begins with a description of Wilhelm Conrad Roentgen's discovery of x-rays in 1895 and the excitement it first caused among members of nineteenth-century society, who feared that private anatomy would be exposed for all to see! This introductory chapter moves into the realm of radiologic science with discussions of x-rays as energy and the unique characteristics of x-rays. Chapter 2 provides a more detailed discussion of the x-ray beam. Chapters follow on radiographic image formation and quality (Chapter 3), exposure technique factors (Chapter 4), scatter control (Chapter 5), image receptors and acquisition (Chapter 6), and image processing and display (Chapter 7). Chapter 8 focuses on the tools available to assist the radiographer in selecting appropriate exposure techniques, such as automatic exposure control devices, anatomically programmed radiography, and exposure technique charts. Chapter 9 helps the reader apply previously gained knowledge to evaluate image quality and to identify factors contributing to poor quality and strategies for improvement. Chapter 10 discusses the components of fluoroscopic units, viewing and recording systems, and finally the digital fluoroscopy process in use today.

Radiation exposure and imaging continues to be a complex subject even in the digital age. The most common reason for repeating a radiograph is improper exposure. This text provides a thorough yet practical level of imaging coverage to equip radiographers with the knowledge they need to produce high-quality images on the first attempt.

DISTINCTIVE FEATURES

Radiographic imaging and exposure is a complex topic, and a mastery of the fundamentals is necessary to become competent, whether you are a student or practicing radiographer. Three special features have been integrated within each chapter to facilitate the understanding and retention of the concepts discussed and to underscore their applicability in a clinical setting. These special features also give the practicing radiographer quick visual access to fundamental information that they need every day. Each feature is distinguished by its own icon for easy recognition.

 Important Relationships summarize the relationships being discussed in the text, as each one occurs, for immediate summary and review. The topic of radiographic imaging and exposure is replete with fundamental, important relationships, and they are emphasized in short, meaningful ways at every opportunity.

 Mathematical Applications demonstrate the importance of mathematical formulas. Radiographic imaging also has a strong quantitative component, and this feature helps accustom the reader to the necessity of mastering mathematical formulas. Because the formulas are presented with clinical scenarios, an immediate application and explanation of the formulas is provided.

 Patient Protection Alerts emphasize the imaging and exposure variables that can have an impact on the patient's radiation exposure. Because computer processing can mask exposure errors, it is even more important for radiographers to comprehend how their exposure technique choices can affect the patient.

NEW TO THIS EDITION

Digital imaging content has been fully integrated in this edition of *Radiographic Imaging & Exposure,* and the reader is able to compare and contrast digital and film-screen radiography. Although digital imaging systems improve the consistency in producing quality radiographic images, the radiographer still ultimately controls the amount of radiation exposure to the patient. This responsibility cannot be overemphasized.

The fourth edition of *Radiographic Imaging & Exposure* includes the following:

- Expanded and in-depth coverage of digital imaging, increased coverage of fluoroscopy including digital fluoroscopy, and x-ray beam coverage with added x-ray emission graphs meet ARRT examination content specifications.
- New content on image receptors and image acquisition that focuses on the construction of image receptors and how the latent (invisible) image is captured instructs students on how to acquire, process, and display digital images and informs them of the advantages and limitations of digital versus film-screen imaging processes.
- Chapter 9, *"Image Evaluation,"* gives students the opportunity to apply the knowledge they have gained from earlier chapters by evaluating image quality and practicing problem-solving skills related to exposure technique factors. This practical application enhances learning and builds on the knowledge students have already acquired.

LEARNING AIDS

One of the primary goals of *Radiographic Imaging & Exposure* is to be a practical textbook that prepares student radiographers for the responsibilities of radiographic imaging in a clinical setting. Every effort has been made to make the material easily accessible and understandable while remaining thorough.

- The writing style is straightforward and concise, and the textbook includes numerous features to aid in the mastery of its content, including *Important Relationships, Mathematical Applications,* and *Patient Protection Alerts.*
- All of the *Important Relationships, Mathematical Applications,* and *Patient Protection Alerts* are also collected in separate appendices for quick reference and review, and appendices are organized by chapters.
- *Radiographic Imaging & Exposure* includes traditional learning aids as well. Each chapter begins with a list of objectives and key terms and concludes with a set of multiple-choice review questions, which help readers to evaluate whether they have achieved the chapter's objectives. An answer key is provided in the back of the book.

ANCILLARIES

For the Instructor

Evolve Resources is an interactive learning environment designed to work in coordination with *Radiographic Imaging & Exposure,* 4th edition. It includes laboratory activities, Power Point slides, mathematical worksheets, an image collection of approximately 210 images, two practice tests with 60 questions each, a Test Bank in Exam View with approximately 550 questions, and web links.

The ancillary material on Evolve is useful for both the practiced and the novice educator. The laboratory exercises accommodate different resources and instructor preferences with recommended laboratory activities. Additional mathematical worksheets are included for educators to provide more practice for students if needed.

Instructors may also use Evolve to provide an Internet-based course component that reinforces and expands the concepts presented in class. Evolve may be used to publish the class syllabus, outlines, and lecture notes; set up "virtual office hours" and e-mail communication; share important dates and information through the online class calendar; and encourage student participation through chat rooms and discussion boards. Evolve allows instructors to post exams and manage their grade books online. For more information, visit *http://evolve.elsevier.com,* or contact an Elsevier sales representative.

Study Aids

Mosby's Radiography Online: Radiographic Imaging, 2nd edition, is a multimedia tool that provides an additional resource to help in the mastery of the topics in *Radiographic Imaging & Exposure.* Elsevier has developed multimedia presentations of basic physics, imaging, radiobiology, and radiation protection. These presentations are available online on Evolve and may be purchased separately.

ACKNOWLEDGMENTS

I am delighted and encouraged by the reception of this textbook by the radiography community throughout the years. The evolution of the fourth edition is a result of numerous individuals who have continued their support and provided valuable feedback on the accuracy of its content. I am truly thankful for Jeanne Olson's many years of commitment to this project and her faith in me as an author. Both Anne Simon and Jan Waters have led me through the convoluted path of publication from pre to post production and demonstrated much perseverance, patience, and, most of all, dedication to a quality product.

Educators, students, and colleagues have challenged me to pursue excellence in producing an imaging textbook that is comprehensible, accurate, and relevant to radiographic imaging. I am also indebted to the many authors before me who have explored complex physics concepts in an effort to explain the theory and practice of radiographic imaging. As digital imaging becomes the reality in radiography, the challenges will only continue. I am thankful for all the imaging professionals who accept these challenges and desire to achieve excellence in radiographic imaging.

Terri L. Fauber

CONTENTS

Radiation and Its Discovery

OBJECTIVES

After completing this chapter, the reader will be able to perform the following:

1. Define all the key terms in this chapter.
2. State all the important relationships in this chapter.
3. Describe the events surrounding the discovery of x-rays.
4. Describe the dual nature of x-ray energy.
5. State the characteristics of electromagnetic radiation.
6. List the properties of x-rays.

KEY TERMS

electromagnetic radiation
fluorescence

frequency
photon

quantum
wavelength

X-rays were discovered in Europe in the late nineteenth century by German scientist Dr. Wilhelm Conrad Roentgen. Although Roentgen discovered x-rays by accident, he proceeded to study them so thoroughly that within a very short time, he had identified all of the properties of x-rays that are recognized today. Roentgen was less interested in the practical use of x-rays than in their characteristics as a form of energy. X-rays are classified as a specific type of energy termed *electromagnetic radiation*, but similar to all other types of electromagnetic energy, x-rays act like both waves and particles.

DISCOVERY

X-rays were discovered on November 8, 1895, by Dr. Wilhelm Conrad Roentgen (Figure 1-1), a German physicist and mathematician. Roentgen studied at the Polytechnic Institute in Zurich. He was appointed to the faculty of the University of Würzburg and was the director of the Physical Institute at the time of his discovery. As a teacher and researcher, his academic interest was the conduction of high-voltage electricity through low-vacuum tubes. A low-vacuum tube is simply a glass tube that has had some of the air evacuated from it. The specific type of tube that Roentgen was working with was called a *Crookes tube* (Figure 1-2).

On ending his workday on November 8, Roentgen prepared his research apparatus for the next experimental session to be conducted when he would return to his workplace. He darkened his laboratory to observe the electrical glow (cathode rays) that occurred when the tube was energized. This glow from the tube would indicate that the tube was receiving electricity and was ready for the next experiment. On this day, Roentgen covered his tube with black cardboard and again electrified the tube. By chance, he noticed a faint glow coming from some material located several feet from his electrified tube. The source was a piece of paper coated with barium platinocyanide. Not believing the cathode rays could reach that far from the

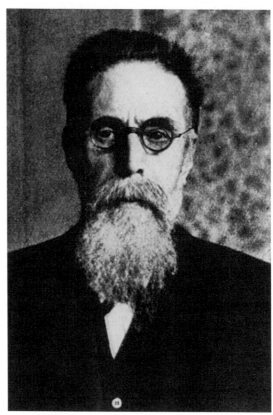

FIGURE 1-1 Dr. Wilhelm Conrad Roentgen.

tube, Roentgen repeated the experiment. Each time Roentgen energized his tube, he observed this glow coming from the barium platinocyanide–coated paper. He understood that energy emanating from his tube was causing this paper to produce light, or fluoresce. *Fluorescence* refers to the instantaneous production of light resulting from the interaction of some type of energy (in this case x-rays) and some element or compound (in this case barium platinocyanide).

Roentgen was understandably excited about this apparent discovery, but he was also cautious not to make any early assumptions about what he had observed. Before sharing information about his discovery with colleagues, Roentgen spent time meticulously investigating the properties of this new type of energy. Of course, this new type of energy was not new at all. It had always existed and was likely produced by Roentgen and his contemporaries who were also involved in experiments with electricity and low-vacuum tubes. Knowing that others were doing similar research, Roentgen worked in earnest to determine just what this energy was.

Roentgen spent the next several weeks working feverishly in his laboratory to investigate as many properties of this energy as he could. He noticed that when he placed his hand between his energized tube and the barium platinocyanide–coated paper, he could see the bones of his hand glow on the paper, with this fluoroscopic image moving as he moved his hand. Curious about this, he produced a static image of his wife Anna Bertha's hand using a 15-minute exposure. This became the world's first radiograph (Figure 1-3). Roentgen gathered other materials and interposed them between his energized tube and the fluorescent paper. Some materials, such as wood, allowed this energy to pass through it and caused the paper to fluoresce. Some, such as platinum, did not.

In December 1895, Roentgen decided that his investigations of this energy were complete enough to inform his physicist colleagues of what he now believed to be a discovery of a new form of energy. He called this energy *x-rays,* with the *x* representing the mathematical symbol of the unknown. On December 28, 1895, Roentgen submitted a scholarly paper on his research activities to his local professional society, the Würzburg Physico-Medical Society. Written in his native German, his article

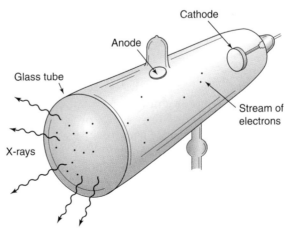

FIGURE 1-2 Crookes tube as used by Roentgen to discover x-rays.

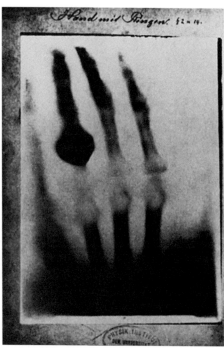

FIGURE 1-3 The first radiograph that demonstrates the bones of the hand of Roentgen's wife, Anna Bertha, with a ring on one finger.

was titled "On a new kind of rays," and it caused a buzz of excitement in the medical and scientific communities. Within a short time, an English translation of this article appeared in the journal *Nature*, dated January 23, 1896.

Roentgen viewed his discovery as an important one, but he also viewed it as one of primarily academic interest. His interest was in the x-ray itself as a form of energy, not in the possible practical uses of it. Others quickly began assembling their own x-ray–producing devices and exposed inanimate objects as well as tissue, both animal and human, both living and dead, to determine the range of use of these x-rays. Their efforts were driven largely by skepticism, not belief that x-rays could do what had been claimed. Skepticism eventually gave way to productive curiosity as investigations concentrated on ways of imaging the living human body for medical benefit.

As investigations into legitimate medical applications of the use of x-rays continued, the nonmedical and nonscientific communities began taking a different view of Roentgen's discovery. X-ray–proof underwear was offered as protection from these rays, which were known to penetrate solid materials. A New Jersey legislator attempted to enact legislation that would ban the use of x-ray–producing devices in opera glasses. Both of these efforts were presumably aimed at protecting one from revealing one's private anatomy to the unscrupulous users of x-rays. The public furor reached such a height that a London newspaper, the *Pall Mall Gazette*, offered the following editorial in 1896: "We are sick of Roentgen rays. Perhaps the best thing would be for all civilized nations to combine to burn all the Roentgen rays, to execute all the discoverers, and to corner all the equipment in the world and to whelm it in the middle of the ocean. Let the fish contemplate each other's bones if they like, but not us."

In a similar vein, but in a more creative fashion, another London newspaper, *Photography,* in 1896 offered the following:

Roentgen Rays, Roentgen Rays?
   What is this craze?
   The town's ablaze
   With this new phase
   Of x-ray ways.
   I'm full of daze, shock and amaze,
   For nowadays
   I hear they'll gaze
   Through cloak and gown and even stays!
   The naughty, naughty Roentgen rays!

Fortunately, the scientific applications of x-rays continued to be investigated for the benefit of society, despite these public distractions. Roentgen's discovery was lauded as one of great significance to science and medicine, and Roentgen received the first Nobel Prize presented for physics in 1901. The branch of medicine that was concerned with using x-rays was called *roentgenology.* A unit of radiation exposure was called the *roentgen.* X-rays were, for a time at least, called *roentgen rays.*

Excitement over this previously undiscovered type of energy was tempered by the realization in 1898 that x-rays could cause biologic damage. This damage was first noticed as a reddening and burning of the skin (called *erythema*) of individuals who were exposed to the large doses of x-rays required at that time. More serious effects, such as the growth of malignant tumors and chromosomal changes, were attributed in later decades to x-ray exposure. Despite these disturbing findings, however, it was also realized that x-rays could be used safely. When radiation protection procedures are followed, which safeguard both radiographer and patient, x-rays assist medical diagnosis by imaging virtually every part of the human body.

X-RAYS AS ENERGY

Energy is the ability to do work and can exist in different forms, such as electrical energy, kinetic energy, thermal energy, and electromagnetic energy. Energy can also be transformed from one form to another. For instance, the electrical energy applied to a stove is changed into heat. The electrical energy applied to an x-ray tube is transformed in to heat and x-rays.

X-radiations, or x-rays, are a type of electromagnetic radiation. *Electromagnetic radiation* refers to radiation that has both electrical and magnetic properties. All radiations that are electromagnetic make up a spectrum (Figure 1-4).

In the academic discipline of physics, energy can generally be described as behaving according to the wave concept of physics or the particle concept of physics. X-rays have a dual nature in that they behave like both waves and particles.

THE ELECTROMAGNETIC SPECTRUM

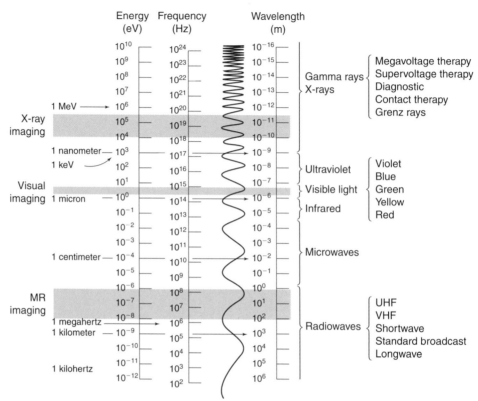

FIGURE 1-4 Electromagnetic spectrum. Radiowaves are the least energetic on the spectrum, and gamma rays are the most energetic.

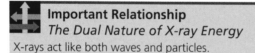

Important Relationship
The Dual Nature of X-ray Energy
X-rays act like both waves and particles.

X-rays can be described as waves because they move in waves that have wavelength and frequency. If a sine wave were to be observed (Figure 1-5), it would be seen that **wavelength** represents the distance between two successive crests or troughs. Wavelength is represented by the Greek letter lambda (λ), and values are given in units of angstroms (Å). An angstrom is a metric unit of length equal to one ten billionth of a meter, or 10^{-10}. X-rays used in radiography range in wavelength from about 0.1 to 1.0 Å. Another unit of measurement for wavelength is nanometer (nm); 1 Å equals 0.1 nm.

The sine wave (Figure 1-5) also demonstrates that **frequency** represents the number of waves passing a given point per given unit of time. Frequency is represented by a lowercase f or by the Greek letter nu (ν), and values are given in units of Hertz (Hz). X-rays used in radiography range in frequency from about 3×10^{19} to 3×10^{18} Hz.

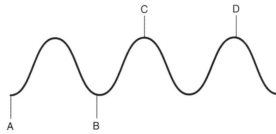

FIGURE 1-5 Sine wave demonstrating wavelength and frequency. One wavelength is equal to the distance between two successive troughs (points *A* to *B*) or the distance between two successive crests (points *C* to *D*).

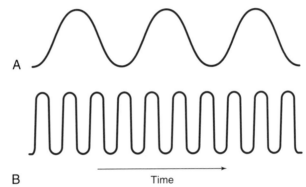

FIGURE 1-6 **A,** Sine wave that demonstrates long wavelength and low frequency. **B,** Sine wave that demonstrates short wavelength and high frequency. Comparison of sine waves **A** and **B** demonstrates the inverse relationship between wavelength and frequency.

Wavelength and frequency are inversely related—that is, as one increases, the other decreases.

Important Relationship
Wavelength and Frequency
Wavelength and frequency are inversely related. Higher-energy x-rays have decreased wavelength and increased frequency. Lower-energy x-rays have increased wavelength and decreased frequency.

This relationship can be observed in Figure 1-6 and is demonstrated by the expression $c = \lambda v$ where *c* represents the speed of light. In this expression, if wavelength increases, frequency must decrease because the speed of light is a constant velocity (3×10^8 m/s or 186,000 miles/s). Conversely, if wavelength decreases, frequency must increase, again because the speed of light is constant. Mathematically, the formulas are $\lambda = c/v$ to solve for wavelength and $v = c/\lambda$ to solve for frequency.

X-rays also behave like particles and move as photons or quanta (plural). A **photon** or **quantum** (singular) is a small, discrete bundle of energy. For most applications in radiography, x-rays are referred to as *photons*. When x-rays interact with matter, they behave more like particles rather than waves. The energy of an individual photon is measured in units of electron volts (eV) and the energy of diagnostic x-rays is approximately between 10^4 and 10^5 eV. Decreasing the wavelength and or increasing the frequency of the x-ray will increase its energy.

PROPERTIES OF X-RAYS

X-rays are known to have several characteristics or properties. These characteristics are briefly explained here and presented in Box 1-1.

- *X-rays are invisible.* In addition to being unable to see x-rays, one cannot feel, smell, or hear them.
- *X-rays are electrically neutral.* X-rays have neither a positive nor a negative charge; they cannot be accelerated or made to change direction by a magnet or electrical field.
- *X-rays have no mass.* X-rays create no resistance to being put into motion and cannot produce force.
- *X-rays travel at the speed of light in a vacuum.* X-rays move at a constant velocity of 3×10^8 m/s or 186,000 miles/s in a vacuum.
- *X-rays cannot be optically focused.* Optical lenses have no ability to focus or refract x-ray photons.
- *X-rays form a polyenergetic or heterogeneous beam.* The x-ray beam that is used in diagnostic radiography is composed of photons that have many different energies. The maximum energy that a photon in any beam may have is expressed by the kilovoltage peak (kVp) that is set on the control panel of the radiographic unit by the radiographer.
- *X-rays can be produced in a range of energies.* These are useful for different purposes in diagnostic radiography. The medically useful diagnostic range of x-ray energies is 30 to 150 kVp.

BOX 1-1	Characteristics of X-rays

Are invisible
Are electrically neutral
Have no mass
Travel at the speed of light in a vacuum
Cannot be optically focused
Form a polyenergetic or heterogeneous beam
Can be produced in a range of energies
Travel in straight lines
Can cause some substances to fluoresce
Cause chemical changes in radiographic and photographic film
Can penetrate the human body
Can be absorbed or scattered in the human body
Can produce secondary radiation
Can cause damage to living tissue

- *X-rays travel in straight lines.* X-rays used in diagnostic radiography form a divergent beam in which each individual photon travels in a straight line.
- *X-rays can cause some substances to fluoresce.* When x-rays strike some substances, those substances produce light. These substances are used in diagnostic radiography, such as image receptors.
- *X-rays cause chemical changes to occur in radiographic and photographic film.* X-rays are capable of causing images to appear on radiographic film and are capable of fogging photographic film.
- *X-rays can penetrate the human body.* X-rays have the ability to pass through the body, based on the energy of the x-rays and on the composition and thickness of the tissues being exposed.
- *X-rays can be absorbed or scattered by tissues in the human body.* Depending on the energy of an individual x-ray photon, that photon may be absorbed in the body or be made to scatter, moving in another direction.
- *X-rays can produce secondary radiation.* When x-rays are absorbed as a result of a specific type of interaction with matter (photoelectric effect), a secondary or characteristic photon is produced.
- *X-rays can cause chemical and biologic damage to living tissue.* Through excitation and ionization (removal of electrons) of atoms comprising cells, damage to the cells can occur.

Since the publication of Roentgen's scientific paper, no other properties of x-rays have been discovered. However, the discussion of x-rays has expanded far beyond the early concerns about modesty or even danger. Today x-rays are accepted as an important diagnostic tool in medicine, and the radiographer is an important member of the health care team. The radiographic imaging professional is responsible for the care of the patient in the radiology department, the production and control of x-rays, and the formation of the radiographic image. Figure 1-7 shows a standard radiographic room that includes the x-ray table, overhead x-ray tube and collimator, and control panel for selection of exposure technique factors. The subsequent chapters of this book uncover the intricate and fascinating details of the art and science of medical radiography.

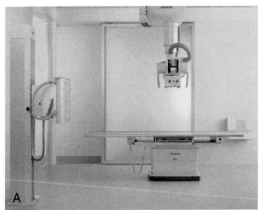
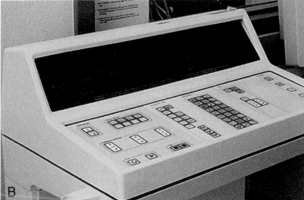

FIGURE 1-7 **A,** Typical radiographic unit showing the x-ray table, overhead x-ray tube, and collimator. **B,** Control panel.

CHAPTER SUMMARY

- X-rays were discovered on November 8, 1895, by Dr. Wilhelm Conrad Roentgen, a German physicist, mathematician, and recipient of the first Nobel Prize for physics.
- The discovery of x-rays was met with skepticism and curiosity and subsequently acceptance of its medical benefit.
- X-rays are a type of electromagnetic radiation with both electrical and magnetic properties.
- Electromagnetic radiation is a form of energy that moves in waves that have wavelength and frequency.
- Wavelength and frequency are inversely related. Higher-energy x-rays have decreased wavelength and increased frequency.
- X-rays act like both waves and particles and have higher energy than other types of electromagnetic radiation, such as visible light.
- X-rays have several important characteristics: They are invisible and electrically neutral, have no mass, travel at the speed of light, penetrate matter, and can cause chemical and biologic changes.

REVIEW QUESTIONS

1. In what year were x-rays discovered?
   A. 1892
   B. 1895
   C. 1898
   D. 1901

2. In what year were some of the biologically damaging effects of x-rays discovered?
   A. 1892
   B. 1895
   C. 1898
   D. 1901

3. X-rays were discovered in experiments dealing with electricity and _____.
   A. ionization
   B. magnetism
   C. atomic structure
   D. vacuum tubes

4. X-rays were discovered when they caused a barium platinocyanide–coated plate to _____.
   A. fluoresce
   B. phosphoresce
   C. vibrate
   D. burn and redden

5. X-radiation is part of which spectrum?
A. Radiation
B. Energy
C. Atomic
D. Electromagnetic

6. X-rays have a dual nature, which means that they behave like both
_____.
A. atoms and molecules
B. photons and quanta
C. waves and particles
D. charged and uncharged particles

7. The wavelength and frequency of x-rays are _____ related.
A. directly
B. inversely
C. partially
D. not

8. X-rays have _____ electrical charge.
A. a positive
B. a negative
C. an alternately positive and negative
D. no

9. X-rays have _____.
A. no mass
B. the same mass as electrons
C. the same mass as protons
D. the same mass as neutrons

10. The x-ray beam used in diagnostic radiography can be described as being
_____.
A. homogeneous
B. monoenergetic
C. polyenergetic
D. scattered

The X-ray Beam

CHAPTER OUTLINE

OBJECTIVES

After completing this chapter, the reader will be able to perform the following:

1. Define all the key terms in this chapter.
2. State all the important relationships in this chapter.
3. Describe construction of the x-ray tube.
4. State the function of each component of the x-ray tube.
5. Describe how x-rays are produced.
6. Explain the role of the primary exposure factors in determining the quality and quantity of x-rays.
7. Explain the line focus principle.
8. State how the anode heel effect can be used in radiography.
9. Differentiate among the types of filtration and explain their purpose.
10. Calculate heat units.
11. Recognize how changing generator output, kVp, mA, and filtration affect the x-ray emission spectrum.
12. List the guidelines followed to extend the life of an x-ray tube.

KEY TERMS

actual focal spot size
added filtration
anode
anode heel effect
bremsstrahlung interactions
cathode
characteristic interactions
compensating filter
dosimeter
effective focal spot size
exposure time
filament

filament current
focusing cup
half-value layer (HVL)
heat unit (HU)
inherent filtration
kilovoltage
leakage radiation
line focus principle
milliamperage
off-focus radiation
rotor
space charge

space charge effect
stator
target
thermionic emission
total filtration
trough filter
tube current
voltage ripple
wedge filter
x-ray emission spectrum

The x-ray tube is the most important part of the x-ray machine because the tube is where the x-rays are produced. Radiographers must understand how the x-ray tube is constructed and how to operate it. The radiographer controls many of the actions that occur within the tube. Kilovoltage peak (kVp), milliamperage (mA), and exposure time all are factors that the radiographer selects on the control panel to produce a quality image. The radiographer also needs to be aware of the amount of heat that is produced during x-ray production because excessive heat can damage the tube.

X-RAY PRODUCTION

The production of x-rays requires a rapidly moving stream of electrons that are suddenly decelerated or stopped. The source of electrons is the cathode, or negative electrode. The negative electrode is heated, and electrons are emitted. The electrons are attracted to the anode, move rapidly toward the positive electrode, and are stopped or decelerated. When the kinetic energy of the electrons is transferred to the anode, x-rays and heat are produced.

Cathode

The **cathode** of an x-ray tube is a negatively charged electrode. It comprises a **filament** and a **focusing cup.** Figure 2-1 shows a double-filament cathode surrounded by a focusing cup. The **filament** is a coiled tungsten wire that is the source of electrons during x-ray production.

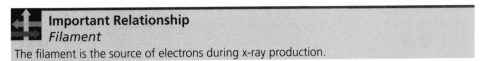

Important Relationship
Filament
The filament is the source of electrons during x-ray production.

Most x-ray tubes are referred to as *dual-focus tubes* because they have two filaments: a large filament and a small filament. Only one filament is energized at any one time during x-ray production. If the radiographer selects a large focal spot when

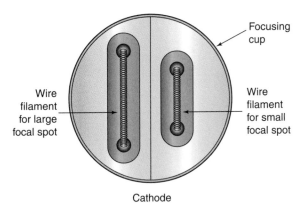

Focusing cup

Wire filament for large focal spot

Wire filament for small focal spot

Cathode

FIGURE 2-1 Most x-ray tubes use a small filament and a large filament, corresponding with a small focal spot size and a large focal spot size, respectively.

setting the control panel, the large filament is energized. If a small focal spot is chosen, the small filament is energized. The **focusing cup** is made of nickel and nearly surrounds the filament. It is open at one end to allow electrons to flow freely across the tube from cathode to anode. It has a negative charge, which keeps the cloud of electrons emitted from the filament from spreading apart. Its purpose is to focus the stream of electrons.

Anode

The **anode** of an x-ray tube is a positively charged electrode composed of molybdenum, copper, tungsten, and graphite. These materials are used for their thermal and electrical conductive properties. The anode consists of a **target** and, in rotating anode tubes, a **stator** and **rotor**. The **target** is a metal that abruptly decelerates and stops electrons in the tube current, allowing the production of x-rays. The target can be either rotating or stationary. Tubes with rotating targets are more common than tubes with stationary ones. Rotating anodes are manufactured to rotate at a set speed ranging from 3000 to 10,000 revolutions per minute (RPM). Figure 2-2 shows how a rotating anode and stationary anode differ in appearance.

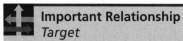

> **Important Relationship**
> *Target*
> The target is the part of the anode that is struck by the focused stream of electrons coming from the cathode. The target stops the electrons and creates the opportunity for the production of x-rays.

The target of rotating anode tubes is made of a tungsten and rhenium alloy. This layer, or track, is embedded in a base of molybdenum and graphite (Figure 2-3). Tungsten generally makes up 90% of the composition of the rotating target, with rhenium making up the other 10%. The face of the anode is angled to help the x-ray photons exit the tube. Rotating targets generally have a target angle ranging from 5 to 20 degrees. Tungsten is used in both rotating and stationary targets because it has a high atomic number of 74 for efficient x-ray production and a high melting point of 3400° C (6152° F). Most of the energy produced by an x-ray tube is heat, so melting of the target can sometimes become a problem, especially with high exposures.

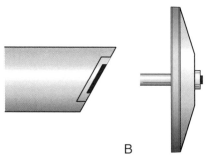

A   B

FIGURE 2-2 Side views of a stationary anode (**A**) and a rotating anode (**B**).

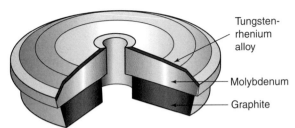

FIGURE 2-3 Typical construction of a rotating anode.

In order to turn the anode during x-ray production, a rotating anode tube requires a stator and rotor (Figure 2-4). The **stator** is an electric motor that turns the rotor at very high speed. The **rotor (made of copper)** is rigidly connected to the target through the anode stem (made of molybdenum), causing the target to rotate rapidly during x-ray production. High-strength ball bearings in the rotor allow it to rotate smoothly at high speeds.

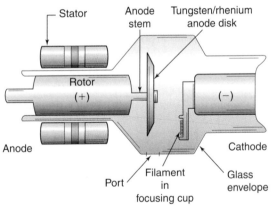

FIGURE 2-4 Structure of a typical x-ray tube, including the major operational parts.

During x-ray production, most of the energy produced at the anode is heat, with x-ray energy being a very small percentage. Heat can pose a problem if allowed to build up, so it is transferred to the envelope and then to the insulating oil surrounding the tube. Many tube assemblies also have a fan that blows air over the tube to help dissipate heat.

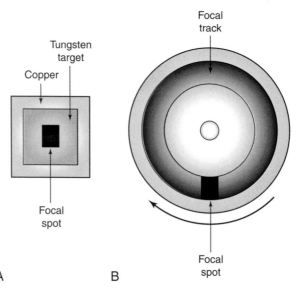

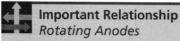

FIGURE 2-5 A, Front view of a stationary anode. **B,** The target area of the rotating anode turns during exposure, and there is an increased physical area—a focal track—that is exposed to electrons.

Rotating anodes can withstand high heat loads. The ability to withstand high heat loads relates to the actual **focal spot,** which is the physical area of the target that is bombarded by electrons during x-ray production. With stationary targets, the focal spot is a fixed area on the surface of the target. With rotating targets, this area is represented by a focal track. Figure 2-5 shows the stationary anode's focal spot and the rotating anode with its focal track. The size of the focal spot is not altered with a rotating anode, but the actual physical area of the target bombarded by electrons is constantly changing, causing a greater area—a focal track—to be exposed to electrons. Because of the larger area of the target being bombarded during an exposure, the rotating anode is able to withstand higher heat loads produced by greater exposure factors. Rotating anode x-ray tubes are used in all applications in radiography, whereas stationary anode tubes are limited to studies of small anatomic structures such as the teeth.

> **Important Relationship**
> *Rotating Anodes*
> Rotating anodes can withstand higher heat loads than stationary anodes because the rotation causes a greater physical area, or focal track, to be exposed to electrons.

X-ray Tube Housing

The components necessary for x-ray production are housed in a glass or metal envelope. Figure 2-6 shows the appearance of a glass x-ray tube. Metal envelopes are more commonly used because of their improved electrical properties.

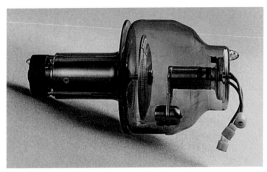

FIGURE 2-6 A glass envelope x-ray tube as it appears before installation in a tube housing.

A disadvantage of a glass envelope x-ray tube is that tungsten evaporated from the filament during exposure can deposit on the inside of the glass, especially in the middle portion of the envelope. This evaporation could affect the flow of electrons and cause the tube to fail. Replacing all of this section of glass with metal prevents these problems and extends the tube life. An additional advantage of a metal envelope is the reduction of **off-focus radiation. Off-focus radiation** occurs when projectile electrons are reflected and x-rays are produced from outside the focal spot. The metal tube envelope can collect these electrons and conduct them away from the anode.

The envelope allows air to be evacuated completely from the x-ray tube, which allows the efficient flow of electrons from cathode to anode. The envelope serves two additional functions: It provides some insulation from electrical shock that may occur because the cathode and anode contain electrical charges, and it dissipates heat in the tube by conducting it to the insulating oil that surrounds the envelope. The purpose of insulating oil is to provide more insulation from electrical shock and to help dissipate heat away from the tube. All of these components are surrounded by metal tube housing except for a port, or window, which allows the primary beam to exit the tube. It is the metal tube housing that the radiographer sees and handles when moving the x-ray tube. The tube housing is lined with lead to provide additional shielding from leakage radiation. **Leakage radiation** refers to any x-rays, other than the primary beam, that escape the tube housing. The tube housing is required to allow no more than 100 mR/hr of leakage radiation to escape when measured at 1 m from the source while the tube operates at maximum output. Electrical current is supplied to the x-ray tube by means of two high-voltage cables that enter the top of the tube assembly.

TARGET INTERACTIONS

The electrons that move from the cathode to the anode travel extremely fast, approximately half the speed of light. The moving electrons, which have kinetic energy, strike the target and interact with the tungsten atoms in the anode to produce x-rays.

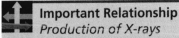

Important Relationship
Production of X-rays
As electrons strike the target, their kinetic energy is transferred to the tungsten atoms in the anode to produce x-rays.

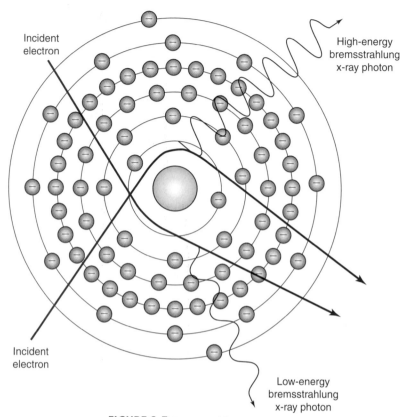

Incident
electron

High-energy
bremsstrahlung
x-ray photon

Incident
electron

Low-energy
bremsstrahlung
x-ray photon

FIGURE 2-7 Bremsstrahlung interaction.

These interactions occur within the top 0.5 mm of the anode surface. Two types of interactions produce x-ray photons: **bremsstrahlung interactions** and **characteristic interactions.**

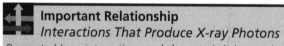

Important Relationship
Interactions That Produce X-ray Photons
Bremsstrahlung interactions and characteristic interactions both produce x-ray photons.

Bremsstrahlung Interactions

Bremsstrahlung is a German word meaning "braking" or "slowing down radiation." **Bremsstrahlung interactions** occur when a projectile electron completely avoids the orbital electrons of the tungsten atom and travels very close to its nucleus. The very strong electrostatic force of the nucleus causes the electron suddenly to "slow down." As the electron loses energy, it suddenly changes its direction, and the energy loss then reappears as an x-ray photon (Figure 2-7).

In the diagnostic energy range, most x-ray interactions are bremsstrahlung. The diagnostic energy range is 30 to 150 kVp. At less than 70 kVp (with a tungsten target), 100% of the x-ray beam consists of bremsstrahlung interactions. At greater than 70 kVp, approximately 85% of the beam consists of bremsstrahlung interactions.

> **Important Relationship**
> *Bremsstrahlung Interactions*
> Most x-ray interactions in the diagnostic energy range are bremsstrahlung.

Characteristic Interactions

Characteristic interactions are produced when a projectile electron interacts with an electron from the inner shell (K-shell) of the tungsten atom. The electron must have enough energy to eject the K-shell electron from its orbit. K-shell electrons in tungsten have the strongest binding energy at 69.5 keV. For a projectile electron to

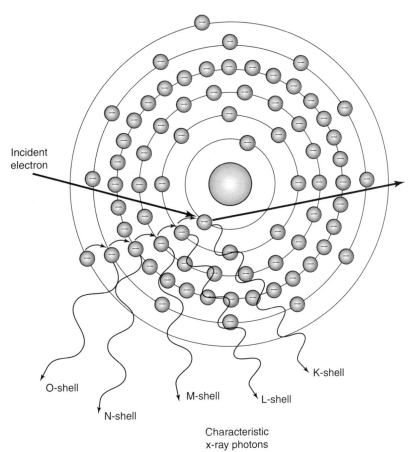

FIGURE 2-8 Characteristic interaction.

remove this orbital electron, it must possess energy equal to or greater than 69.5 keV. When the K-shell electron is ejected from its orbit, an outer-shell electron drops into the open position and creates an energy difference. The energy difference is emitted as an x-ray photon (Figure 2-8). Electrons from the L-, M-, O-, and P-shells of the tungsten atom are also ejected from their orbits. However, the photons created from these interactions have very low energy and, depending on filtration, may not even reach the patient. K-shell characteristic x-rays have an average energy of approximately 69 keV; therefore, they contribute significantly to the useful x-ray beam. At less than 70 kVp (with a tungsten target), no characteristic x-rays are present in the beam. At greater than 70 kVp, approximately 15% of the beam consists of characteristic x-rays. X-rays produced through these interactions are termed ***characteristic x-rays*** because their energies are characteristic of the tungsten target element.

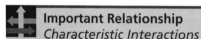
Important Relationship
Characteristic Interactions
Characteristic x-rays can be produced in a tungsten target only when the kVp is set at 70 or greater because the binding energy of the K-shell electron is 69.5 keV.

To summarize, when bremsstrahlung and characteristic interactions are compared, most x-ray interactions produced in diagnostic radiology result from bremsstrahlung. There is no difference between a bremsstrahlung x-ray and a characteristic x-ray at the same energy level; they are simply produced by different processes.

X-RAY EMISSION SPECTRUM

X-ray energy is measured in kiloelectron-volts (keV) (1000 electron volts). The x-ray beam is polyenergetic (many energies) and consists of a wide range of energies known as the **x-ray emission spectrum**. The lowest energies are always approximately 15 to 20 keV, and the highest energies are always equal to the kVp set on the control

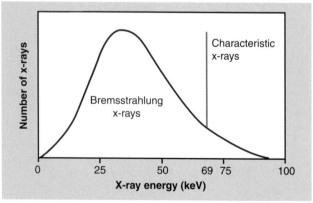

FIGURE 2-9 An 80-kVp x-ray emission spectrum from a tungsten target. Most x-rays occur between 30 keV and 40 keV. Characteristic x-ray energies are discrete and are represented by the line at 69 keV.

panel. For example, an 80-kVp x-ray exposure technique produces x-ray energies ranging from 15 to 80 keV (Figure 2-9). The smallest number of x-rays occurs at the extreme low and high ends of the spectrum. The greatest number of x-ray energies occurs between 30 keV and 40 keV for an 80-kVp exposure. The **x-ray emission spectrum,** or the range and intensity of x-rays emitted, changes with different exposure technique settings on the control panel.

X-RAY EXPOSURE

A radiographic exposure is produced by a radiographer using two switches located on the control panel of the x-ray unit. These are sometimes combined into a single switching device that has two levels of operation corresponding with the rotor preparation and x-ray exposure. In either case, the switches that are used to make an x-ray exposure are considered *deadman switches*. Deadman switches require positive pressure to be applied during the entire x-ray exposure process. If the radiographer lets off of either switch, releasing positive pressure, the exposure process is immediately terminated.

The first switch is usually called the *rotor,* or *prep button,* and the second switch is usually called the *exposure,* or *x-ray button.* The activation of the exposure switch by the radiographer produces specific reactions inside the x-ray tube. The rotor must be activated before the x-ray exposure is activated to produce an x-ray exposure properly.

Pushing the rotor, or prep button, causes an electrical current to be induced across the filament in the cathode. This **filament current** is approximately 3 to 5 amps and operates at about 10 V. The amount of current flowing through the filament depends on the mA set at the control panel. The **filament current** heats the tungsten filament. This heating of the filament causes thermionic emission to occur. **Thermionic emission** refers to the boiling off of electrons from the filament.

Important Relationship
Thermionic Emission
When the tungsten filament gains enough heat *(therm),* the outer-shell electrons *(ions)* of the filament atoms are boiled off, or emitted, from the filament.

The electrons liberated from the filament during thermionic emission form a cloud around the filament called the **space charge.** This term is descriptive because there is an actual negative charge from these electrons that exists in space around the filament. **Space charge effect** refers to the tendency of the space charge not to allow more electrons to be boiled off of the filament. The focusing cup, with its own negative charge, forces the electrons in the space charge to remain together.

By pushing the rotor, or prep button, the radiographer also activates the stator that drives the rotor and rotating target (Box 2-1). While thermionic emission is occurring and the space charge is forming, the stator starts to turn the anode, accelerating it to top speed in preparation for x-ray production. If an exposure could be made before the target is up to speed, the heat produced would be too great for the slowly rotating target, causing serious damage. The machine does not allow the exposure to occur until the target is up to full speed, even if the exposure switch is activated. The radiographer can press the rotor and exposure switches one after the other, and the machine makes the exposure as soon as it is ready, with no damage to the tube. It takes only a few seconds for the space charge to be produced and for the rotating target to reach its top speed (Figure 2-10).

BOX 2-1 | Preparing the Tube for Exposure

When the rotor, or prep button, is activated:

On the Cathode Side of the X-ray Tube
1. Filament current heats up the filament.
2. This heat boils electrons off the filament (thermionic emission).
3. These electrons gather in a cloud around the filament (space charge).
4. The negatively charged focusing cup keeps the electron cloud focused together.
5. The number of electrons in the space charge is limited (space charge effect).

On the Anode Side of the X-ray Tube
1. The rotating target begins to turn rapidly, quickly reaching top speed.

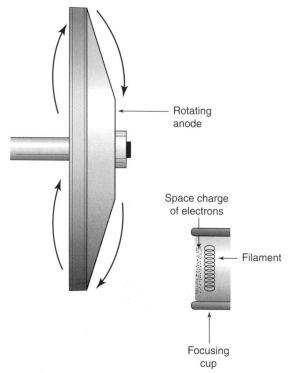

Rotating anode

Space charge of electrons

Filament

Focusing cup

FIGURE 2-10 When the radiographer activates the rotor, or prep button, a filament current is induced across the filament, causing electrons to be burned off and gather in a cloud around the filament. At the same time, the rotating anode begins to turn.

BOX 2-2 | **Making an X-ray Exposure**

After activation of the rotor and the exposure is initiated:

On the Cathode Side of the X-ray Tube
1. High negative charge strongly repels electrons.
2. These electrons stream away from the cathode and toward the anode (tube current).

On the Anode Side of the X-ray Tube
1. High positive charge strongly attracts electrons in the tube current.
2. These electrons strike the anode.
3. X-rays and heat are produced.

When the radiographer pushes the exposure, or x-ray, button, the x-ray exposure begins (Box 2-2). The kVp level, which depends on the actual kVp value set on the control panel by the radiographer, is applied across the tube from cathode to anode. This creates potential difference, and the cathode becomes highly negatively charged, strongly repelling the also negatively charged electrons. The anode becomes positively charged, strongly attracting the electrons.

Electrons that comprised the space charge now flow quickly from cathode to anode in a current. **Tube current** refers to the flow of electrons from cathode to anode and is measured in units called *milliamperes* (mA). It is important to note that electrons flow in only one direction in the x-ray tube—from cathode to anode.

Important Relationship
Tube Current
Electrons flow in only one direction in the x-ray tube—from cathode to anode. This flow of electrons is called the *tube current* and is measured in milliamperes (mA).

As these electrons strike the anode target, they are converted to either x-rays or heat. In other words, an energy conversion occurs. The kinetic energy of the moving electrons is changed to electromagnetic energy (x-rays) and thermal energy (heat). Most of the electrons in the tube current (approximately 99%) are converted to heat, whereas only 1% (approximately) of these electrons are converted to x-rays. These events are illustrated in Figure 2-11.

Important Relationship
Energy Conversion in the X-ray Tube
As electrons strike the anode target, approximately 99% of their kinetic energy is converted to heat, whereas only 1% (approximately) of their energy is converted to x-rays.

X-RAY QUALITY AND QUANTITY

The radiographer initiates and controls the production of x-rays. Manipulating the prime exposure factors on the control panel (kVp, mA, and exposure time) allows both the quantity and the quality of the x-ray beam to be altered. The quantity of

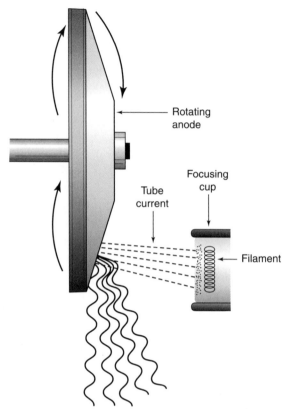

FIGURE 2-11 After activation of the rotor and the exposure is initiated, a high voltage, or kilovoltage, is applied across the tube, making the cathode highly negative and the anode highly positive. Electrons are repelled from the cathode side and attracted to the anode side. The negatively charged focusing cup focuses the electrons into a stream, and they quickly cross the tube gap in a tube current. Electrons interacting with the target are converted into x-rays and heat.

the x-ray beam indicates the number of x-ray photons in the primary beam, and the quality of the x-ray beam indicates its penetrating power. Knowledge of the prime exposure factors and their effect on the production of x-rays assists the radiographer in producing quality radiographs.

Kilovoltage

The **kilovoltage** (kVp) that is set by the radiographer and applied across the x-ray tube at the time the exposure is initiated determines the speed at which the electrons in the tube current move.

 Important Relationship
Kilovoltage and the Speed of Electrons
The speed of the electrons traveling from the cathode to the anode increases as the kilovoltage applied across the x-ray tube increases.

Selecting a higher voltage results in greater repulsion of electrons from the cathode and greater attraction of electrons toward the anode. The speed at which the electrons in the tube current move determines the quality or energy of the x-rays that are produced. The higher the energy of the x-ray photon, the greater the penetrability, or ease with which it moves through tissue. Whether addressing the x-ray photons themselves or the primary beam, *quality* refers to the energy level of the radiation (Box 2-3).

Important Relationship
Speed of Electrons and Quality of X-rays
The speed of the electrons in the tube current determines the quality or energy of the x-rays that are produced. The quality or energy of the x-rays that are produced determines the penetrability of the primary beam.

Important Relationship
kVp and Beam Penetrability
As kVp increases, beam penetrability increases; as kVp decreases, beam penetrability decreases.

In addition to kVp having an effect on the quality of x-ray photons produced, kVp also has an effect on the quantity or number of x-ray photons produced (Figure 2-12). Increased kVp results in more x-rays being produced because increased kVp

BOX 2-3	kVp and X-ray Quality

1. Higher kVp results in electrons that move faster in the tube current from cathode to anode.
2. The faster the movement of the electrons in the tube current the greater the energy of the x-rays produced.
3. The greater the energy of x-rays produced, the greater the penetrability of the primary beam.
4. The quality of the x-ray beam refers to its energy level, so adjusting the kVp affects the quality of the x-ray beam.

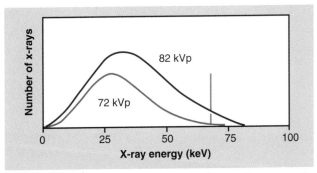

FIGURE 2-12 Increasing the kVp from 72 to 82 shows an increase in the quantity of x-rays (amplitude), and the x-ray emission shifts toward the right, indicating an increase in the energy or quality of the beam.

increases the efficiency of x-ray production. (Box 2-4 describes quality control methods for evaluating kilovoltage accuracy.)

In order to provide sufficient potential difference (kVp) to allow x-ray production, a generator is required to convert low voltage (volts) to high voltage (kilovolts). Three basic types of x-ray generators are available: single phase, three phase, and high frequency. Each generator produces a different voltage waveform (Figure 2-13). These waveforms are a reflection of the consistency of the voltage supplied to the x-ray tube during an x-ray exposure. The term **voltage ripple** describes voltage waveforms in terms of how much the voltage varies during x-ray production. From Figure 2-13 it can be seen that for single-phase generation, voltage varies from the peak to a value of zero. Voltage ripple for single-phase generators is said to be 100% because there is total variation in the voltage waveform, from peak voltage to zero voltage. For three-phase generators, voltage ripple is 13% for 6-pulse and 4% for 12-pulse. High-frequency generators produce a voltage ripple of less than 1%. Voltage used in the x-ray tube is the most consistent with high-frequency generators. The more consistent the voltage applied to the x-ray tube throughout the exposure, the greater the quantity and energy level (quality) of the x-ray beam. Figure 2-14 shows x-ray emission for different types of generators.

BOX 2-4 | Quality Control Check: Kilovoltage Accuracy

- X-ray quality can be affected if the actual kilovoltage used is inaccurate.
  A digital kVp meter measures the actual kilovoltage, and a Wisconsin Test Cassette estimates the kilovoltage by measuring densities (blackness) produced on a film.
- The maximum variability of the kilovoltage is ±5%.

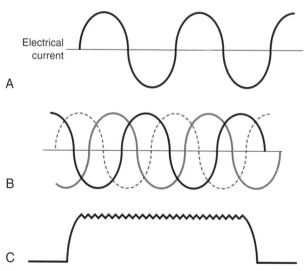

FIGURE 2-13 Voltage waveforms produced by various x-ray generators. **A,** Single phase. **B,** Three phase. **C,** High frequency.

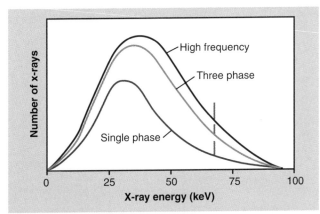

FIGURE 2-14 The quantity (amplitude) and the quality (shift to the right) of the x-ray beam are increased when using high-frequency and three-phase generators because they are more efficient in x-ray production.

BOX 2-5	mA and X-ray Quantity

1. Higher mA results in more electrons that move in the tube current from cathode to anode.
2. The more electrons in the tube current, the more x-rays produced.
3. The number of x-rays that are produced is directly proportional to the mA.

Milliamperage

Milliamperage (mA) is the unit used to measure the tube current. Tube current is the number of electrons flowing per unit time between the cathode and anode. For example, at 200 mA, there is a specific amount of current applied to the filament, causing a certain amount of thermionic emission. Based on the amount of thermionic emission, there is a space charge consisting of a certain number of electrons; 200 mA indicates the number of electrons (based on the space charge) flowing in the tube per second. Generally, changing to the 400-mA station on the control panel causes twice as much thermionic emission, twice as big a space charge, and twice as many electrons to flow per second. The milliamperage that is set by the radiographer determines the number of electrons flowing in the tube and the quantity of x-rays produced (Box 2-5). The quantity of electrons in the tube current is directly proportional to the milliamperage. If the milliamperage increases, the quantity of electrons and the quantity of x-rays increase proportionally. If the milliamperage decreases, the quantity of electrons and the quantity of x-rays decrease by the same proportion. Milliamperage does not affect the quality, or energy, of the x-rays produced (Figure 2-15).

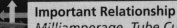

Important Relationship
Milliamperage, Tube Current, and X-ray Quantity
The quantity of electrons in the tube current and quantity of x-rays produced are directly proportional to the milliamperage.

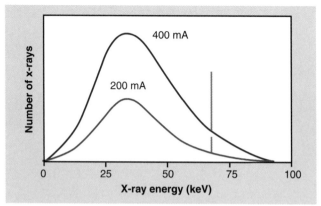

FIGURE 2-15 Changing the mA results in a proportional change in the quantity (amplitude) of x-rays produced.

Exposure Time

Exposure time determines the length of time that the x-ray tube produces x-rays. The exposure time set by the radiographer can be expressed in seconds or milliseconds, as either a fraction or a decimal. This exposure time determines the length of time that the tube current is allowed to flow from cathode to anode. The longer the exposure time, the greater the quantity of electrons that flow from the cathode to the anode and the greater the quantity of x-rays produced (Box 2-6). For example, if 400 mA at an exposure time of 0.25 second produces 5000 x-rays, then doubling the exposure time to 0.50 second at 400 mA would produce 10,000 x-rays. Changes in exposure time produce the same effect on the number of x-rays produced as do changes in milliamperage. (Box 2-7 describes quality control methods for evaluating exposure timer accuracy.)

BOX 2-6 | **Exposure Time and X-ray Quantity**

1. Longer exposure time results in more electrons that move in the tube current from cathode to anode.
2. The more electrons in the tube current, the more x-rays produced.
3. The number of x-rays that are produced is directly proportional to the exposure time.

BOX 2-7 | **Quality Control Check: Exposure Timer Accuracy**

- X-ray quantity can be affected if the actual exposure time used is inaccurate. A digital timer device measures the actual exposure time. A synchronous spinning top test device estimates the actual time by measuring the density (blackness) arc produced on film with a timer protractor or by counting the number of black dots expected for the type of x-ray generator.
- The maximum variability of the exposure timer is ±5% for times >10 ms and ±10% for times <10 ms.

>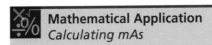
> **Important Relationship**
> *Exposure Time, Tube Current, and X-ray Quantity*
> The quantity of electrons that flows from cathode to anode and the quantity of x-rays produced are directly proportional to the exposure time.

Milliamperage and Time

When milliamperage is multiplied by exposure time, the result is known as *mAs*, which the radiographer may be able to set at the control panel. Mathematically, mAs is simply expressed as follows: mA × s = mAs, where *s* represents exposure time in fractions of a second (as actual fractions or in decimal form) or in seconds.

> **Mathematical Application**
> *Calculating mAs*
>
> $$mAs = mA \times seconds$$
>
> Examples:
>
> $$200 \text{ mA} \times 0.25 \text{ s} = 50 \text{ mAs}$$
> $$500 \text{ mA} \times 2/5 \text{ s} = 200 \text{ mAs}$$
> $$800 \text{ mA} \times 100 \text{ ms (milliseconds or 0.1 second)} = 80 \text{ mAs}$$

The quantity of electrons that flow from cathode to anode is directly proportional to mAs (Box 2-8). The quantity of x-ray photons produced is directly proportional to the quantity of electrons that flow from cathode to anode. An increase or decrease in mA, exposure time, or mAs directly affects the quantity of x-rays produced; mAs has no effect on the quality of x-rays produced. (Box 2-9 describes quality control methods for evaluating radiation output.)

> **Important Relationship**
> *Quantity of Electrons, X-rays, and mAs*
> The quantity of electrons flowing from the cathode to the anode and the quantity of x-rays produced are directly proportional to mAs.

> **BOX 2-8** | **mAs and X-ray Quantity**
>
> 1. Higher mAs results in more electrons that move in the tube current from cathode to anode.
> 2. The more electrons in the tube current, the more x-rays produced.
> 3. The number of x-rays that are produced is directly proportional to the mAs.
> 4. mAs affects only the quantity of x-rays produced; it has no effect on the quality of the x-rays.

LINE FOCUS PRINCIPLE

The **line focus principle** describes the relationship between the actual and effective focal spots in the x-ray tube.

BOX 2-9 | **Quality Control Check: Radiation Output**

- Variations in the generator or x-ray tube performance may cause inconsistent exposures and affect x-ray quantity. Three quality control tests are typically performed with a **dosimeter** (a device that measures x-ray exposure) to evaluate radiation output by measuring the radiation intensity: reproducibility of exposure, mAs reciprocity, and milliamperage and exposure time linearity.
- **Reproducibility of exposure:** Verifies the consistency of radiation output for a given set of exposure factors. The maximum variability of reproducibility of radiation exposures is ±5%.
- **mAs reciprocity:** Verifies the consistency of radiation intensity for changes in mA and exposure time with constant mAs. The maximum variability of reciprocity is ±10%.
- **Milliamperage and exposure time linearity:** Verifies that proportional changes in mA or exposure time or both likewise change the radiation intensity. Doubling the mA or exposure time should double the radiation intensity. The maximum variability of linearity is ±10%.

Important Relationship
Line Focus Principle
The line focus principle describes the relationship between the actual focal spot, where the electrons in the tube current bombard the target, and the effective focal spot, that same area as seen from directly below the tube.

Actual focal spot size refers to the size of the area on the anode target that is exposed to electrons from the tube current. Actual focal spot size depends on the size of the filament producing the electron stream. **Effective focal spot size** refers to focal spot size as measured directly under the anode target (Figure 2-16).

A tube's focal spot is an important factor because a large focal spot can withstand the heat produced by large exposures, whereas a small focal spot produces better image quality. The line focus principle demonstrates how, by angling the face of the anode, the actual focal spot can remain relatively large, while the effective focal spot is reduced in size. Greater heat capacity can be achieved while maintaining good image quality.

When manufactured, every tube has a specific anode angle, typically ranging from 5 to 20 degrees. Based on the line focus principle, the amount of anode angle determines the size of the effective focal spot.

A larger target angle produces a larger effective focal spot, and a smaller target angle produces a smaller effective focal spot. The relationship among target angle, effective focal spot size, and actual focal spot size is illustrated in Figure 2-17.

Important Relationship
Anode Angle and Effective Focal Spot Size
Based on the line focus principle, the smaller the anode angle, the smaller the effective focal spot size.

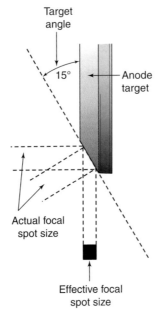

FIGURE 2-16 The line focus principle addresses the relationship between the size of the actual focal spot (where the electrons actually bombard the target) and the effective focal spot (the same area as viewed and measured directly below the target).

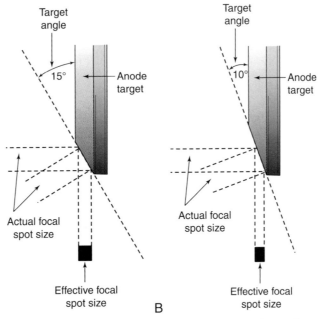

FIGURE 2-17 Based on the line focus principle, a large target angle produces a large effective focal spot size (**A**), and a small target angle produces a small effective focal spot size (**B**). Both actual focal spot sizes are the same, meaning that they can withstand the same heat loading. The smaller effective focal spot results in improved image quality.

ANODE HEEL EFFECT

A phenomenon known as the **anode heel effect** occurs because of the angle of the target. The heel effect describes how the x-ray beam has greater intensity (number of x-rays) on the cathode side of the tube, with the intensity diminishing toward the anode side (Figure 2-18).

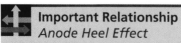
Important Relationship
Anode Heel Effect
X-rays are more intense on the cathode side of the tube. The intensity of the x-rays decreases toward the anode side.

As x-rays are produced, they leave the anode in all directions. The x-rays that are emitted toward the anode side of the tube have farther to travel, and some are absorbed by the anode itself (anode heel) and are reduced in number compared with the photons that are emitted in the direction of the cathode. The difference in the intensities between the two ends can be as much as 45%. The heel effect can be used to advantage in radiography because the cathode end of the tube can be placed over the thicker body part, resulting in more even exposure to the image receptor.

The anode heel effect can be used in imaging the thoracic spine, which has small vertebrae at the top and large vertebrae at the bottom. By placing the patient's head

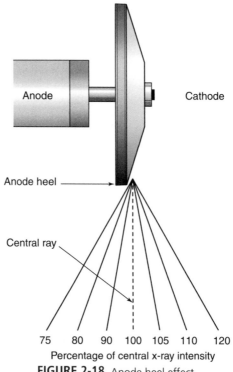

FIGURE 2-18 Anode heel effect.

under the anode end of the tube, the more intense radiation is directed toward the lower, larger portion of the spine, and less intense radiation exposes the upper, smaller vertebrae.

BEAM FILTRATION

The x-ray beam produced at the anode exits the tube housing to become the primary beam. This is the x-ray beam that eventually records the body part onto the image receptor. The x-rays that exit the tube are polyenergetic. They consist of low-energy, medium-energy, and high-energy photons. The low-energy photons are unable to penetrate the anatomic part and do not contribute to image formation. They contribute only to patient dose.

> **Important Relationship**
> *Low-Energy Photons, Patient Dose, and Image Formation*
> Low-energy photons serve only to increase patient dose and do not contribute to image formation.

Reduction of the low-energy photons requires that filtration be added to the x-ray beam to attenuate or absorb these photons. **Added filtration** describes the filtration that is added to the port of the x-ray tube. Aluminum is the material primarily used for this purpose because it absorbs more of the low-energy photons while the useful higher-energy photons can exit (Figure 2-19).

Various components within the x-ray tube assembly also contribute to the attenuation of low-energy x-rays. **Inherent filtration** refers to the filtration that is permanently in the path of the x-ray beam. Three components contribute to inherent filtration: (1) the envelope of the tube, (2) the oil that surrounds the tube, and (3) the window in the tube housing. The mirror inside the collimator (beam restrictor located just below the x-ray tube) adds additional filtration (see Figure 2-19). **Total filtration** in the x-ray beam is the sum of the added filtration and the inherent filtration. The U.S. government sets standards for total filtration to ensure that patients receive minimum doses of radiation. The current guidelines state that x-ray tubes operating at greater than 70 kVp must have a minimum total filtration of 2.5 mm of aluminum or its equivalent. Increasing the amount of tube filtration increases the x-ray beam quality because there is a greater percentage of high-energy x-rays compared with low-energy x-rays. In addition, increasing tube filtration decreases the quantity of x-rays or x-ray emission (Figure 2-20). (Box 2-10 describes quality control methods for evaluating filtration.)

> **Patient Protection Alert**
> *Beam Filtration*
> Low-energy photons, created during x-ray production, are unable to penetrate the patient. Patients are protected from unnecessary exposure to this low-energy radiation by having inherent and added filtration in the path of the x-ray beam.

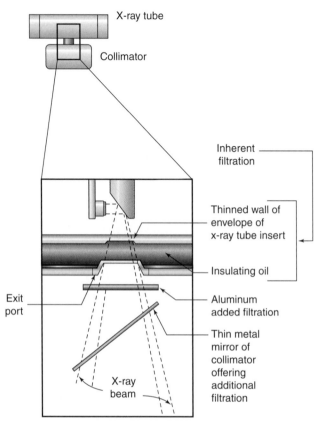

FIGURE 2-19 Aluminum (Al) added filtration is shown at the port, or window, of the x-ray tube and the collimator mirror. The inherent filtration of the envelope and the oil are shown.

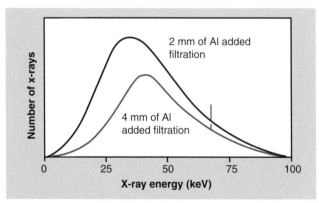

FIGURE 2-20 Increasing beam filtration decreases the quantity (amplitude) and increases the quality (shift to the right) of the x-ray beam.

BOX 2-10	**Quality Control Check: Beam Filtration**

- **Half-value layer (HVL)**, the amount of filtration that reduces the intensity of the x-ray beam to one-half its original value, is considered the best method for describing x-ray quality.
- The HVL can be used as an indirect measure of the total filtration in the path of the x-ray beam. It is expressed in millimeters of aluminum (mm-Al).
- During the HVL test, a radiation measuring device, such as a dosimeter, is used to measure both radiation intensity of the original exposure and radiation intensity following the addition of aluminum filtration in the path of the primary beam.
- According to the NCRP Report #102, for equipment operated at 70 kVp and greater, the minimum HVL should be at least 2.5 mm. An HVL <2.5 mm indicates insufficient filtration.
- If the HVL is at the appropriate level, the total filtration in the x-ray tube is adequate to protect patients from unnecessary low-energy radiation.

COMPENSATING FILTERS

Compensating filters can be added to the primary beam to alter its intensity. These types of filters are used to image anatomic areas that are nonuniform in makeup and assist in producing more consistent exposure to the image receptor.

The most common type of compensating filter is a simple **wedge filter** (Figure 2-21A). The thicker part of the wedge filter is lined up with the thinner portion of the anatomic part that is being imaged, allowing fewer x-ray photons to reach that end of the part. A wedge filter may be used for an anteroposterior (AP) projection of the femur, where the hip end is considerably larger than the knee end. A **trough filter** performs a function similar to the wedge filter; however, it is designed differently (Figure 2-21B). The trough filter has a double wedge. A trough filter may be used for an AP projection of the thorax to compensate for the easily penetrated air-filled lungs.

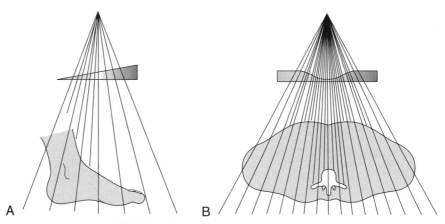

FIGURE 2-21 A, Wedge filter. B, Trough filter.

TABLE 2-1	Generator Factor
Generator Type	**Factor**
Single phase	1.00
Three phase	1.35
High frequency	1.40

HEAT UNITS

During x-ray production, most of the kinetic energy of the electrons is converted to heat. This heat can damage the x-ray tube and the anode target. The amount of heat produced from any given exposure is expressed by the **heat unit (HU)**. The number of HUs produced depends on the type of x-ray generator being used and the exposure factors selected for a particular exposure and can be expressed mathematically as:

$$HU = mA \times time \times kVp \times generator\ factor$$

The generator factor (Table 2-1) takes into account that the use of more consistent x-ray generators results in more heat.

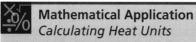 **Mathematical Application**
Calculating Heat Units
An exposure is made with a three-phase x-ray unit using 600 mA, and 0.05 second, 75 kVp. How many heat units are produced from this exposure?

$$HU = mA \times time \times kVp \times generator\ factor$$

$$HU = 600 \times 0.05 \times 75 \times 1.35$$

$$= 3037.5\ HU$$

Different models of x-ray tubes vary in their ability to withstand the heat produced by x-ray exposures. Prior to modern x-ray tubes, radiographers were responsible for evaluating their exposure technique selection to avoid excessive heat load. Box 2-11 explains the use of tube rating charts to avoid heat damage. Manufacturers of current x-ray units build their equipment so that tube-damaging exposures cannot be made. Generally, if an inappropriate technique is set, the radiographer sees a message such as "Technique Overload," or the machine may simply not expose after the rotor button is activated. Routine use of high-exposure techniques, although within the x-ray tube's limit, can potentially damage the x-ray tube.

EXTENDING X-RAY TUBE LIFE

X-ray tubes are expensive devices that can fail because of radiographer error or carelessness. Not only do failed tubes result in an expense for purchasing a new tube, but there is also down time for a radiographic room when a failed tube is being replaced, decreasing productivity of the room. A few simple but important guidelines

BOX 2-11 | Tube Rating Charts

Prior to today's x-ray tubes, manufacturers used instantaneous load tube rating charts, also called *single-exposure rating charts,* to describe the exposure limits of x-ray tubes. An instantaneous load tube rating chart is used to determine whether a particular exposure would be safe to make and to determine what limits on kVp, mA, and exposure time must be made to make a safe exposure. Violation of these limits as indicated by the tube rating chart would almost certainly result in permanent and irreparable damage to the x-ray tube. Figure 2-22 shows a typical instantaneous load tube rating chart. For example, the maximum kVp that can be used with 700 mA and 0.3 second exposure time is 90 kVp. The maximum mA that can be used with 105 kVp and 0.2 second exposure time is 600 mA. The maximum exposure time that can be used with 85 kVp and 900 mA is 0.05 s. Although 130 kVp, 500 mA, and 0.1 s would produce a safe exposure, 130 kVp, 500 mA, and 0.2 s would not.

In addition to tube rating charts, manufacturers provided anode and housing cooling charts. Based on the quantity of heat units, these charts provided radiographers with information about the amount of time that must elapse before initiating another exposure.

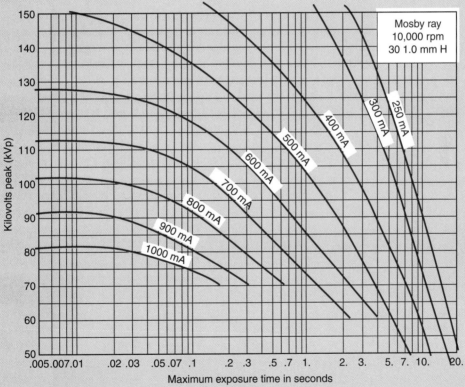

FIGURE 2-22 Typical instantaneous load tube rating chart that can be used to determine safe and unsafe exposures.

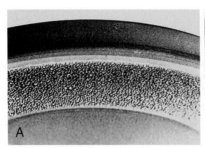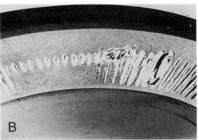

FIGURE 2-23 Two heat-damaged anode targets. **A,** Target shows pitting of the anode track caused by consistent overloading of exposure factors. **B,** Target shows melting of the focal track caused by failure of the rotor to rotate the anode. This failure usually is due to heat damage to the rotor bearings from overloading the exposure factors.

of x-ray tube operation should be adhered to consistently by the radiographer to extend tube life:

- If applicable, warm up the tube according to the manufacturer's specifications, especially if it has not been energized for 2 hours or more.
- Avoid excessive heat unit generation. Repeatedly using exposure techniques near an x-ray tube's limit increases the total heat units. Figure 2-23 shows anode targets that have been damaged as a result of excessive heat loading.
- Do not hold down the rotor button without making an exposure. Holding down the rotor button unnecessarily causes excessive wear on both the filament and the rotor.
- Use lower tube currents with longer exposure times when possible to minimize wear on the filament.
- Do not move the tube while it is energized. This movement can cause damage to the anode and anode stem as a result of torque, the force that acts to produce rotation.
- If the rotor makes noticeable noise, stop using the tube until it has been inspected by a qualified service person. Noises can be indicative of a potentially serious problem.

Radiographers create diagnostic images by producing an x-ray beam that provides visualization of anatomic structures. The x-rays produced by the radiographer affect not only the quality of the image but also the life of the x-ray tube. Understanding the prime exposure factors and their effect on the x-ray beam and knowing what happens inside the x-ray tube are important considerations in radiography.

CHAPTER SUMMARY

- X-rays are produced when electrons are boiled off (thermionic emission) the cathode filament, accelerated across to the anode target, and suddenly stopped. Heat is also produced.
- The anode, containing the tungsten-rhenium alloy target, typically rotates, allowing for larger exposures.

- X-rays are produced by bremsstrahlung (primarily) and characteristic interactions, which occur as the electrons interact with the tungsten atoms in the target.
- Manipulation of the primary factors affects the quality and quantity of radiation. kVp affects both the quality (energy, penetrability) and the quantity of x-rays, whereas mA and exposure time (or mAs when combined) affect only quantity.
- The line focus principle describes the relationship between the anode angle and the effective focal spot. The anode heel effect results in more intense radiation exiting the tube toward the cathode side.
- Added and inherent beam filtration ensures that minimal low-energy x-ray photons reach the patient. The half value layer (HVL) is an indirect measure of total filtration and is used to describe x-ray quality.
- There are numerous methods for extending tube life, including attending to the amount of heat produced during x-ray production. Heat units are the measure of the amount of heat produced using specific exposure factors.

REVIEW QUESTIONS

1. Which x-ray tube component serves as a source of electrons for x-ray production?
   A. Focusing cup
   B. Filament
   C. Stator
   D. Target

2. Electrons interact with the _____ to produce x-rays and heat.
   A. focusing cup
   B. filament
   C. stator
   D. target

3. The cloud of electrons that forms before x-ray production is referred to as _____.
   A. thermionic emission
   B. space charge
   C. space charge effect
   D. tube current

4. The burning or boiling off of electrons at the cathode is referred to as _____.
   A. thermionic emission
   B. space charge
   C. space charge effect
   D. tube current

5. Which primary exposure factor influences both the quantity and the quality of x-ray photons?
   A. mA
   B. mAs
   C. kVp
   D. Exposure time

6. The unit used to express tube current is _____.
   A. mA
   B. mAs
   C. kVp
   D. s

7. What percentage of the kinetic energy is converted to heat when moving electrons strike the anode target?
   A. 1%
   B. 25%
   C. 59%
   D. 99%

8. The intensity of the x-ray beam is greater on the _____.
   A. cathode side of the tube
   B. anode side of the tube
   C. short axis of the beam
   D. long axis of the beam

9. According to the line focus principle, as the target angle decreases, the _____.
   A. actual focal spot size decreases
   B. actual focal spot size increases
   C. effective focal spot size decreases
   D. effective focal spot size increases

10. _____ extends x-ray tube life.
    A. Selecting higher tube currents
    B. Using small focal spots when possible
    C. Producing exposures with a wide range of kVp values
    D. Warming up the tube after 2 hours of nonuse

11. Which type of target interaction is responsible for most of the x-rays in the diagnostic beam?
    A. Characteristic interaction
    B. Thermionic emission
    C. Bremsstrahlung interaction
    D. None of the above

12. How much mAs is produced when the radiographer sets 70 kVp, 600 mA, and 50 ms?
   A. 3.5 mAs
   B. 30 mAs
   C. 300 mAs
   D. 350 mAs

13. Increasing the kVp results in _____.
   A. x-rays with higher energy
   B. x-rays with lower energy
   C. more x-rays
   D. A and C
   E. B and C

14. Total filtration in the x-ray beam includes _____.
   A. compensating filters
   B. inherent filtration
   C. added filtration
   D. B and C
   E. all of the above

15. How many heat units result from an exposure made on a single-phase x-ray unit using 400 mA, 0.2 second, and 70 kVp?
   A. 5600 HU
   B. 7560 HU
   C. 7896 HU
   D. 8120 HU

Image Formation and Radiographic Quality

CHAPTER OUTLINE

Image Formation
  Differential Absorption
Radiographic Quality
  Image Brightness or Density
  Image Contrast

Spatial Resolution
  and Recorded Detail
Distortion
Scatter
Quantum Noise

Image Artifacts
Image Characteristics
  Digital Imaging
  Film-Screen Imaging

OBJECTIVES

After completing this chapter, the reader will be able to perform the following:

1. Define all the key terms in this chapter.
2. State all the important relationships in this chapter.
3. Describe the process of radiographic image formation.
4. Explain the process of beam attenuation.
5. Identify the factors that affect beam attenuation.
6. Describe the x-ray interactions termed *photoelectric effect* and *Compton effect*.
7. Define the term *ionization*.
8. State the composition of exit radiation.
9. State the effect of scatter radiation on the radiographic image.
10. Explain the process of creating the various shades of image brightness and densities.
11. Describe the necessary components of radiographic quality.
12. Explain the importance of brightness and density to image quality.
13. Explain the importance of contrast to image quality.
14. Differentiate between high-contrast and low-contrast images.
15. Explain the importance of spatial resolution and recorded detail to image quality.
16. Explain the importance of both size and shape distortion to image quality.
17. Compare and contrast attributes of a digital and film image.
18. Explain the digital characteristics of matrix and pixels.
19. Compare the dynamic range capabilities between digital and film-screen imaging.
20. Recognize the effect of quantum noise and scatter on image quality.
21. Discuss the effects of image artifacts on radiographic quality.
22. Differentiate between the characteristics of a digital and film image.

KEY TERMS

absorption	elongation	photoelectric effect
active layer	emulsion	photoelectron
artifact	exit radiation	pixel density
attenuation	exposure intensity	pixel pitch
binary number system	fog	pixels
bit	foreshortening	quantum noise
bit depth	grayscale	recorded detail
brightness	high contrast	remnant radiation
byte	image receptor	scale of contrast
coherent scattering	intensity of radiation exposure	scattering
Compton effect	invisible image	secondary electron
Compton electron	ionization	shape distortion
contrast resolution	latent image	short-scale contrast
densitometer	long-scale contrast	size distortion
density	low contrast	spatial resolution
diagnostic densities	magnification	subject contrast
differential absorption	manifest image	tissue density
distortion	matrix	transmission
dynamic range	optical density	visible image

To produce a radiographic image, x-ray photons must pass through tissue and interact with an **image receptor (IR)** (a device that receives the radiation leaving the patient), such as an imaging plate in computed radiography (CR). Both the quantity and the quality of the primary x-ray beam affect its interaction within the various tissues that make up the anatomic part. In addition, the composition of the anatomic tissues affects the x-ray beam interaction. The absorption characteristics of the anatomic part are determined by its thickness, atomic number, and tissue density or compactness of the cellular structures. Finally, the radiation that exits the patient is composed of varying energies and interacts with the image receptor to form the latent or invisible image and must be processed.

A visible radiographic image is produced following processing of the latent or invisible image. Depending on the type of imaging system, acquiring, processing, and displaying of the image can vary significantly. However, the attributes of a quality radiographic image are similar regardless of the type of imaging system. This chapter focuses on how the image is formed and its quality after processing.

IMAGE FORMATION

Differential Absorption

The process of image formation is a result of **differential absorption** of the x-ray beam as it interacts with the anatomic tissue. Differential absorption is a process whereby some of the x-ray beam is absorbed in the tissue and some passes through (transmits) the anatomic part. The term *differential* is used because varying anatomic parts do not *absorb* the primary beam to the same degree. Anatomic parts composed of bone absorb more x-ray photons than parts filled with air. Differential absorption of the primary x-ray beam creates an image that structurally represents the anatomic area of interest (Figure 3-1).

> **Important Relationship**
> *Differential Absorption and Image Formation*
> A radiographic image is created by passing an x-ray beam through the patient and interacting with an image receptor, such as an imaging plate in computed radiography (CR). The variations in absorption and transmission of the exiting x-ray beam structurally represent the anatomic area of interest.

Creating a radiographic image by differential absorption requires that several processes occur: beam attenuation, absorption, and transmission.

Beam Attenuation. As the primary x-ray beam passes through anatomic tissue, it loses some of its energy. Fewer x-ray photons remain in the beam after it interacts with anatomic tissue. This reduction in the energy or number of photons in the primary x-ray beam is known as **attenuation.** Beam attenuation occurs as a result of the photon interactions with the atomic structures that comprise the tissues. Two distinct processes occur during beam attenuation: absorption and scattering.

Absorption. As the energy of the primary x-ray beam is deposited within the atoms comprising the tissue, some x-ray photons are completely absorbed. Complete **absorption** of the incoming x-ray photon occurs when it has enough energy to remove (eject) an inner-shell electron. The ejected electron is called a **photoelectron** and quickly loses energy by interacting with nearby tissues. The ability to remove (eject) electrons, known as **ionization,** is one of the characteristics of x-rays. In the diagnostic range, this x-ray interaction with matter is known as the **photoelectric effect.**

With the photoelectric effect, the ionized atom has a vacancy, or electron hole, in its inner shell. An electron from an outer shell drops down to fill the vacancy. Because of the difference in binding energies between the two electron shells, a

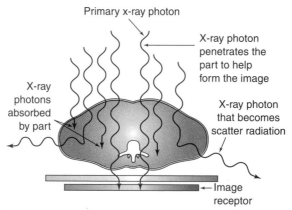

FIGURE 3-1 As the primary x-ray beam interacts with the anatomic part, photons are absorbed, scattered, and transmitted. The differences in the absorption characteristics of the anatomic part create an image that structurally represents the anatomic part.

secondary x-ray photon is emitted (Figure 3-2). This secondary x-ray photon typically has very low energy and is unlikely to exit the patient.

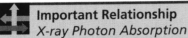

Important Relationship
X-ray Photon Absorption
During attenuation of the x-ray beam, the photoelectric effect is responsible for total absorption of the incoming x-ray photon.

The probability of total photon absorption during the photoelectric effect depends on the energy of the incoming x-ray photon and the atomic number of the anatomic tissue. The energy of the incoming x-ray photon must be at least equal to the binding energy of the inner-shell electron. After absorption of some of the x-ray photons,

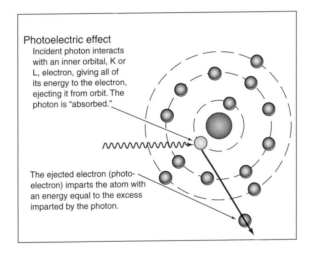

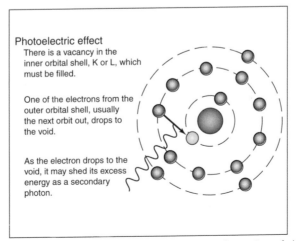

FIGURE 3-2 The photoelectric effect is responsible for total absorption of the incoming x-ray photon.

the overall energy or quantity of the primary beam decreases as it passes through the anatomic part.

Scattering. Some incoming photons are not absorbed but instead lose energy during interactions with the atoms comprising the tissue. This process is called **scattering**. It results from the diagnostic x-ray interaction with matter known as the **Compton effect**. The loss of energy of the incoming photon occurs when it ejects an outer-shell electron from a tissue atom. The ejected electron is called a **Compton electron** or **secondary electron**. The remaining lower-energy x-ray photon changes direction and may leave the anatomic part to interact with the image receptor (Figure 3-3).

> ⬍ **Important Relationship**
> *X-ray Beam Scattering*
> During attenuation of the x-ray beam, the incoming x-ray photon may lose energy and change direction as a result of the Compton effect.

Compton interactions can occur within all diagnostic x-ray energies and are an important interaction in radiography. The probability of a Compton interaction occurring depends on the energy of the incoming photon. It does not depend on the atomic number of the anatomic tissue. For example, a Compton interaction is just as likely to occur in soft tissue as in tissue composed of bone.

When a higher kVp is used, the overall number of x-ray interactions with matter decrease because of increased photon transmission. However, the percentage of photoelectric interactions generally decreases at higher kilovoltages within the diagnostic range, whereas the percentage of Compton interactions is likely to increase at higher kilovoltages within the diagnostic range. Box 3-1 compares photoelectric and Compton interactions.

Coherent scattering is an interaction that occurs with low-energy x-rays, typically below the diagnostic range. The incoming photon interacts with the atom, causing it

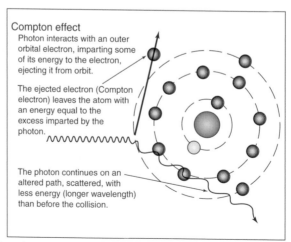

Compton effect
Photon interacts with an outer orbital electron, imparting some of its energy to the electron, ejecting it from orbit.

The ejected electron (Compton electron) leaves the atom with an energy equal to the excess imparted by the photon.

The photon continues on an altered path, scattered, with less energy (longer wavelength) than before the collision.

FIGURE 3-3 During the Compton effect, the incoming photon loses energy and changes its direction.

| BOX 3-1 | **Comparing Photoelectric and Compton Effects** |

Photoelectric Effect
- Incoming photon has sufficient energy to eject an inner-shell electron and be completely absorbed.
- An electron from an upper-level shell fills the electron hole or vacancy.
- A secondary photon is created because of the difference in the electrons' binding energies.
- The probability of this effect depends on the energy of the incoming x-ray photon and the composition of the anatomic tissue.
- Fewer photon interactions occur at higher kVp, but of those interactions, a smaller percentage are photoelectric interactions.

Compton Effect
- Incoming photon loses energy when it ejects an outer shell electron and changes direction.
- The scattered photon may be absorbed within the patient tissues, leave the anatomic part, interact with the image receptor, or expose anyone near the patient.
- Scattered photons that strike the image receptor provide no useful information.
- The probability of this effect depends on the energy of the incoming x-ray photon but not the composition of the anatomic tissue.
- Fewer photon interactions occur at higher kVp, but a greater percentage of those interactions are Compton interactions.

to become excited. The x-ray does not lose energy, but it changes direction. Coherent scattering could occur within the diagnostic range of x-rays and may interact with the image receptor, but it is not considered an important interaction in radiography.

If a scattered photon strikes the image receptor, it does not contribute any useful information about the anatomic area of interest. If scattered photons are absorbed within the anatomic tissue, they contribute to the radiation exposure to the patient. In addition, if the scattered photon leaves the patient and does not strike the image receptor, it could contribute to the radiation exposure of anyone near the patient.

The preceding discussion focused on photon interactions that occur in radiography when using x-ray energies within the moderate range. Higher-energy x-rays, beyond the diagnostic range, result in other interactions: pair production and photodisintegration. X-ray interactions beyond the diagnostic range are important in radiation therapy.

Factors Affecting Beam Attenuation. The amount of x-ray beam attenuation is affected by the thickness of the anatomic part, its atomic number and tissue density, and the energy of the x-ray beam.

Tissue Thickness. For a given anatomic tissue, increasing its thickness increases beam attenuation by either absorption or scattering. X-rays are attenuated exponentially and generally reduced by approximately 50% for each 4 to 5 cm (1.6 to 2 inches) of tissue thickness (Figure 3-4). More x-rays are needed to produce a radiographic image for a thicker anatomic part. Fewer x-rays are needed to produce a radiographic image for a thinner anatomic part.

Type of Tissue. Tissue composed of a higher atomic number, such as bone, attenuates the x-ray beam more than tissue composed of a lower atomic number, such as fat. The higher atomic number indicates there are more atomic particles to absorb or scatter the x-ray photon. X-ray absorption is more likely to occur in tissues composed of a higher atomic number compared with tissues composed of a lower atomic number.

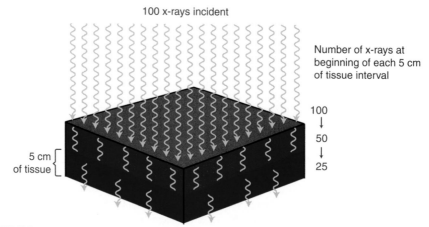

FIGURE 3-4 X-rays are attenuated exponentially and generally reduced by approximately 50% for each 4 to 5 cm (1.6 to 2 inches) of tissue thickness.

Tissue density (matter per unit volume), or the compactness of the atomic particles comprising the anatomic part, also affect the amount of beam attenuation. For example, muscle and fat tissue are similar in atomic number; however, their atomic particles differ in compactness, and tissue density varies. Muscle tissue has atomic particles that are more dense or compact and therefore attenuate the x-ray beam more than fat cells. Bone is composed of tissue with a higher atomic number, and the atomic particles are more compacted or dense. Anatomic tissues are typically ranked based on their attenuation properties. Four substances account for most of the beam attenuation in the human body: bone, muscle, fat, and air. Bone attenuates the x-ray beam more than muscle, muscle attenuates the x-ray beam more than fat, and fat attenuates the x-ray beam more than air. The atomic number of the anatomic part and its tissue density affect x-ray beam attenuation.

X-ray Beam Quality. The quality of the x-ray beam or its penetrating ability affects its interaction with anatomic tissue. Higher-penetrating x-rays (shorter wavelength with higher frequency) are more likely to be transmitted through anatomic tissue without interacting with the tissues' atomic structures. Lower-penetrating x-rays (longer wavelength with lower frequency) are more likely to interact with the atomic structures and be either absorbed or scattered. The kilovoltage selected during x-ray production determines the energy or penetrability of the x-ray photon, and this affects its attenuation in anatomic tissue. Beam attenuation is decreased with a higher-energy x-ray beam and increased with a lower-energy x-ray beam (Table 3-1).

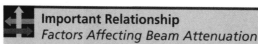

Important Relationship
Factors Affecting Beam Attenuation
Increasing tissue thickness, atomic number, and tissue density increase x-ray beam attenuation because more x-rays are absorbed by the tissue. Increasing the quality of the x-ray beam decreases beam attenuation because the higher-energy x-rays penetrate the tissue.

TABLE 3-1	Factors Affecting Attenuation		
Factor	Beam Attenuation	Absorption	Transmission
Tissue Thickness			
• Increasing thickness	↑	↑	↓
• Decreasing thickness	↓	↓	↑
Tissue Atomic Number			
• Increasing atomic no.	↑	↑	↓
• Decreasing atomic no.	↓	↓	↑
Tissue Density			
• Increasing tissue density	↑	↑	↓
• Decreasing tissue density	↓	↓	↑
X-ray Beam Quality			
• Increasing beam quality	↓	↓	↑
• Decreasing beam quality	↑	↑	↓

Transmission If the incoming x-ray photon passes through the anatomic part without any interaction with the atomic structures, it is called **transmission** (Figure 3-5). The combination of absorption and transmission of the x-ray beam provides an image that structurally represents the anatomic part. Because scatter radiation is also a process that occurs during interaction of the x-ray beam and anatomic part, the quality of the image created is compromised if the scattered photon strikes the image receptor.

Exit Radiation. When the attenuated x-ray beam leaves the patient, the remaining x-ray beam, referred to as **exit radiation** or **remnant radiation,** is composed of both transmitted and scattered radiation (Figure 3-6). The varying amounts of transmitted and absorbed radiation (differential absorption) create an image that structurally represents the anatomic area of interest. Scatter exit radiation (Compton interactions) that reach the image receptor do not provide any diagnostic information about the anatomic area. Scatter radiation creates unwanted exposure on the image called **fog.** Methods used to decrease the amount of scatter radiation reaching the image receptor are discussed in Chapter 5.

Important Relationship
X-ray Interaction with Matter
When the diagnostic primary x-ray beam interacts with anatomic tissues, three processes occur: absorption, scattering, and transmission.

The areas within the anatomic tissue that absorb incoming x-ray photons (photoelectric effect) create the white or clear areas (more brightness or low density) on the displayed image. The incoming x-ray photons that are transmitted create areas of less brightness or high density on the displayed image. Anatomic tissues that vary in absorption and transmission create a range of brightness or shades of gray (Figure 3-7). The various shades of gray recorded in the radiographic image make anatomic

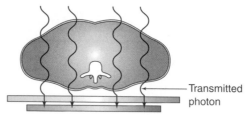

FIGURE 3-5 Some incoming x-ray photons pass through the anatomic part without any interactions.

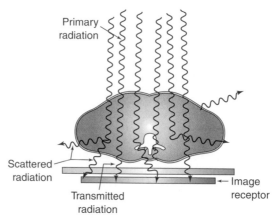

FIGURE 3-6 Radiation that exits the anatomic part comprises transmitted and scattered radiation.

tissue visible. Skeletal bones are differentiated from the air-filled lungs because of their differences in absorption and transmission.

Less than 5% of the primary x-ray beam interacting with the anatomic part actually reaches the image receptor, and an even lower percentage is used to create the radiographic image. The exit radiation that interacts with an image receptor creates the **latent image,** or **invisible image.** This latent image is not visible until it is processed to produce the **manifest image,** or **visible image.**

 Important Relationship
Image Brightness or Densities
The range of image brightness or densities visible after processing is a result of the variation in x-ray absorption and transmission as the x-ray beam passes through anatomic tissues.

RADIOGRAPHIC QUALITY

A quality radiographic image accurately represents the anatomic area of interest, and information is well visualized for diagnosis. It is important to identify the attributes of a quality radiographic image before comprehending all the factors that affect its quality. Radiographic images can be acquired from two different types of image receptors: digital and film-screen. The process of creating the latent image by

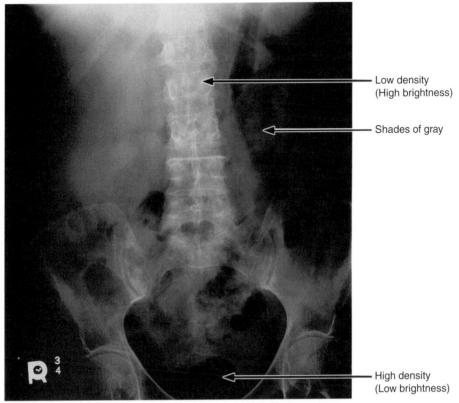

Low density
(High brightness)

Shades of gray

High density
(Low brightness)

FIGURE 3-7 A radiographic image represents the various absorption characteristics of the anatomic part. An area of high density (low brightness) is where the x-ray beam was transmitted, and an area of low density (high brightness) is where the x-ray beam was absorbed. Anatomic tissues that vary in absorption and transmission create the shades of gray on the image.

differential absorption is the same for both digital and film image receptors, but the acquisition, processing, and display vary greatly.

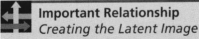

Important Relationship
Creating the Latent Image

The process of differential absorption for image formation is the same for digital and film-screen imaging. The varying x-ray intensities exiting the anatomic area of interest form the latent image.

The *visibility* of the anatomic structures and the *accuracy* of their structural lines recorded (sharpness) determine the overall quality of the radiographic image. Visibility of the recorded detail refers to the *brightness* or *density* of the image, and the accuracy of the structural lines is achieved by maximizing the amount of *spatial resolution* or *recorded detail* and minimizing the amount of *distortion*. Visibility of the recorded detail is achieved by the proper balance of image brightness or density and contrast.

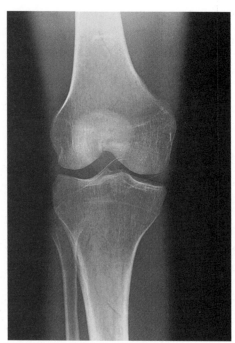

FIGURE 3-8 Radiograph with diagnostic density (brightness).

Image Brightness or Density

How the radiograph is displayed determines whether to evaluate the image in terms of brightness or density. Digital images are typically displayed on a computer monitor, whereas film-screen images are displayed on film. Digital images can also be printed on specialized film. Brightness and density refer to the same image quality attribute but are defined differently. **Brightness** is the amount of luminance (light emission) of a display monitor. **Density** is the amount of overall blackness on the processed image. An area of increased brightness viewed on a computer monitor shows decreased density on a film image. An area of decreased brightness visualized on a computer monitor has increased density on a film image.

A radiograph must have sufficient brightness or density to visualize the anatomic structures of interest (Figure 3-8). A radiograph that is too light has excessive brightness or insufficient density to visualize the structures of the anatomic part (Figure 3-9). Conversely, a radiograph that is too dark has insufficient brightness or excessive density, and the anatomic part cannot be well visualized (Figure 3-10). The radiographer must evaluate the overall brightness or density on the image to determine whether it is sufficient to visualize the anatomic area of interest. He or she then decides whether the radiograph is diagnostic or unacceptable.

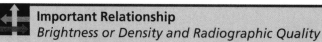

Important Relationship
Brightness or Density and Radiographic Quality
A radiographic image must have sufficient brightness or density to visualize the anatomic structures of interest.

> **Important Relationship**
> *Differentiating Among Anatomic Tissues*
> The ability to distinguish among types of tissues is determined by the differences in brightness levels or densities in the image or contrast. Anatomic tissues that attenuate the beam similarly have low subject contrast. Anatomic tissues that attenuate the beam very differently have high subject contrast.

Brightness or density is easily measurable; however, contrast is a more complex attribute. Evaluating radiographic quality in terms of contrast is more subjective (it is affected by individual preferences). The level of radiographic contrast desired in an image is determined by the composition of the anatomic tissue to be radiographed and the amount of information needed to visualize the tissue for an accurate diagnosis. For example, the level of contrast desired in a chest radiograph is different from the level of contrast required in a radiograph of an extremity.

Radiographic or *image contrast* is a term used in both digital and film-screen imaging to describe variations in brightness and density. In digital imaging, the number of different shades of gray that can be stored and displayed by a computer system is termed **grayscale**. Because the digital image is processed and reconstructed in the computer as digital data, its grayscale or contrast can be altered.

Radiographic film images are typically described by their **scale of contrast,** or the range of densities visible. A film image with few densities but great differences among them is said to have **high contrast;** this is also described as **short-scale contrast** (Figure 3-16). A radiograph with a large number of densities but few differences among them is said to have **low contrast;** this is also described as **long-scale contrast** (Figure 3-17).

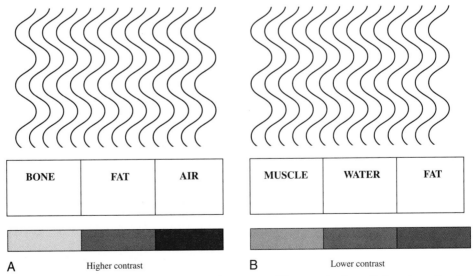

A   Higher contrast   B   Lower contrast

FIGURE 3-13 A, Higher contrast resulting from great differences in the radiation absorption for tissues that vary greatly in composition. **B,** Lower contrast resulting from fewer differences in the radiation absorption for tissues that are more similarly composed.

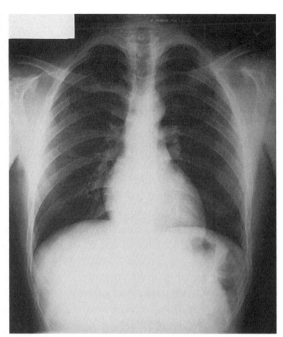

FIGURE 3-14 The thorax is an anatomic area of high subject contrast because there is great variation in tissue composition.

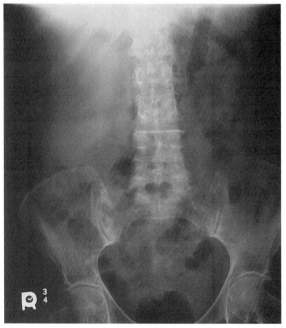

FIGURE 3-15 The abdomen is an anatomic area of low subject contrast because it is composed of similar tissue types.

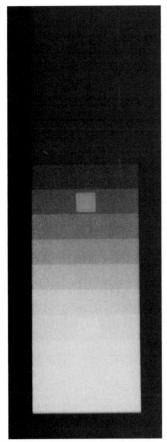

FIGURE 3-16 High-contrast (short-scale) image showing fewer gray levels and greater differences between individual densities.

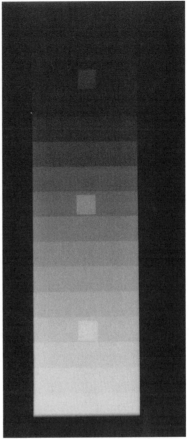

FIGURE 3-17 Low-contrast (long-scale) image showing many gray levels and few difference between individual densities.

The term **contrast resolution** is used to describe the ability of an imaging receptor to distinguish between objects having similar subject contrast. Digital image receptors have improved contrast resolution compared with film-screen image receptors.

Spatial Resolution and Recorded Detail

The quality of a radiographic image depends on both the visibility and the accuracy of the anatomic structural lines recorded (sharpness). Adequate visualization of the anatomic area of interest (brightness/density and contrast) is just one component of radiographic quality. To produce a quality radiograph, the anatomic details must be recorded accurately and with the greatest amount of sharpness. Spatial resolution and recorded detail are terms used to evaluate accuracy of the anatomic structural lines recorded. **Spatial resolution** refers to the smallest object that can be detected in an image and is the term typically used in digital imaging. **Recorded detail** refers to

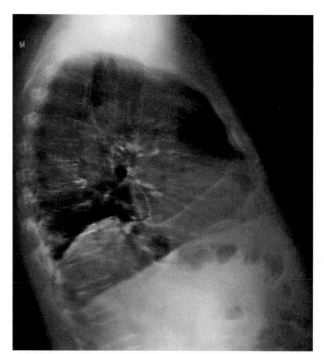

FIGURE 3-18 Image showing motion unsharpness.

the distinctness or sharpness of the structural lines that make up the recorded image and is the term used in film-screen imaging.

The ability of a radiographic image to demonstrate sharp lines determines the quality of the spatial resolution or recorded detail. The imaging process makes it impossible to produce a radiographic image without some degree of unsharpness. A radiographic image that has a greater amount of spatial resolution or recorded detail minimizes the amount of unsharpness of the anatomic structural lines.

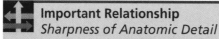

Important Relationship
Sharpness of Anatomic Detail
The accuracy of the anatomic structural lines recorded in the radiographic image is determined by its spatial resolution and recorded detail.

A radiographic image cannot be an exact reconstruction of the anatomic structure. Some information is always lost during the process of image formation. In addition, factors such as patient motion increase the amount of unsharpness recorded in the image (Figure 3-18). It is the radiographer's responsibility to minimize the amount of information lost by manipulating the factors that affect the sharpness of the recorded image. Diagnostic quality is achieved by maximizing the amount of spatial resolution or recorded detail and minimizing the amount of image distortion.

Sharpness of recorded detail and visibility of recorded detail have typically been discussed as two separate qualities of the radiographic image. Generally, this separation remains true except when imaging small anatomic structures. A small anatomic structure is best visualized when its brightness or density varies significantly from the background. If unsharpness is increased, the visibility of small anatomic detail is compromised. An increase in the amount of unsharpness recorded on the image decreases the contrast of small anatomic structures, reducing the overall visibility of the structural lines. The spreading of the structural lines with increased unsharpness decreases the differences in brightness or density between the structural lines of the area of interest and the background. As a result, the difference in brightness or density between the area of interest and the background becomes less (low contrast), and the visibility of the anatomic structure is reduced (Figure 3-19).

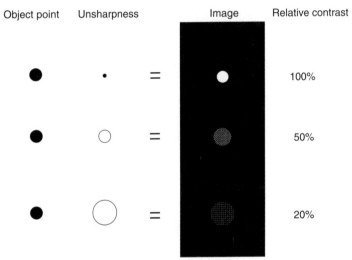

FIGURE 3-19 Unsharpness and image contrast. Increasing the amount of unsharpness decreases the brightness or density difference (contrast) between the area of interest and its surrounding background.

Distortion

Distortion results from the radiographic misrepresentation of either the size (magnification) or the shape of the anatomic part. When the image is distorted, spatial resolution or recorded detail is also reduced.

Size Distortion (Magnification).   The term **size distortion** (or **magnification**) refers to an increase in the image size of an object compared with its true, or actual, size. Radiographic images of objects are always magnified in terms of the true object size. The source-to-image receptor distance (SID) and object-to-image receptor distance (OID) play an important role in minimizing the amount of size distortion of the radiographic image.

Because radiographers produce radiographs of three-dimensional objects, some size distortion always occurs as a result of OID. The parts of the object that are farther away from the image receptor are represented radiographically with more size distortion than parts of the object that are closer to the image receptor. Even if the object is in close contact with the image receptor, some part of the object is farther away from the image receptor than other parts of the object. SID also influences the total amount of magnification on the image. As SID increases, size distortion (magnification) decreases; as SID decreases, size distortion (magnification) increases.

> **Important Relationship**
> *Size Distortion*
> Radiographic images of objects are always magnified in terms of the true object size. The SID and OID play an important role in minimizing the amount of size distortion or magnification created.

Shape Distortion. In addition to size distortion, objects that are being imaged can be misrepresented radiographically by distortion of their shape. **Shape distortion** can appear in two different ways radiographically: elongation or foreshortening. **Elongation** refers to images of objects that appear longer than the true objects. **Foreshortening** refers to images that appear shorter than the true objects. Examples of elongation and foreshortening can be seen in Figure 3-20.

Shape distortion can occur from inaccurate central ray (CR) alignment of the tube, the part being radiographed, or the image receptor. Any misalignment of the CR among these three factors—tube, part, or image receptor—alters the shape of the part recorded in the image.

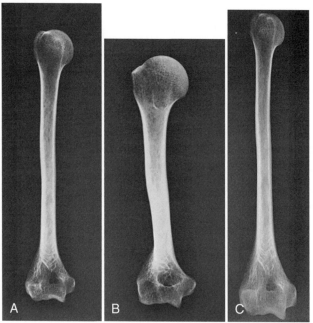

FIGURE 3-20 A, No distortion. B, Foreshortened. C, Elongated.

> **Important Relationship**
> *Shape Distortion*
> Shape distortion can occur from inaccurate central ray (CR) alignment of the tube, the part being radiographed, or the image receptor. Elongation refers to images of objects that appear longer than the true objects. Foreshortening refers to images that appear shorter than the true objects.

Sometimes shape distortion is used to advantage in particular projections or positions. For example, CR angulation is sometimes required to elongate a part so that a particular anatomic structure can be visualized better. Also, rotating the part (and therefore creating shape distortion) is sometimes required to eliminate superimposition of objects that normally obstruct visualization of the area of interest. In general, shape distortion is not a necessary or desirable characteristic of radiographs.

The factors that determine the amount of image distortion are equally important for digital and film-screen imaging. Both SID and OID determine the amount of magnification of the anatomic structures on the image. In addition, improper alignment of the CR, anatomic part, image receptor, or a combination of these components distorts the shape of the image, whether obtained with a digital or film-screen image receptor.

Scatter

Scatter radiation, as described previously, can add unwanted exposure to the radiographic image as a result of Compton interactions. Unwanted exposure or fog on the image does not provide information about the anatomic area of interest. Scatter degrades or decreases the visibility of the anatomic structures. The scatter or unwanted exposure recorded on the image has the effect of decreasing the contrast by masking the desired brightness or densities on the image and changing the degree of differences (Figure 3-21).

Fog produced as a result of scatter reaching the image receptor can be visualized on both a digital and a film image. Even though the computer can change the contrast or gray levels displayed in the digital image, scatter radiation reaching the image receptor does not provide any information about the area of interest. Because digital image receptors can detect low levels of radiation intensity, they are more sensitive to scatter radiation than film.

Quantum Noise

Image noise contributes no useful diagnostic information and serves only to detract from the quality of the image. **Quantum noise** is a concern in digital and film-screen imaging and is photon dependent. Quantum noise is visible as brightness or density fluctuations on the image. *Quantum mottle* is the term typically used when referring to noise on a film image. The fewer the photons reaching the image receptor to form the image, the greater the quantum noise visible on the digital image.

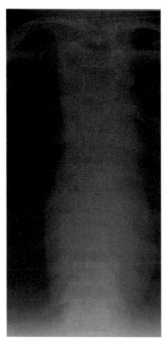

FIGURE 3-21 Scatter and fog.

> ### Important Relationship
> *Number of Photons and Quantum Noise*
> Decreasing the number of photons reaching the image receptor may increase the amount of quantum noise within the radiographic image; increasing the number of photons reaching the image receptor may decrease the amount of quantum noise within the radiographic image.

Although quantum noise can be a problem for both digital and film-screen imaging, it is more likely to occur in digital imaging. As mentioned previously, the digital computer system can adjust for low or high x-ray exposures during image acquisition. When the x-ray exposure to the image receptor is too low (decreased number of photons), computer processing alters the appearance of the digital image to make the brightness acceptable, but the image displays increased quantum noise (Figure 3-22). Certain postprocessing options may render quantum noise more or less noticeable.

The exposure technique should be selected based on the requirements for the type of radiographic procedure performed. A factor that differentiates digital from film-screen imaging is the ability of the computer to adjust the brightness of the image after exposure technique errors. Although the computer can adjust for both low-exposure and high-exposure technique errors, the radiographer is still responsible for selecting exposure techniques that produce acceptable image quality, while simultaneously maintaining patient exposure as low as reasonably achievable (ALARA). In particular, exposures that are too low adversely affect the quantum

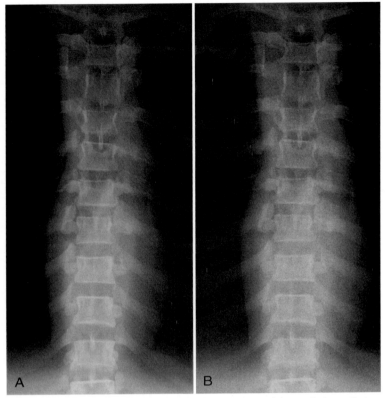

FIGURE 3-22 A, Image created using an appropriate x-ray exposure technique. **B,** Image shows increased quantum noise as a result of insufficient x-ray exposure to the image receptor.

noise of the image even though the computer can adjust the brightness. Exposures that are too high result in excessive radiation exposure to the patient. It is recommended that radiographers continue to select exposure techniques that produce diagnostic-quality radiographic images, regardless of whether the imaging system is digital or film-screen.

Image Artifacts

An **artifact** is any unwanted image on a radiograph. Artifacts are detrimental to radiographs because they can make visibility of anatomy, a pathologic condition, or patient identification information difficult or impossible. They decrease the overall quality of the radiographic image. Various methods are used to classify artifacts. Generally, artifacts can be classified as *plus-density* and *minus-density*. Plus-density artifacts are greater in density than the area of the image immediately surrounding them. Minus-density artifacts are of less density than the area of the image immediately surrounding them.

Errors such as double exposing an image receptor or the improper use of equipment can result in image artifacts and must be avoided. Foreign bodies are a

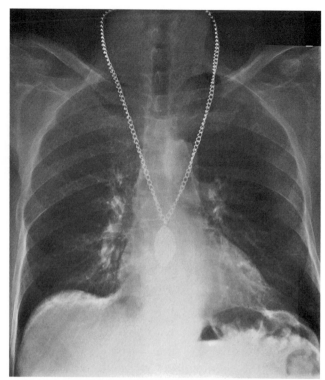

FIGURE 3-23 Image artifact.

classification of artifacts imaged within the patient's body. Variation in exposure techniques may be necessary when imaging for a suspected foreign body.

Although the causes of some artifacts are the same regardless of the type of imaging system, others are specific to digital or film imaging. Artifacts from patient clothing and items imaged that are not a part of the area of interest are the same for both film and digital systems. The radiographer must be diligent in removing clothing or items that could obstruct visibility of the anatomic area of interest (Figure 3-23). Scatter radiation or fog and image noise have also been classified as radiographic artifacts because they add unwanted information on the image.

Artifacts specific to film-screen imaging are typically a result of film storage, handling, and chemical processing. Digital image artifacts can be a result of errors during extraction of the latent image from the image receptor, inadequate CR imaging plate erasure, or performance of the electronic detectors.

IMAGE CHARACTERISTICS

As discussed previously, several attributes are evaluated to determine the quality of a radiographic image. Because imaging systems can acquire, process, and display the image differently, image characteristics also vary. The following discussion focuses on the major differences between digital and film images.

Digital Imaging

In digital imaging, the latent image is stored as digital data and must be processed by the computer for viewing on a display monitor. Digital imaging can be accomplished by using a specialized image receptor that can produce a computerized radiographic image. Two types of digital radiographic systems are in use today: computed radiography (CR) and direct digital radiography (DR). Regardless of whether the imaging system is CR or DR, the computer can manipulate the radiographic image in various ways after the image has been created digitally.

A unique characteristic of digital image receptors is their wide dynamic range. **Dynamic range** refers to the range of exposure intensities an image receptor can accurately detect; this means that moderately underexposed or overexposed images may still be of acceptable diagnostic quality. Because the image is constructed of digital data and is viewed on a display monitor, it can exhibit a wider range of brightness or densities. As a result, anatomic areas of widely different x-ray attenuation, such as soft tissues and bony structures, can be more easily visualized on a digital image.

> **Important Relationship**
> *Dynamic Range and Digital Image Receptors*
> Digital image receptors can accurately detect a wide range of exit radiation intensities (wide dynamic range), and therefore anatomic tissues can be better visualized.

Digital images are composed of numeric data that can be easily manipulated by a computer. When displayed on a computer monitor, there is tremendous flexibility in terms of altering the brightness (density) and contrast of a digital image. The practical advantage of such capability is that, regardless of the original exposure technique factors (within reason), any anatomic structure can be independently and well visualized. Computers can also perform various postprocessing image manipulations to improve visibility of the anatomic region further.

A digital image is recorded as a **matrix** or combination of rows and columns (array) of small, usually square, "picture elements" called **pixels**. The size of the pixel is measured in microns (0.001 mm). Each pixel is recorded as a single numeric value, which is represented as a single brightness level on a display monitor. The location of the pixel within the image matrix corresponds to an area within the patient or volume of tissue (Figure 3-24).

For a given anatomic area, or field of view (FOV), a matrix size of 1024 × 1024 has 1,048,576 individual pixels; a matrix size of 2048 × 2048 has 4,194,304 pixels. Digital image quality is improved with a larger matrix size that includes a greater number of smaller pixels (Figure 3-25 and Box 3-2). Although image quality is improved for a larger matrix size and smaller pixels, computer processing time, network transmission time, and digital storage space increase as the matrix size increases.

The numeric value assigned to each pixel is determined by the relative attenuation of x-rays passing through the corresponding volume of tissue. Pixels representing highly attenuating tissues, such as bone, are usually assigned a low value for higher brightness than pixels representing tissues of low x-ray attenuation (Figure 3-26).

1 Pixel

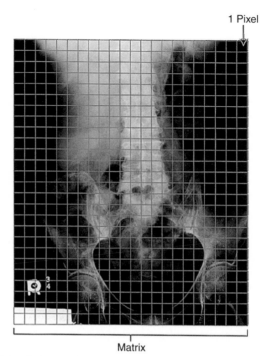

Matrix

FIGURE 3-24 Location of the pixel within the image matrix corresponds to an area within the patient or volume of tissue. *Note:* Pixel size not to scale and used for illustration only.

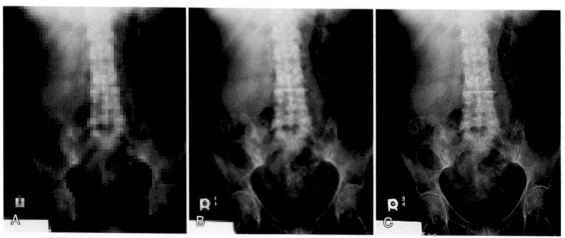

FIGURE 3-25 For a given field of view (FOV), the larger the matrix size, the greater the number of smaller individual pixels. Increasing the number of pixels improves the quality of the image. **A,** Matrix size is 64 × 64. **B,** Matrix size is 215 × 215. **C,** Matrix size is 2048 × 2048.

BOX 3-2	**Digital Imaging Terminology**

Matrix—image displayed as a combination of rows and columns (array); a larger matrix size improves digital spatial resolution

Pixel—smallest component of the matrix; a greater number of smaller pixels improves digital spatial resolution

Pixel bit depth—number of bits that determines the precision with which the exit radiation is recorded and controls the exact pixel brightness that can be specified

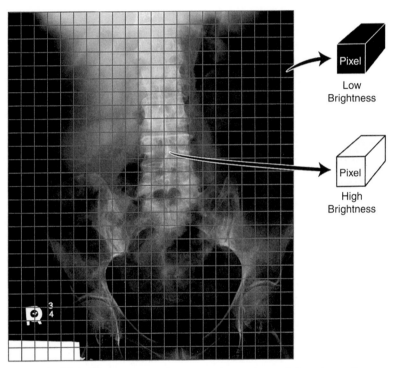

FIGURE 3-26 Each pixel value represents a volume of tissue imaged.

Each pixel also has a **bit depth,** or number of bits (Box 3-3) that determines the amount of precision in digitizing the analog signal and therefore the number of shades of gray that can be displayed in the image. Bit depth is determined by the analog-to-digital converter that is an integral component of every digital imaging system. Because the binary system is used, bit depth is expressed as 2 to the power of n, or the number of bits (2^n). A larger bit depth allows a greater number of shades of gray to be displayed on a computer monitor. For example, a 12-bit depth (2^{12}) can display 4096 shades of gray, a 14-bit depth can display 16,384 shades of gray, and a 16-bit depth can display 65,536 shades of gray. A system that can digitize and display a greater number of shades of gray has better contrast resolution. An image with increased contrast resolution increases the visibility of recorded detail and the ability to distinguish among small anatomic areas of interest.

BOX 3-3 | Binary Digits

Computers operate and communicate through the **binary number system,** which uses combinations of zeros and ones to process and store information. A digital transistor can be operated in two states, either off (0) or on (1). Each 0 and 1 is called a **bit** and refers to the computer's basic unit of information. When 8 bits are combined, they form a **byte,** and 2 bytes form a word.

Binary digits are used to display the brightness level (shades of gray) of the digital image. The greater the number of bits, the greater the number of shades of gray, and the quality of the image is improved.

Important Relationship
Pixel Bit Depth and Contrast Resolution

The greater the pixel bit depth (i.e., 14-bit), the more precise the digitization of the analog signal, and the greater the number of shades of gray available for image display. Increasing the number of shades of gray available to display on a digital image improves its contrast resolution.

A digital image is composed of discrete information in the form of pixels that display various shades of gray. As mentioned previously, the greater the number of pixels in an image matrix, the smaller their size. An image consisting of a greater number of pixels per unit area, or **pixel density,** provides improved spatial resolution. In addition to its size, the pixel spacing or distance measured from the center of a pixel to an adjacent pixel determines the **pixel pitch** (Figure 3-27).

Important Relationship
Pixel Density and Pitch and Spatial Resolution

Increasing the pixel density and decreasing the pixel pitch increases spatial resolution. Decreasing pixel density and increasing pixel pitch decreases spatial resolution.

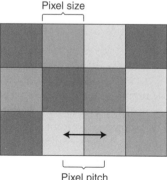

FIGURE 3-27 The distance measured from the center of a pixel to an adjacent pixel determines the pixel pitch or pixel spacing.

Different types of digital image receptors use various methods of transforming the continuous exit radiation intensities into the array of discrete pixels for image display. Some digital image receptors use a sampling technique, whereas others have fixed detector elements that are used to capture the exit radiation intensities. Regardless of the type used, a major determinant of spatial resolution of digital images is the pixel size and its spacing.

The device used for digital image display also affects the ability to view anatomic details. High-resolution monitors are required to maximize the amount of spatial resolution viewed in the digital image.

Film-Screen Imaging

A major difference between digital and film-screen imaging is that film is used as the medium for acquiring, processing, and displaying the radiographic image. In order to create and display the radiographic image, an **active layer** or **emulsion** is adhered to a sheet of polyester plastic. The emulsion contains crystals suspended in gelatin that serve as the latent imaging centers. To reduce patient exposure, radiographic film is placed between two intensifying screens. The intensifying screens convert the exit radiation intensities into visible light, and the light exposes the crystals in the emulsion.

The film must be processed chemically in an automatic processor before it is visualized on the sheet of polyester plastic. Once it is chemically processed, the film image displays densities ranging from dark to light that correspond to the variations in the intensities of radiation exiting the anatomic tissues. The dark densities are created when the exposed crystals are converted to black metallic silver. The light or clear areas on the film result from removal of the unexposed crystals during chemical processing. The resulting image represents a range of densities created as a result of the x-ray attenuation characteristics of the anatomic structures. Anatomic tissues that transmitted radiation are visualized as dark densities and anatomic tissues that absorbed radiation are visualized as light or clear areas on the film.

Optical density. Density on the radiographic film image can be quantified and is therefore an objective measure that can be used for comparison. A **densitometer** is a device used to numerically determine the amount of blackness on the radiograph (i.e., it measures radiographic density).

This device is constructed to emit a constant intensity of light (incident) onto an area of the film and then measure the amount of light transmitted (Figure 3-28). The densitometer determines the amount of light transmitted and calculates a measurement known as *optical density (OD)*. **Optical density** is a numeric calculation that compares the intensity of light transmitted through an area on the film (I_t) to the amount of light originally striking (incident) the area (I_0). The ratio of these intensities is called *transmittance*. Box 3-4 shows the mathematical formula used to calculate *percent transmittance*. Because the range of radiographic densities is large, the calculation of radiographic densities is compressed into a logarithmic scale (Table 3-2) for easier management.

As shown in Box 3-5, optical density is defined as the logarithm (Log_{10}) of the inverse of transmittance. For example, an area of the image that allows 10% of the original incident light to be transmitted has a transmittance of 1/10 or 0.1. The

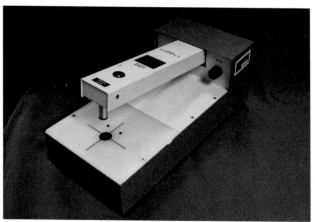

FIGURE 3-28 A densitometer is used to measure optical densities.

BOX 3-4 | **Light Transmittance Formula**

$$\frac{I_t}{I_o} \times 100$$

where I_t represents the amount of light transmitted and I_o represents the amount of original light incident on the film.

---

inverse of transmittance is therefore 10, and the logarithm of 10 (the optical density) is 1. Similarly, an area that allows only 1% of the original incident light through has an optical density of 2.0.

 Important Relationship
Light Transmittance and Optical Density
As the percentage of light transmitted decreases, the optical density increases; as the percentage of light transmitted increases, the optical density decreases.

Notice the relationship between light transmittance and optical density (Table 3-2). When 100% of the light is transmitted, the optical density equals 0.0. When 50% of the light is transmitted, the optical density is equal to 0.3, and when 25% of the light is transmitted, the optical density equals 0.6. When a logarithmic scale base 10 is used, every 0.3 change in optical density corresponds to a change in the percentage of light transmitted by a factor of 2 ($\log_{10}$ of 2 = 0.3).

Important Relationship
Optical Density and Light Transmittance
For every 0.3 change in optical density, the percentage of light transmitted has changed by a factor of 2. A 0.3 increase in optical density results from a decrease in the percentage of light transmitted by half, whereas a 0.3 decrease in optical density results from an increase in the percentage of light transmitted by a factor of 2.

TABLE 3-2	Percentage of Light Transmittance and Calculated Optical Densities	
Percentage of Light Transmitted ($I_t/I_o \times 100$)	Fraction of Light Transmitted (I_t/I_o)	Optical Density (log I_o/I_t)
100	1	0
50	1/2	0.3
32	8/25	0.5
25	1/4	0.6
12.5	1/8	0.9
10	1/10	1
5	1/20	1.3
3.2	4/125	1.5
2.5	1/40	1.6
1.25	1/80	1.9
1	1/100	2
0.5	1/200	2.3
0.32	2/625	2.5
0.125	1/800	2.9
0.1	1/1000	3
0.05	1/2000	3.3
0.032	1/3125	3.5
0.01	1/10,000	4

BOX 3-5	Optical Density Formula

$$\text{Optical density} = \text{Log}_{10} \frac{I_o}{I_t}$$

where I_o represents the amount of original light incident on the film and I_t represents the amount of transmitted light.

Diagnostic Range. Optical densities can range from 0.0 to 4.0 OD. However, the diagnostic range of optical densities for general radiography usually falls between 0.50 and 2.0 OD. This desired range of optical densities is found between the extreme low and high densities produced on the radiograph.

The radiation exposure to the image receptor primarily determines the amount of optical density created on the film after processing. The **intensity of radiation exposure** or **exposure intensity** is a measurement of the amount and energy of the x-rays reaching an area of the film. When all other factors remain the same, increasing the exposure intensity will increase the optical density.

Important Relationship
Exposure Intensity and Optical Density
Increasing the exposure intensity to the film-screen image receptor will increase the optical density, while decreasing the exposure intensity to the film-screen image receptor will decrease the exposure intensity.

In film-screen imaging the optical densities created on the processed radiograph cannot be altered. As a result, choosing the proper exposure intensity to create an appropriate range of optical densities (or **diagnostic densities**) during film-screen imaging is critical to producing a quality radiographic image. In order to visualize the anatomic area of interest, a film image must display diagnostic densities.

Although film-screen served as a good medium for radiographic images for many decades, it has many limitations that can be overcome with digital imaging. One major deficiency is the limited dynamic range (the range of exposure intensities an image receptor can accurately detect) of film-screen. This limitation renders a film-screen radiograph very sensitive to underexposure or overexposure, which may necessitate image retakes. A limited dynamic range also restricts visibility of structures that differ greatly in x-ray attenuation. An example is the difficulty of optimally visualizing both soft tissue and bony structures within a given film image.

Important Relationship
Dynamic Range and Film-Screen Imaging
The range of exposure intensities that film can accurately detect is limited (limited dynamic range). This renders film more susceptible to overexposure and underexposure and restricts its ability to display tissues that vary greatly in x-ray attenuation.

Other drawbacks of film-screen imaging involve the cost of film itself, the necessity of developing the latent image into a manifest image via chemical processing, and potential artifacts related to film handling and chemical processing. The time required to process the film before viewing the radiograph can delay the progress of an examination or the diagnosis. Automatic film processors incur considerable equipment and maintenance costs and demand frequent quality control procedures.

Another restriction associated with a film image is that once the film has been processed, the image is permanent, and further adjustments cannot be made. There is no option to alter the density or contrast of the manifest image. Therefore, the anatomic area that is to be optimally imaged must be selected at the time of exposure. For example, when an image is taken in the thoracic region, the exposure technique must be selected depending on whether the area of interest is the lungs or the ribs. A related issue is the limited contrast resolution, which is the ability to distinguish tissues of similar subject contrast, of film-screen receptors. Even if technique factors are chosen to optimize soft tissue contrast, the differential absorption among various soft tissues is slight and not well differentiated using film-screen.

In addition, film images cannot be electronically stored or duplicated, displayed on computer monitors, or transmitted over computer networks. Traditional film archives consume significant space and are frequently prone to loss of films. In addition, personnel costs associated with maintaining the archive and the expense of storing radiographs and then retrieving them when needed for comparison is prohibitive.

Digital imaging overcomes many of the limitations of conventional film radiography. Digital radiographic images can be acquired and displayed quickly and can be efficiently transmitted, processed, interpreted on a display monitor, stored, and retrieved via electronic means. Digital image receptors eliminate the need for film and film processing hardware and generally exhibit greater dynamic range and contrast resolution than film-screen image receptors. Image acquisition, processing, and display are discussed more thoroughly in later chapters.

CHAPTER SUMMARY

- A radiographic image is a result of the differential absorption of the primary x-rays that interact with the varying tissue composition of the anatomic area of interest.
- Beam attenuation occurs when the primary x-ray beam loses energy as it interacts with anatomic tissues.
- X-rays have the ability to eject electrons (ionization) from atoms within anatomic tissue.
- Three primary processes occur during x-ray interaction with anatomic tissues: absorption, transmission, and scattering.
- Total absorption of the incoming x-ray photon is a result of the photoelectric effect.
- Scattering of the incoming x-ray photon is a result of the Compton effect.
- Scatter radiation reaching the image receptor provides no useful information and creates unwanted exposure or fog on the radiograph.
- The process of differential absorption remains the same for image formation regardless of the type of image receptor.
- A radiographic image is composed of varying amounts of brightness or densities that structurally represent the anatomic area of interest.
- The visibility and accuracy of the anatomic structural lines recorded determine the overall quality of the radiographic image.
- Visibility of the recorded details is achieved by the proper balance of image brightness or density and contrast.
- Image contrast provides the ability to distinguish among the types of tissues irradiated.
- Grayscale is the number of different shades of gray that can be stored and displayed in a digital image.
- Short-scale contrast and long-scale contrast describe the number of and difference between densities visible in film-screen imaging.
- Digital images have improved contrast resolution compared with film-screen images.
- Spatial resolution and recorded detail refer to the accuracy of the anatomic structural lines recorded.
- Distortion describes the amount of magnification or misrepresentation in shape of the anatomic structures.
- Scatter radiation produces unwanted exposure on the image, known as fog.
- Quantum noise is a result of too few photons reaching the image receptor and is more of a concern in digital imaging.
- An artifact is any unwanted image on a radiograph.
- A digital image having a larger matrix and smaller-sized pixels has improved quality.
- A pixel's bit depth determines the shades of gray available to display the digital image or its contrast resolution.
- Spatial resolution is improved by increasing the pixel density and decreasing the pixel pitch.

- A film image is displayed on a polyester sheet of plastic composed of densities resulting from exposed crystals converted to black metallic silver after chemical processing.
- Optical density is a measurement of the amount of light transmitted through an area on the film.
- Digital image receptors have wider dynamic range compared with film-screen image receptors.

REVIEW QUESTIONS

1. The process whereby a radiographic image is created by variations in absorption and transmission of the exiting x-ray beam is known as _____.
A. attenuation
B. the photoelectric effect
C. the Compton effect
D. differential absorption

2. Which of the following processes occur during the x-ray beam interaction with tissue?
(1) Absorption
(2) Photon transmission
(3) Scattering
A. 1 and 2 only
B. 1 and 3 only
C. 2 and 3 only
D. 1, 2, and 3

3. The ability of an x-ray photon to remove an atom's electron is a characteristic known as _____.
A. attenuation
B. scattering
C. ionization
D. absorption

4. The x-ray interaction responsible for absorption is _____.
A. differential
B. photoelectric
C. attenuation
D. Compton

5. The x-ray interaction responsible for scattering is _____.
A. differential
B. photoelectric
C. attenuation
D. Compton

6. Remnant radiation is composed of which of the following?
   (1) Transmitted radiation
   (2) Absorbed radiation
   (3) Scattered radiation
   A. 1 and 2 only
   B. 1 and 3 only
   C. 2 and 3 only
   D. 1, 2, and 3

7. What interaction creates unwanted exposure to the image, known as fog?
   A. Compton
   B. Transmitted
   C. Photoelectric
   D. Absorption

8. Which of the following factors would affect beam attenuation?
   (1) Tissue atomic number
   (2) Beam quality
   (3) Fog
   A. 1 and 2 only
   B. 1 and 3 only
   C. 2 and 3 only
   D. 1, 2, and 3

9. The low-density or high brightness areas on a radiographic image are created by _____.
   A. transmitted radiation
   B. scattered radiation
   C. absorbed radiation
   D. primary radiation

10. An anatomic part that transmits the incoming x-ray photon would create an area of _____ on the radiographic image.
    A. fog
    B. low density or high brightness
    C. high density or low brightness
    D. gray

11. The process of creating a radiographic image by differential absorption varies for film-screen and digital imaging.
    A. True
    B. False

12. An attribute (or attributes) of a radiographic image that affects the *visibility* of sharpness is _____.
A. distortion
B. contrast
C. density
D. contrast and density

13. A radiographic film image with many densities but little differences among them is said to have _____.
A. high contrast
B. low contrast
C. short-scale contrast
D. excessive density

14. Which of the following is defined as the range of exposure intensities an image receptor can accurately detect?
A. Long-scale contrast
B. Spatial resolution
C. Quantum noise
D. Dynamic range

15. Which of the following would improve digital image quality?
A. Small matrix and large pixel size
B. Decreased pixel density and increased pixel pitch
C. Large matrix and large pixel size
D. Large matrix and increased pixel density

Exposure Technique Factors

OBJECTIVES

After completing this chapter, the reader will be able to perform the following:

1. Define all the key terms in this chapter.
2. State all the important relationships in this chapter.
3. Explain the relationship between milliamperage and exposure time with radiation production and image receptor (IR) exposure.
4. Calculate changes in milliamperage and exposure time to change or maintain exposure to the IR.
5. Compare the effect of changes in milliamperage (mA) and exposure time on digital and film-screen images.
6. Recognize how to correct exposure factors for a density error.
7. Explain how kilovoltage peak (kVp) affects radiation production and IR exposure.
8. Calculate changes in kVp to change or maintain exposure to the IR.
9. Compare the effect of changes in kVp on digital and film-screen images.
10. Recognize the factors that affect recorded detail and distortion.
11. Calculate changes in mAs for changes in source-to-image receptor distance.
12. Calculate the magnification factor, and determine image and object size.
13. Describe the use of grids and beam restriction and their effect on IR exposure and image quality.
14. Calculate changes in mAs when adding or removing a grid.
15. Recognize patient factors that may affect IR exposure.
16. Identify the exposure factors that can affect patient radiation exposure.
17. State exposure technique modifications for the following considerations: body habitus, pediatric patients, projections and positions, soft tissue, casts and splints, and pathologic conditions.

In Chapter 2, variables that affect both the quantity and the quality of the x-ray beam were presented. Milliamperage and time affect the quantity of radiation produced, and kilovoltage affects both the quantity and the quality. Chapter 3 emphasized that a good-quality radiographic image accurately represents the anatomic area of interest. The characteristics evaluated for image quality are density or brightness, contrast, recorded detail or spatial resolution, distortion, and noise. This chapter focuses on exposure techniques and the use of accessory devices and their effect on the radiation reaching the image receptor (IR) and the image produced. Radiographers have the responsibility of selecting the combination of exposure factors to produce a good-quality image. Knowledge of how these factors affect the image individually and in combination assists the radiographer to produce a radiographic image with the amount of information desired for a diagnosis.

Because various types of IRs respond differently to the radiation exiting the patient, these differences are noted throughout this chapter. Digital IRs separate acquisition from processing and image display; their response to changes in radiation exposure does not affect the amount of brightness displayed on the image. The level of brightness and contrast can be altered during computer processing and image display. However, the amount of exposure to the digital IR needs to be carefully selected, as with film-screen IRs, to produce a quality image with the least amount of exposure to the patient. Radiographic film acquires the latent image and needs to be chemically processed before the image can be displayed. Changes in the quantity and the quality of radiation exposure to a film-screen IR affect the amount of density and contrast visible on the processed radiograph. This chapter discusses all the primary and secondary factors and their effects on the radiation reaching the IR.

PRIMARY FACTORS

The primary exposure technique factors the radiographer selects on the control panel are milliamperage (mA), time of exposure, and kilovoltage peak (kVp). Depending on the type of control panel, milliamperage and exposure time may be selected separately or combined as one factor, milliamperage/second (mAs). Regardless, it is important to understand how changing each separately or in combination affects the radiation reaching the IR and the radiographic image.

Milliamperage and Exposure Time

The quantity of radiation reaching the patient affects the amount of remnant radiation reaching the IR. The product of milliamperage and exposure time has a direct proportional relationship with the quantity of x-rays produced. Once the

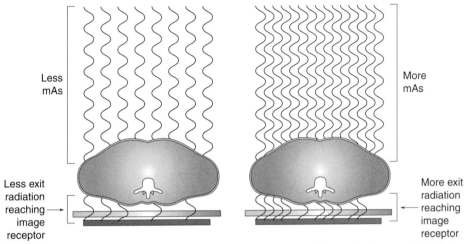

FIGURE 4-1 The mAs and radiation exposure. As the quantity of x-rays is increased (mAs), the exposure to the image receptor proportionally increases.

anatomic part is adequately penetrated, as the quantity of x-rays is increased, the exposure to the IR proportionally increases (Figure 4-1). Conversely, when the quantity of x-rays is decreased, the exposure to the IR decreases. Therefore, exposure to the IR can be increased or decreased by adjusting the amount of radiation (mAs).

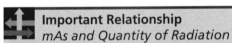

Important Relationship
mAs and Quantity of Radiation
As the mAs is increased, the quantity of radiation reaching the IR is increased. As the mAs is decreased, the amount of radiation reaching the IR is decreased.

Because the mAs is the product of milliamperage and exposure time, increasing milliamperage or time has the same effect on the radiation exposure.

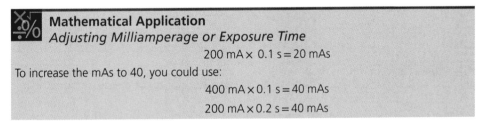

Mathematical Application
Adjusting Milliamperage or Exposure Time
$$200 \text{ mA} \times 0.1 \text{ s} = 20 \text{ mAs}$$
To increase the mAs to 40, you could use:
$$400 \text{ mA} \times 0.1 \text{ s} = 40 \text{ mAs}$$
$$200 \text{ mA} \times 0.2 \text{ s} = 40 \text{ mAs}$$

As demonstrated in the Mathematical Application, mAs can be doubled by doubling the milliamperage or doubling the exposure time. A change in either milliamperage or exposure time proportionally changes the mAs. To maintain the same mAs, the radiographer must increase the milliamperage and proportionally decrease the exposure time.

Important Relationship
Milliamperage and Exposure Time

Milliamperage and exposure time have an inverse proportional relationship when maintaining the same mAs.

Mathematical Application
Adjusting Milliamperage and Exposure Time to Maintain mAs

200 mA × 100 ms (0.1 s) = 20 mAs

To maintain the mAs, use:

400 mA × 50 ms (0.05 s) = 20 mAs

100 mA × 200 ms (0.2 s) = 20 mAs

It is important for the radiographer to determine the amount of mAs needed to produce a diagnostic image. This is not an easy task because there are so many variables that can affect the amount of mAs required. For example, single-phase generators produce less radiation for the same mAs compared with a high-frequency generator. A patient's age, the general condition of the patient, and the presence of a pathologic condition also affect the amount of mAs required for the procedure. In addition, IRs respond differently for a given mAs. Digital IRs can detect a wide range of radiation intensities (wide dynamic range) exiting the patient and are not as dependent on the mAs as film-screen IRs. However, exposure errors can adversely affect the quality of the digital image. If the mAs is too low (low exposure to the digital IR), image brightness is adjusted during computer processing to achieve the desired level. Although the level of brightness has been adjusted, there may be increased quantum noise visible within the image (Figure 4-2). If the mAs selected is too high (high exposure to the digital IR), the brightness can also adjusted, but the patient has received more radiation than necessary.

Important Relationship
mAs and Digital Image Brightness

The amount of mAs does not have a direct effect on image brightness when using digital IRs. During computer processing, image brightness is maintained when the mAs is too low or too high. A lower-than-needed mAs produces an image with increased quantum noise, and a higher-than-needed mAs exposes the patient to unnecessary radiation.

Because the brightness of a digital image can be altered during image processing, information about the exposure to the IR is important. Manufacturers of each type of digital system specify the expected range of x-ray exposure sufficient to produce a quality image. A numeric value (**exposure indicator**) is displayed on the processed image to indicate the level of x-ray exposure received (incident exposure) to the digital IR. It is important for the radiographer to consider the indicated value because exposure errors, as stated previously, affect the quality of the digital image and the radiation dose to the patient. Exposure errors are not obvious by simply looking at the digital image because the digital data are normalized to provide images with

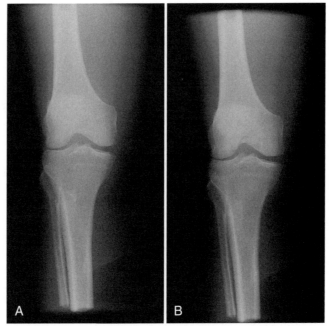

FIGURE 4-2 A, Radiograph obtained with low mAs showing increased quantum noise. B, Radiograph obtained with high mAs showing decreased quantum noise.

diagnostic density or brightness. Most manufacturers of digital IRs suggest a range for the exposure indicator based on the radiographic procedure. If the exposure indicator value falls outside of this range, image quality or patient exposure or both could be compromised.

> **Important Relationship**
> *Exposure Indicator Value*
> A numeric value or exposure indicator is displayed on the processed digital image that indicates the level of x-ray exposure received (incident exposure) to the IR. If the exposure indicator value falls outside of the manufacturer's suggested range, image quality or patient exposure or both could be compromised.

For film-screen IRs, the mAs controls the density produced in the image. There is a direct relationship between the amount of mAs and the amount of density produced when using film-screen IRs. When the mAs is increased, density is increased; when the mAs is decreased, density is decreased (Figure 4-3).

When a film image is too light (insufficient density), a greater increase in mAs may be needed to correct the density, or the mAs may need to be decreased to correct a film image that has excessive density. When using a film-screen IR, radiographers need to assess the level of density produced on the processed image and determine whether the density is sufficient to visualize the anatomic area of interest. The radiographer must decide how much of a change in mAs is needed to correct for the density error.

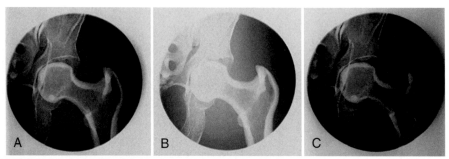

FIGURE 4-3 Changes in mAs have a direct effect on density. **A,** Original image. **B,** Decrease in density when the mAs is decreased by half. **C,** Increase in density when the mAs is doubled.

Generally, for repeat radiographs necessitated by density errors, the mAs is adjusted by a factor of 2; therefore, a minimum change involves doubling or halving the mAs. This change typically brings the film densities back to visualize the anatomic area of interest best. Radiographs that have sufficient but not optimal density usually are not repeated. If a radiograph must be repeated because of another error, such as positioning, the radiographer may also use the opportunity to make an adjustment in density to produce a radiograph of optimal quality. Making a visible change in radiographic density requires that the minimum amount of change in mAs be approximately 30% (depending on equipment, this may vary between 25% and 35%). Radiographic images generally are not repeated to make only a slight visible change. A radiographic image repeated because of insufficient or excessive density requires a change in mAs by a factor of at least 2.

> **Important Relationship**
> *mAs and Film-Screen Density*
> The amount of mAs has a direct effect on the amount of radiographic density produced when using a film-screen IR. The minimum change needed to correct for a density error is determined by multiplying or dividing the mAs by 2.

To visualize the anatomic area of interest best, the mAs selected must produce a sufficient amount of radiation reaching the IR, regardless of type. An excessive or insufficient amount of mAs adversely affects image quality and patient radiation exposure.

Kilovoltage Peak

The kVp affects the exposure to the IR because it alters the amount and penetrating ability of the x-ray beam. The area of interest must be adequately penetrated before the mAs can be adjusted to produce a quality radiographic image. When adequate penetration is achieved, increasing the kVp further results in more radiation reaching the IR. In addition to affecting the amount of radiation exposure to the IR, the kVp also affects image contrast.

Important Relationship
kVp and the Radiographic Image
Increasing or decreasing the kVp changes the amount of radiation exposure to the IR and the contrast produced within the image.

Kilovoltage Peak and Exposure to the Image Receptor. Because kVp affects the amount of radiation reaching the IR, its effect on the digital image is similar to the effect of mAs. Assuming that the anatomic part is adequately penetrated, too much radiation reaching the IR (within reason) produces a digital image with the appropriate level of brightness as a result of computer adjustment during image processing; however, the patient has been overexposed. Similarly, too little radiation reaching the IR (within reason) produces a digital image with the appropriate level of brightness, but the increased quantum noise decreases image quality. Excessive or insufficient radiation exposure to the digital IR, as a result of the mAs or kVp, should be reflected in the exposure indicator value.

 Important Relationship
Exposure Errors in Digital Imaging
kVp and mAs exposure errors should be reflected in the exposure indicator value; however, image brightness can be maintained during computer processing.

 Patient Protection Alert
Excessive Radiation Exposure and Digital Imaging
Although the computer can adjust image brightness for technique exposure errors, routinely using more radiation than required for the procedure in digital radiography unnecessarily increases patient exposure. Even though the digital system can adjust for overexposures, it is an unethical practice to overexpose a patient knowingly.

The kVp has a greater effect on the image when using film-screen IRs. Increasing the kVp increases IR exposure and the density produced on a film image, and decreasing the kVp decreases IR exposure and the density produced on a film image (Figure 4-4).

For film-screen IRs, kVp has a direct relationship with density; however, the effect of the kVp on density is not equal throughout the range of kVp (low, middle, and high). A greater change in the kVp is needed when operating at a high kVp (>90) compared with operating at a low kVp (<70) (Figure 4-5).

 Important Relationship
Exposure Errors and Film-Screen Imaging
kVp directly affects the density produced on a film-screen image; however, its effect is not equal throughout the range of kVp (low, middle, and high).

Kilovoltage is not a factor typically manipulated to vary the amount of IR exposure because the kVp also affects contrast. However, it is sometimes necessary to manipulate the kVp to maintain the required exposure to the IR. For example, using

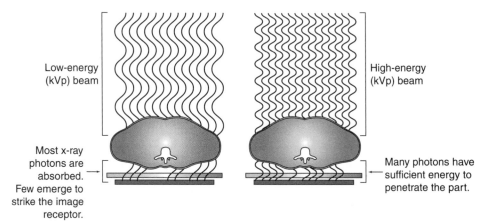

Low-energy
(kVp) beam

High-energy
(kVp) beam

Most x-ray
photons are
absorbed.
Few emerge to
strike the image
receptor.

Many photons have
sufficient energy to
penetrate the part.

FIGURE 4-4 The kVp and radiation exposure. Increasing the kVp increases the penetrating power of the radiation and increases the exposure to the image receptor.

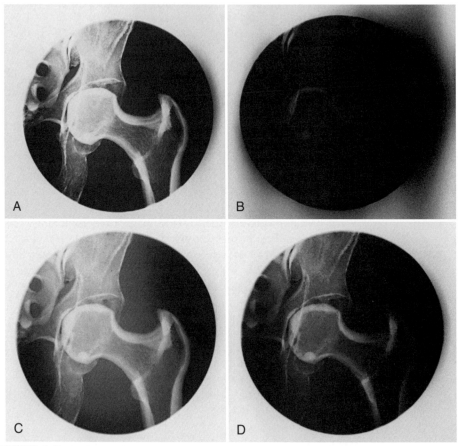

A   B

C   D

FIGURE 4-5 The kVp range and radiographic density. A-D, Radiographs produced at 50 kVp (**A**) and produced at 90 kVp with the mAs adjusted to maintain radiographic density (**C**); a 10-kVp increase at 50 kVp (**B**) produces a greater change in density than a 10-kVp increase at 90 kVp (**D**).

portable or mobile x-ray equipment may limit choices of mAs settings, and the radiographer must adjust the kVp to maintain sufficient exposure to the IR.

Maintaining or adjusting exposure to the IR can be accomplished with kVp by using the **15% rule**. The 15% rule states that changing the kVp by 15% has the same effect as doubling the mAs or reducing the mAs by 50%; for example, increasing the kVp from 82 to 94 (15%) produces the same exposure to the IR as increasing the mAs from 10 to 20.

Important Relationship
kVp and the 15% Rule
A 15% increase in kVp has the same effect on exposure to the IR as doubling the mAs. A 15% decrease in kVp has the same effect on exposure to the IR as decreasing the mAs by half.

Increasing the kVp by 15% increases the exposure to the IR, unless the mAs is decreased. Also, decreasing the kVp by 15% decreases the exposure to the IR, unless the mAs is increased. As mentioned earlier, the effects of changes in the kVp are not uniform throughout the range of kVp. When a low or high kVp is used, the amount of change in the kVp required to maintain the exposure to the IR may be greater than or less than 15%.

Mathematical Application
Using the 15% Rule
To increase exposure to the IR, multiply the kVp by 1.15 (original kVp + 15%):
$$75 \text{ kVp} \times 1.15 = 86 \text{ kVp}$$
To decrease exposure to the IR, multiply the kVp by 0.85 (original kVp − 15%):
$$75 \text{ kVp} \times 0.85 = 64 \text{ kV}p$$
To maintain exposure to the IR, when increasing the kVp by 15% (kVp × 1.15), divide the original mAs by 2:
$$75 \text{ kVp} \times 1.15 = 86 \text{ kVp and mAs/2}$$
When decreasing the kVp by 15% (kVp × 0.85), multiply the mAs by 2:
$$75 \text{ kVp} \times 0.85 = 64 \text{ and mAs} \times 2$$

Patient Protection Alert
kVp/mAs
Whenever possible, a higher kilovoltage and lower mAs should be used to reduce patient exposure. Increasing kilovoltage requires less mAs to maintain the desired exposure to the IR and decreases the radiation dose to the patient. For example, changing from 75 to 86 when imaging a pelvis is a 15% increase in kVp and would require half the mAs needed for the original 75 kVp. Higher kVp increases the beam penetration, and therefore less radiation is needed to achieve a desired exposure to the IR.

Kilovoltage Peak and Radiographic Contrast. Altering the penetrating power of the x-ray beam affects its absorption and transmission through the anatomic tissue being radiographed. Higher kVp increases the penetrating power of the x-ray beam and results in less absorption and more transmission in the anatomic tissues, which results in less variation in the x-ray intensities exiting the patient (lower subject contrast). As a result, images with lower contrast (more shades of gray) are produced (Figure 4-6). When a low kVp is used, the x-ray beam penetration is decreased, resulting in more absorption and less transmission, which results in greater variation in the x-ray intensities exiting the patient (higher subject contrast). A high-contrast (fewer shades of gray) radiographic image is produced (Figure 4-7).

Important Relationship
kVp and Radiographic Contrast

A high kVp results in less absorption and more transmission in the anatomic tissues, which results in less variation in the x-ray intensities exiting the patient (lower subject contrast), producing a low-contrast image. A low kVp results in more absorption and less x-ray transmission but with more variation in the x-ray intensities exiting the patient (higher subject contrast), resulting in a high-contrast image.

In digital imaging, the kVp affects the variation in radiation intensities exiting the patient and image contrast; however, image brightness and contrast are primarily controlled during computer processing. When a kVp that is too low is selected, the brightness and contrast are adjusted, but quantum noise may be visible. Additionally, when a kVp that is too high is selected, the image brightness and contrast are adjusted, but patient exposure may be increased. Although image contrast can be

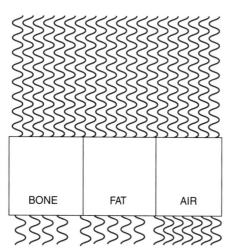
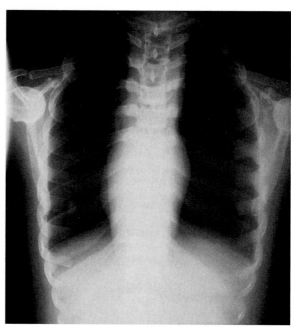

BONE   FAT   AIR

FIGURE 4-6 The kVp and exit-beam intensities. Higher kVp increases the penetrating power of the x-ray beam and results in less absorption and more transmission in the anatomic tissues, which results in less variation in the x-ray intensities exiting the patient. As a result, images with lower contrast are produced.

adjusted when using a kVp that is too high, increased scatter radiation reaches the IR and may adversely affect image quality.

> ### Important Relationship
> #### *Kilovoltage and Digital Image Quality*
> Assuming that the anatomic part is adequately penetrated, changing the kVp affects the radiation exposure to the digital IR similarly to changing the mAs, but dissimilar to mAs, kVp also affects image contrast. However, image brightness and contrast are primarily controlled during computer processing.

Changing the kVp affects its absorption and transmission as it interacts with anatomic tissue; however, using a higher kVp reduces the total number of interactions and increases the amount of x-rays transmitted. In these interactions, more Compton scattering than x-ray absorption occurs (photoelectric effect), and more scatter exits the patient. It is important to understand that in addition to kVp changing the subject contrast, it also affects the amount of scatter reaching the IR and therefore radiographic contrast.

> ### Important Relationship
> #### *Kilovoltage, Scatter Radiation, and Radiographic Contrast*
> At higher kVp, a greater proportion of Compton scattering occurs compared with x-ray absorption (photoelectric effect), which decreases radiographic contrast. Decreasing the kVp decreases the proportion of Compton scattering and increases radiographic contrast.

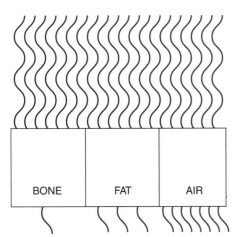

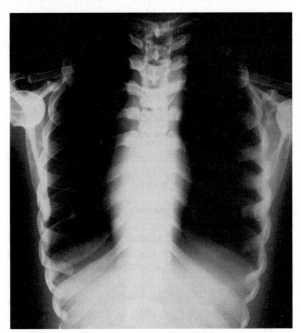

FIGURE 4-7 The kVp peak and exit-beam intensities. Lower kVp decreases the x-ray beam penetration, resulting in more absorption and less transmission, which results in greater variation in the x-ray intensities exiting the patient. As a result, images with higher contrast are produced.

The level of radiographic contrast desired—and therefore the kVp selected—depends on the type and composition of the anatomic tissue, the structures that must be visualized, and to some extent the type of IR. These factors make achieving a desired level of radiographic contrast more complex than achieving a desired level of exposure to the IR, especially for film-screen imaging. Radiographic film can be manufactured to display different levels of contrast. In addition to the type of film used, the kVp selected controls the level of contrast produced in the image.

For most anatomic regions, an accepted range of kVp provides an appropriate level of radiographic contrast. As long as the kVp selected is sufficient to penetrate the anatomic part, the kVp can be manipulated further to alter the radiographic contrast.

Radiographs generally are not repeated because of contrast errors. More often, the radiographer evaluates the level of contrast achieved to improve the contrast for additional radiographs or similar circumstances that arise with a different patient. If a repeat radiograph is necessary and kVp is to be adjusted either to increase or to decrease the level of contrast, the 15% rule provides an acceptable method of adjustment. In addition, whenever a 15% change is made in the kVp to maintain the exposure to the IR, the radiographer must adjust the mAs by a factor of 2. Remember that a 15% change in kVp does not produce the same effect across the entire range of kVp used in radiography. A greater increase is needed for a high kVp ($\geq$90) than for a low kVp (<70).

The selection of kVp alters its absorption and transmission through the anatomic part regardless of the type of IR used, and therefore kVp must be selected wisely. Exposure techniques using higher kVp with lower mAs exposure techniques are recommended in digital imaging because contrast is primarily controlled during computer processing. Higher kVp and lower mAs values are not recommended as a general rule during film-screen imaging because of the contrast required to visualize the anatomic structures best.

SECONDARY FACTORS

Many secondary or influencing factors affect the radiation reaching the IR and image quality. It is important for the radiographer to understand their effects individually and in combination.

Focal Spot Size

On the control panel, the radiographer can select whether to use a small or large focal spot size. The physical dimensions of the focal spot on the anode target in x-ray tubes used in standard radiographic applications usually range from 0.5 to 1.2 mm. Small focal spot sizes are usually 0.5 mm or 0.6 mm, and large focal spot sizes are usually 1 mm or 1.2 mm. Focal spot size is determined by the filament size. When the radiographer selects a particular focal spot size, he or she is actually selecting a filament size that is energized during x-ray production. Focal spot size is an important consideration for the radiographer because the focal spot size affects recorded detail (Figure 4-8).

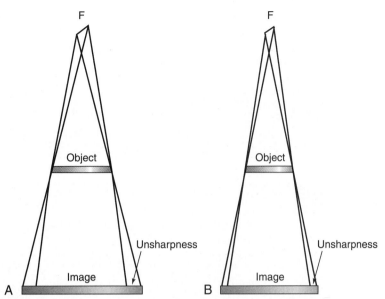

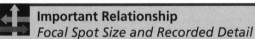

FIGURE 4-8 Focal spot size and recorded detail. Focal spot size influences the amount of unsharpness recorded in the image. As focal spot size changes, so does the amount of unsharpness. **A,** Larger focal spot. **B,** Smaller focal spot.

> **Important Relationship**
> *Focal Spot Size and Recorded Detail*
> As focal spot size increases, unsharpness increases, and recorded detail decreases; as focal spot size decreases, unsharpness decreases, and recorded detail increases.

Generally, the smallest focal spot size available should be used for every exposure. However, exposure is limited with a small focal spot size. When a small focal spot is used, the heat created during the x-ray exposure is concentrated in a smaller area and could cause tube damage. The radiographer must weigh the importance of improved recorded detail for a particular examination or anatomic part against the amount of radiation exposure used. Modern radiographic x-ray generators are equipped with safety circuits that prevent an exposure from being made if that exposure exceeds the tube loading capacity for the focal spot size selected. Repeated exposures made just under the limit over a long period can still jeopardize the life of the x-ray tube.

Source-to-Image Receptor Distance

The distance between the source of the radiation and the IR, **source-to-image receptor distance (SID)**, affects the amount of radiation reaching the patient. Because of the divergence of the x-ray beam, the intensity of the radiation varies at different distances.

This relationship between distance and x-ray beam intensity is best described by the inverse square law. The **inverse square law** states that the intensity of the x-ray beam is inversely proportional to the square of the distance from the source.

Because beam intensity varies as a function of the square of the distance, SID affects the quantity of radiation reaching the IR. As SID is increased, the x-ray intensity is spread over a larger area; this decreases the overall intensity of the x-ray beam reaching the IR (Figure 4-9).

Important Relationship
SID and X-ray Beam Intensity
As SID increases, the x-ray beam intensity is spread over a larger area. This decreases the overall intensity of the x-ray beam reaching the IR.

Mathematical Application
Inverse Square Law Formula
$$\frac{I_1}{I_2} = \frac{(D_2)^2}{(D_1)^2}$$
The intensity of radiation at an SID of 40 inches is equal to 400 mR. What is the intensity of radiation when the distance is increased to 72 inches?
$$\frac{400 \text{ mR}}{X} = \frac{(72)^2}{(40)^2} \quad 400 \text{ mR} \times 1600 = 640,000 = 5184 \text{ X}; \quad \frac{640,000}{5184} = X; \quad 123.5 \text{ mR} = X$$

Because increasing the SID decreases x-ray beam intensity, the mAs must be increased accordingly to maintain the proper exposure to the IR. When the SID

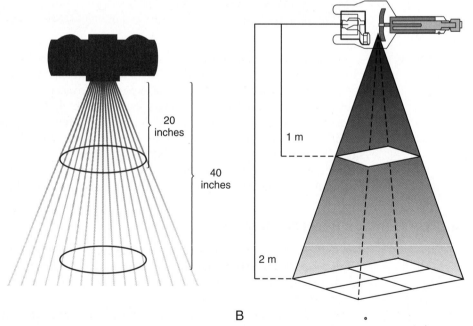

A   B

FIGURE 4-9 SID and radiation intensity. **A** and **B,** Changing SID and its effect on the divergence of the beam **(A)** and its effect on the intensity of the x-ray beam reaching the image receptor **(B).**

is decreased, the beam intensity increases; therefore, the mAs must be decreased accordingly to maintain proper exposure to the IR.

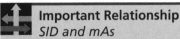

Important Relationship
SID and mAs
Increasing the SID requires that the mAs be increased to maintain exposure to the IR, and decreasing the SID requires a decrease in the mAs to maintain exposure to the IR.

Maintaining consistent radiation exposure to the IR when the SID is altered requires that the mAs be adjusted to compensate. The **mAs/distance compensation formula** provides a mathematical calculation for adjusting the mAs when changing the SID.

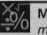

Mathematical Application
mAs/Distance Compensation Formula
$$\frac{mAs_1}{mAs_2} \frac{(SID_1)^2}{(SID_2)^2}$$
Optimal exposure to the IR is achieved at an SID of 40 inches using 25 mAs. The SID must be increased to 72 inches. What adjustment in mAs is needed to maintain exposure to the IR?
$$\frac{25}{X} = \frac{(40)^2}{(72)^2}; \; 1600\,X = 129{,}600; \; \frac{129{,}600}{1600}; X = 81\;mAs_2$$

Standard distances are used in radiography to provide more consistency in radiographic quality. Most diagnostic radiography is performed at an SID of 40 inches, 48 inches, or 72 inches. Certain circumstances, such as trauma or mobile radiography, do not allow for standard distances to be used. In these circumstances, the radiographer must determine the change needed in the mAs to obtain a quality radiograph. When a 72-inch (180-cm) SID cannot be used, adjusting the SID to 56 inches (140 cm) requires half the mAs. When a 40-inch (100-cm) SID cannot be used, adjusting the SID to 56 inches (140 cm) requires twice the mAs. This quick method of calculating mAs changes should produce sufficient exposure to the IR.

In addition to altering the intensity of radiation, SID affects image distortion and recorded detail or spatial resolution regardless of the type of IR. As the distance between the source and IR increases, the diverging x-rays become more perpendicular to the object radiographed and influence the amount of size distortion produced on a radiograph (Figure 4-10).

Important Relationship
SID, Size Distortion, and Recorded Detail
As SID increases, size distortion (magnification) decreases, and recorded detail or spatial resolution increases; as SID decreases, size distortion (magnification) increases, and recorded detail or spatial resolution decreases.

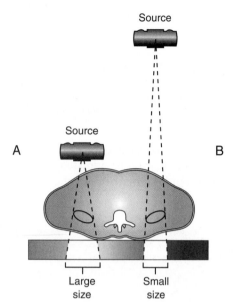

FIGURE 4-10 SID and size distortion. **A** and **B,** A long SID creates less magnification than a short SID. The image in **A** is larger than the image in **B** because the object is closer to the source.

Standard distances for SID are used in radiography to accommodate equipment limitations. Except for chest and cervical spine radiography, a 40-inch (100-cm) or 48-inch (120-cm) SID is standard. A larger 72-inch (180-cm) SID, such as used for chest imaging, decreases the magnification of the heart and records its size more accurately.

Object-to-Image Receptor Distance

When distance is created between the object radiographed and the IR, known as **object-to-image receptor distance (OID)**, decreased beam intensity may result. As the exit radiation continues to diverge, less overall intensity of the x-ray beam reaches the IR. Decreasing the exposure to the IR may require an increase in the mAs to compensate.

When sufficient distance between the object and IR exists, an air gap is created, also preventing the scatter radiation from striking the IR (Figure 4-11). Whenever the amount of scatter radiation reaching the IR is reduced, the radiographic contrast is increased. This effect on contrast is more visible for anatomic areas that produce a high percentage of scatter radiation exiting the patient. Reducing the scatter reaching the IR by increased OID has a greater effect on contrast for film-screen compared with digital IRs.

In addition to affecting the intensity of radiation reaching the IR, the OID also affects the amount of image distortion and recorded detail or spatial resolution. Optimal recorded detail or spatial resolution is achieved when the OID is zero. However, this OID cannot realistically be achieved in radiographic

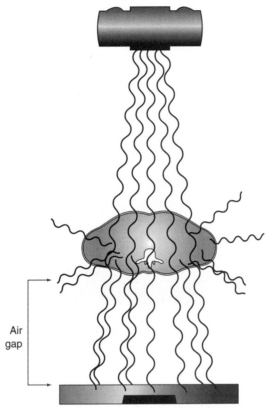

Air
gap

FIGURE 4-11 OID and air gap. Distance created between the object and the image receptor reduces the amount of scatter radiation reaching the image receptor.

imaging because there is always some distance created between the area of interest and the IR. As the exit beam leaves the patient, it continues to diverge. When distance is created between the area of interest and the IR, the diverging exit beam records the anatomic part with increased size distortion or magnification (Figure 4-12).

Important Relationship
OID, Size Distortion, and Recorded Detail or Spatial Resolution
Increasing the OID increases magnification and decreases the recorded detail or spatial resolution, whereas decreasing the OID decreases magnification and increases the recorded detail or spatial resolution.

OID is the only factor that affects the intensity of radiation reaching the IR, image contrast, magnification, and recorded detail or spatial resolution. The distance between the area of interest and the IR has the greatest effect on the amount of size distortion. The radiographer must position the area of interest as close to the IR as possible to minimize the amount of distortion. Although the amount of

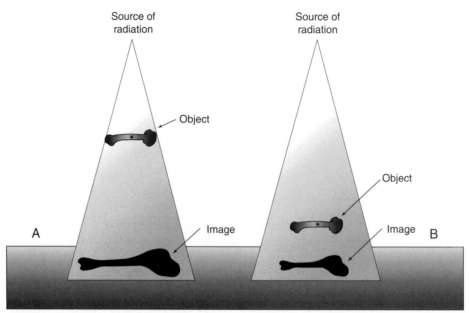

FIGURE 4-12 OID and size distortion. **A** and **B,** A long OID creates more magnification than a short OID. The image in **A** is larger than the image in **B** because the object is farther from the image receptor.

OID necessary to affect image quality adversely has not been standardized, the radiographer should minimize the amount of OID whenever possible. In some situations, it is difficult to minimize OID because of factors or conditions beyond the radiographer's control. In these instances, size distortion can still be reduced by increasing SID.

Calculating Magnification

To observe the effect of distance (SID and OID) on size distortion, it is necessary to consider the magnification factor. The **magnification factor (MF)** indicates how much size distortion or magnification is demonstrated on a radiograph. The MF can be expressed mathematically by the following formula:

$$MF = SID \div SOD$$

Source-to-object distance (SOD) refers to the distance from the x-ray source (focal spot) to the object being radiographed. SOD can be expressed mathematically as follows:

$$SOD = SID - OID$$

SOD is demonstrated in Figure 4-13.

MF of 1 indicates no magnification, which means that the image size matches the true object size. True object size on a radiograph is impossible to achieve because some magnification exists on every radiograph. MF greater than 1 can be expressed

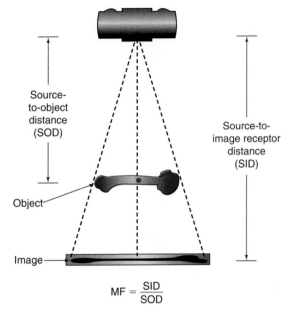

$$MF = \frac{SID}{SOD}$$

FIGURE 4-13 SOD. The SOD is the distance between the source of the x-ray and the object radiographed.

as a percentage of magnification. For example, MF of 1.15 indicates the image size is 15% larger than the object size.

> **Mathematical Application**
> *Magnification Factor*
> An anteroposterior projection (AP) of the knee is produced with an SID of 40 inches and an OID of 3 inches (SOD is equal to 37 inches). What is the MF?
> $$SOD = SID - OID \quad MF = \tfrac{40}{37}; \; MF = 1.081$$
> $$37 = 40 - 3$$

In the case of the Mathematical Application for MF, MF of 1.081 means that the image size is 8.1% larger than the true object size. It should be noted that the MF computed here is a minimum. A 3-inch OID implies that the posterior surface of the patient's knee was 3 inches away from the IR for an anteroposterior (AP) projection. Anatomy that is anterior to the posterior surface of the knee, such as the patella, is farther away from the IR and is magnified even more.

It may be helpful to know the measurement of the true object size in comparison with its size on a radiographic image. Once the MF is known, the object size can be determined. This requires the use of another formula:

$$Object\ size = \frac{Image\ size}{MF}$$

> ### Mathematical Application
> *Determining Object Size*
> On an AP image of a knee taken with an SID of 40 inches and an OID of 3 inches (SOD = 37 inches), the size of a lesion measures 0.5 inch in diameter on the radiograph. The MF has been determined to be 1.081. What is the object size of this lesion?
>
> $$\frac{40}{37} = 1.081 \text{ MF} \quad \text{Object size} = \frac{0.5 \text{ inch}}{1.081}$$
>
> The object size is 0.463 inch.

Perhaps the most practical use of these formulas is to observe how changing the SID and OID affects the image size. Size distortion or magnification can be increased by decreasing the SID or by increasing the OID. This increase in magnification can be demonstrated mathematically by using the MF, then calculating the change in the size of the object on the radiographic image. Any time magnification is increased, recorded detail or spatial resolution decreases.

Central Ray Alignment

Shape distortion of the anatomic area of interest can occur from inaccurate central ray (CR) alignment of the tube, the part being radiographed, or the IR. Any misalignment of the CR among these three factors alters the shape of the part recorded on the image.

For example, Figure 4-14 demonstrates shape distortion when the anatomic part and IR are misaligned. In addition, shape distortion can occur if the CR of the primary beam is not directed to enter or exit the anatomy as required for the particular projection or position (off centering). This shape distortion occurs because the path of individual photons in the primary beam becomes more divergent as the distance increases from the CR. The radiographer must properly control alignment of the tube, part, and IR, and he or she must properly direct the CR to minimize shape distortion. In addition to creating shape distortion, CR angulation and misalignment of the tube, part, and IR could affect the exposure to the IR. For example, when the CR is angled, the distance between the source of the radiation and the IR is increased. Generally, when the CR is angled, the SID is decreased accordingly to maintain exposure to the IR. If misalignment occurs among the tube, part, or IR, the distance between the source of radiation and the IR or the part and the IR could be increased or decreased. This change could affect the amount of exposure to the IR, and the mAs may need adjustment.

Grids

A radiographic grid is a device that is placed between the anatomic area of interest and the IR to absorb scatter radiation exiting the patient. Limiting the amount of scatter radiation that reaches the IR improves the quality of the image. Much of the scatter radiation exiting the patient does not reach the IR when absorbed by a grid (Figure 4-15). The effect of less scatter, or unwanted exposure, on the image is to increase the radiographic contrast (Figure 4-16).

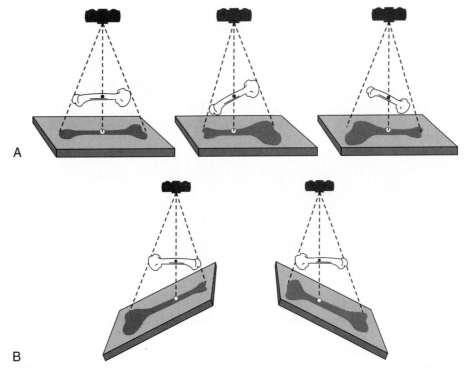

A

B

FIGURE 4-14 Misalignment and shape distortion. **A,** Part not parallel to image receptor. **B,** Image receptor not parallel to part.

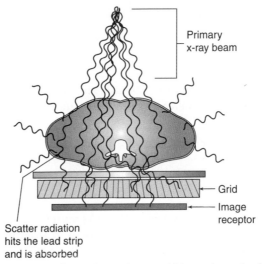

FIGURE 4-15 Grids and scatter absorption. When a grid is used, much of the scatter radiation toward the image receptor is absorbed.

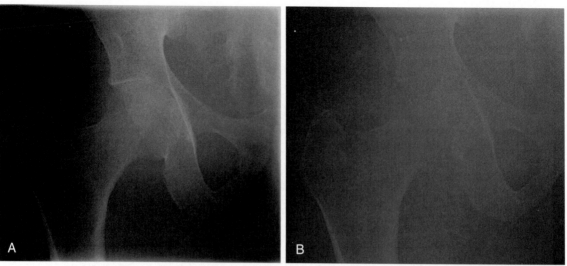

FIGURE 4-16 A, Radiograph obtained using a grid. B, Radiograph obtained without a grid.

TABLE 4-1	Grid Conversion Chart
Grid Ratios	**Grid Conversion Factor (GCF)**
No grid	1
5:1	2
6:1	3
8:1	4
12:1	5
16:1	6

> **Important Relationship**
> *Grids, Scatter, and Contrast*
> Placing a grid between the anatomic area of interest and the IR absorbs scatter radiation exiting the patient and increases radiographic contrast.

The more efficient a grid is in absorbing scatter, the greater is its effect on radiographic contrast. Grids also absorb some of the transmitted radiation exiting the patient and therefore reduce the amount of radiation reaching the IR.

> **Important Relationship**
> *Grids and Image Receptor Exposure*
> Adding, removing, or changing a grid requires an adjustment in mAs to maintain radiation exposure to the IR.

When grids are used, the mAs must be adjusted to maintain exposure to the IR. In addition, the more efficient a grid is in absorbing scatter, the greater is the increase in mAs. The grid conversion formula is a mathematical formula for adjusting the mAs for changes in the type of grid.

When a grid is added, the radiographer must use the correct grid conversion factor (Table 4-1) to multiply by the mAs to compensate for the decrease in exposure.

When a grid is removed, the correct conversion grid factor must be divided into the mAs to compensate for the increase in exposure. When the grid ratio is changed, the following formula should be used to adjust the exposure:

$$\frac{mAs_1}{mAs_2} = \frac{Grid\ conversion\ factor_1}{Grid\ conversion\ factor_2}$$

Grid construction and efficiency are discussed in greater detail in Chapter 5.

Mathematical Application
Adjusting mAs for Changes in Grid

A quality radiograph is obtained using 5 mAs at 70 kVp without using a grid. What new mAs is needed when adding a 12:1 grid to maintain the same exposure to the IR?

$$\frac{5\ mAs}{X} = \frac{1}{5}; \ 1\ X = 25; \ X = 25\ mAs$$

The new mAs produces an exposure comparable with the IR.

! **Patient Protection Alert**
Grid Selection

Decisions regarding the use of a grid and grid ratio should be made by balancing image quality and patient protection. To keep patient exposure as low as possible, grids should be used only when appropriate, and the grid ratio should be the lowest that would provide sufficient contrast improvement.

Beam Restriction

Any change in the size of the x-ray field alters the amount of tissue irradiated. A larger field size (decreasing collimation) increases the amount of tissue irradiated, causing more scatter radiation to be produced, and increases the amount of radiation reaching the IR. The increased amount of scatter reaching the IR results in less radiographic contrast. Conversely, a smaller field size (increasing collimation) reduces the amount of tissue irradiated, the amount of scatter radiation produced, and the amount of radiation reaching the IR. The decreased amount of scatter radiation reaching the IR results in higher radiographic contrast but requires an increase in the mAs. The effect of collimation is greater when imaging large anatomic areas, performing examinations without a grid, and using a high kVp.

Important Relationship
Beam Restriction and Image Receptor Exposure

Changes in beam restriction alter the amount of tissue irradiated and therefore affect the amount of exposure to the IR. The effect of collimation is greater when imaging large anatomic areas, performing examinations without a grid, and using a high kVp.

! **Patient Protection Alert**
Beam Restriction

In performing a radiographic examination, the radiographer should be aware of the anatomic area of interest and limit the x-ray field size to just beyond this area. Collimating to the appropriate field size is a basic method for protecting the patient from unnecessary exposure.

Generator Output

Exposure techniques and the amount of radiation output depend on the type of generator used. Generators with more efficient output, such as three-phase or high-frequency units, require lower exposure technique settings to produce an image comparable with single-phase units. The radiographer must be aware of the generator output when using different types of equipment, especially when performing examinations in different departments. For example, imaging a knee using a single-phase generator requires more mAs than imaging a knee using a three-phase generator. In addition, x-ray generators must be calibrated periodically to ensure that they are producing consistent radiation output.

Tube Filtration

Small variations in the amount of tube filtration should not have any effect on radiographic quality. Variability of the x-ray tube filtration should be checked as a part of routine quality control checks on the radiographic equipment. X-ray tubes that have excessive or insufficient filtration may begin to affect image quality. Increasing the amount of tube filtration increases the percentage of higher-penetrating x-rays to lower-penetrating x-rays. As a result, the x-ray beam has increased energy and can increase the amount of scatter radiation reaching the IR. The increased x-ray energy (kVp) and scatter production decrease radiographic contrast. The amount of tube filtration should not vary greatly, and therefore small changes do not have a visible effect on radiographic contrast.

Compensating Filters

When imaging an anatomic area that varies greatly in tissue thickness, a compensating filter can be placed in the primary beam to produce a more uniform exposure to the IR. The use of compensating filters requires an increase in the mAs to maintain the overall exposure to the IR. The amount of increase in the mAs depends on the thickness and type of compensating filter. Additionally, the use of a compensating filter increases the exposure to the patient.

PATIENT FACTORS

Body Habitus

Body habitus refers to the general form or build of the body, including size. It is important for the radiographer to consider body habitus when establishing exposure techniques. There are four types of body habitus: sthenic, hyposthenic, hypersthenic, and asthenic (Figure 4-17).

The sthenic body habitus accounts for approximately 50% of the adult population and is commonly called a *normal* or *average* build. The hyposthenic type accounts for approximately 35% of adults and refers to a similar type of body habitus as sthenic, but with a tendency toward a more slender and taller build. Together, the sthenic and hyposthenic types of body habitus are, in terms of establishing radiographic techniques, classified as *normal* or *average* for the adult population. These two types of body habitus account for approximately 85% of adults.

Hypersthenic and asthenic body habitus types are more extreme and are less common. The hypersthenic body habitus—a large, stocky build—accounts for only 5% of adults. These individuals have thicker part sizes compared with sthenic or hyposthenic individuals, so exposure factors for their radiographic examinations are higher.

Asthenic refers to a very slender body habitus and accounts for only 10% of adults. Exposure factors for asthenic individuals are at the low end of technique charts because their respective part sizes are thinner than those of sthenic and hyposthenic individuals.

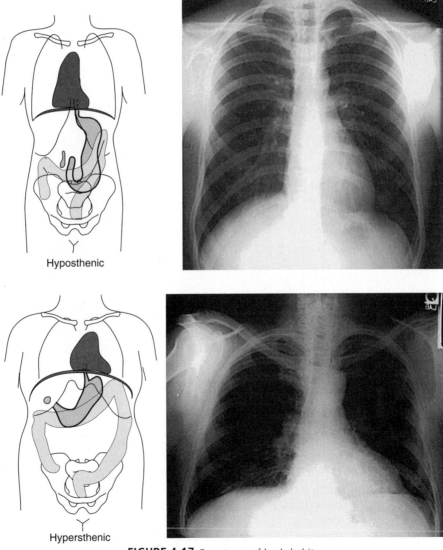

Hyposthenic

Hypersthenic

FIGURE 4-17 Four types of body habitus.

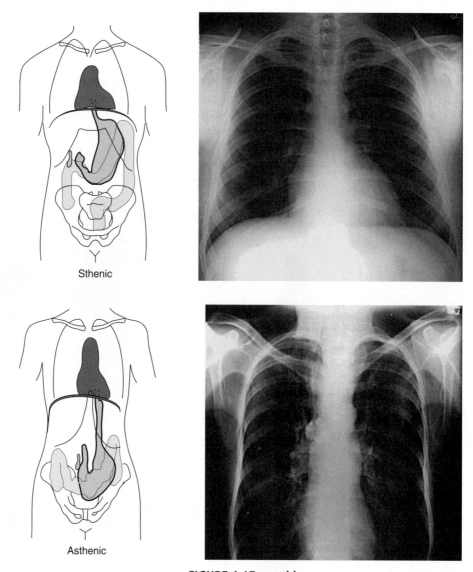

Sthenic

Asthenic

FIGURE 4-17, cont'd

Part Thickness

The thickness of the anatomic part being imaged affects the amount of x-ray beam attenuation that occurs. A thick part absorbs more radiation, whereas a thin part transmits more radiation. Maintaining the exposure to the IR when imaging a thicker part requires the mAs to be increased accordingly. In addition, when a thinner anatomic part is being radiographed, the mAs must be decreased accordingly.

Because x-rays are attenuated exponentially, a general guideline is that for every change in part thickness of 4 to 5 cm (1.6 to 2 inches), the radiographer should adjust the mAs by a factor of 2. For example, an optimal radiograph is obtained using 20 mAs on an anatomic part that measures 18 cm (7 inches). The same anatomic part is radiographed in another patient, and it measures 23 cm (9 inches). What new mAs is needed to the expose the IR? Because the part thickness increased by 5 cm (2 inches), the original mAs is multiplied by 2, yielding 40 mAs. If the same part in another patient measures 28 cm (11 inches), what new mAs is needed? Because the part thickness increased by another 5 cm (2 inches), the mAs is multiplied by 2, yielding 80 mAs. This mAs is four times greater than that for the original patient who measured 10 cm (4 inches) less.

As the thickness of a given type of anatomic tissue increases, the amount of scatter radiation also increases, and radiographic contrast decreases. Using a higher kVp for a thicker part only adds to the increase in scatter radiation. Increased scatter radiation would continue to degrade the quality of the image because it creates fog, which decreases the contrast.

The amount of radiographic contrast achieved is also influenced by the composition of the anatomic part to be radiographed. As mentioned in Chapter 3, subject contrast is one of the categories of radiographic contrast. The thickness of the tissue, atomic number, and cell compactness (tissue density) affect its absorption characteristics. The absorption characteristics of the anatomic tissue create the range of densities and brightness produced on a radiograph. Tissues that have a higher atomic number absorb more radiation than tissues with a lower atomic number.

Anatomic structures that have a wide range of tissue composition, such as atomic number and tissue density, demonstrate high subject contrast. Anatomic structures that consist of similar type tissue demonstrate low subject contrast. The radiographer cannot control the composition of the anatomic part to be radiographed. Changing the kVp alters its absorption and transmission within anatomic tissues. Knowledge of the absorption characteristics of anatomic tissues and the effect of kVp helps the radiographer produce a desired level of radiographic contrast. The selection of kVp to produce a desired level of contrast is more crucial when using film-screen IRs. Acquiring the image using digital IRs allows for changes in image contrast during computer processing.

Pediatric Patients

Pediatric patients are a technical challenge for radiographers for many reasons. Pediatric patients, because of their smaller size, require lower kVp and mAs values compared with adults.

Pediatric chest radiography requires the technologist to choose fast exposure times to stop diaphragm motion in patients who cannot or will not voluntarily suspend their breathing. A fast exposure time may eliminate the possibility of using automatic exposure control (AEC) systems for pediatric chest radiography.

Exposure factors used for the adult skull can be used for pediatric patients 6 years and older because the bone density of these children has developed to an adult level. However, exposure factors must be modified for patients younger than 6 years. It is recommended that the radiographer decrease the kVp by at least 15% to compensate for this lack of bone density. Radiographic examination of all other parts of pediatric patients' anatomy requires an adjustment in exposure techniques.

SPECIAL CONSIDERATIONS

Appropriate exposure factor selection and its modification for variability in the patient are critical to the production of a quality radiograph. The radiographer must be able to recognize a multitude of patient and equipment variables and have a thorough understanding of how these variables affect the resulting radiograph to make adjustments to produce a quality image.

Projections and Positions

Different radiographic projections and patient positions of the same anatomic part often require modification of exposure factors. For example, an oblique position of the lumbar spine requires more exposure than an AP projection because of an increase in the amount of tissue through which the primary beam must pass. However, an oblique ankle radiograph requires slightly less exposure than the AP for comparable exposure to the IR.

General guidelines, based on variations in radiographic projection or patient position, can be followed to change exposure factors. When compared with an AP projection, an increase or a decrease in the amount of tissue should determine any changes in exposure factors for oblique and lateral patient positions.

Casts and Splints

Casts and splints can be produced with materials that attenuate x-rays differently. Selecting appropriate exposure factors can be challenging because of the wide variation of materials used for these devices. The radiographer should pay close attention to both the type of material and how the cast or splint is used.

Casts. Casts can be made of either fiberglass or plaster. Fiberglass generally requires no change in exposure factors from the values used for the same anatomic part without a cast.

Plaster presents a problem in terms of exposure factors. Plaster casts require an increase in exposure factors compared with that needed to radiograph the same part without a cast. However, the method and amount of increase in exposure have not been standardized.

Exposure factor adjustments for cast materials may be based on the part thickness using a technique chart. For example, if an AP ankle measured through the CR is 4 inches (10 cm) without the cast and 8 inches (20 cm) with the cast, the radiographer simply increases the exposure technique to that of an ankle measuring 8 inches (20 cm) to obtain an acceptable radiograph.

Splints. Splints present less of a problem in determining appropriate exposure factors than casts. Inflatable (air) and fiberglass splints do not require any increase in exposure. Wood, aluminum, and solid plastic splints may require that exposure factors be increased, but only if they are in the path of the primary beam. For example, if two pieces of wood are bound to the sides of a lower leg, no increase in exposure is necessary for an AP projection because the splint is not in the path of the primary beam and does not interfere with the radiographic image. Using the same example, if a lateral projection is produced, the splint is in the path of the primary beam and interferes with the radiographic imaging of the part. An increase in exposure technique is required to produce a properly exposed radiograph.

Pathologic Conditions

Pathologic conditions that can alter the absorption characteristics of the anatomic part being examined are divided into two categories. *Additive diseases* are diseases or conditions that increase the absorption characteristics of the part, making the part more difficult to penetrate. *Destructive diseases* are diseases or conditions that decrease the absorption characteristics of the part, making the part less difficult to penetrate. Table 4-2 lists additive and destructive diseases. Generally, it is necessary to increase the kVp when radiographing parts that have been affected by additive diseases and to decrease the kVp when radiographing parts affected by destructive diseases.

However, it is not necessary to compensate for all additive and destructive diseases. It is often desirable to image diseases with exposure factors that would normally be used for a specific anatomic part so that the effect of that disease on that part can be visualized clearly.

TABLE 4-2	Common Additive and Destructive Diseases and Conditions by Anatomic Area
Additive Conditions	**Destructive Conditions**
Abdomen	
Aortic aneurysm	Bowel obstruction
Ascites	Free air
Cirrhosis	
Hypertrophy of some organs (e.g., splenomegaly)	
Chest	
Atelectasis	Emphysema
Congestive heart failure	Pneumothorax
Malignancy	
Pleural effusion	
Pneumonia	
Skeleton	
Hydrocephalus	Gout
Metastases (osteoblastic)	Metastases (osteolytic)
Osteochondroma (exostoses)	Multiple myeloma
Paget's disease (late stage)	Paget's disease (early stage)
	Osteoporosis
Nonspecific Sites	
Abscess	Atrophy
Edema	Emaciation
Sclerosis	Malnutrition

When it is necessary or desirable to compensate for additive or destructive diseases or conditions, it is best to make changes in the kVp. Changing the kVp is fundamentally correct because the kVp affects the penetrating ability of the primary beam, and it is the penetrability of the anatomic part that is affected by these particular diseases and conditions. It is impossible to state an exact amount or percentage of kVp that should be changed because the state or severity of the disease or condition is different with each patient. However, a minimum change of 15% in kVp is recommended. There are some instances in which a change in mAs may be more appropriate to the type of pathologic condition. For example, if the anatomic area has significant increases in gas, such as in bowel obstruction, a large decrease in mAs is best.

Soft Tissue

Objects such as small pieces of wood, glass, or swallowed bones are difficult to visualize radiographically using the normal exposure factors for a particular anatomic part. Several situations in which a soft tissue technique may be needed are visualization of the larynx in a young child with croup, possible foreign body obstruction in the throat, and foreign body location in the extremities (Figure 4-18). Exposure factors must be altered to demonstrate these soft tissues for film-screen imaging. When the area of interest requires less density to visualize the soft tissue, the mAs should

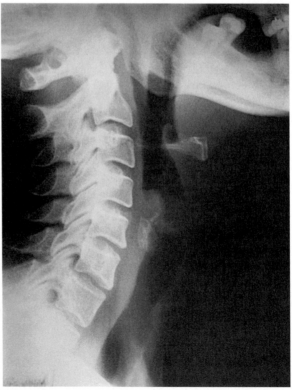

FIGURE 4-18 Soft tissue imaging. Lateral soft tissue neck radiograph.

be decreased accordingly. Digital imaging systems allow visualization of soft tissues without changing the exposure technique.

Contrast Media

A contrast medium (also called *contrast agent*) is used when imaging anatomic tissues that have low subject contrast. A **contrast medium** is a substance that can be instilled into the body by injection or ingestion. The type of contrast medium used changes the absorption characteristics of the tissues by either increasing or decreasing the attenuation of the x-ray beam. Positive contrast agents, such as barium and iodine, have a high atomic number and absorb more x-rays (increase attenuation) than the surrounding tissue (Figure 4-19). Negative contrast agents, such as air, decrease the attenuation of the x-ray beam and transmit more radiation than the surrounding tissue (Figure 4-20). Positive contrast agents produce less radiographic density or more brightness than the adjacent tissues. Negative contrast agents produce more radiographic density or less brightness than the adjacent tissues.

Although negative contrast agents decrease the attenuation characteristics of the part being examined, their use does not require a change in exposure factors. Negative contrast agents can also be used in conjunction with positive contrast agents. Positive contrast media studies require an increase in exposure factors compared with imaging the same part without a positive contrast medium.

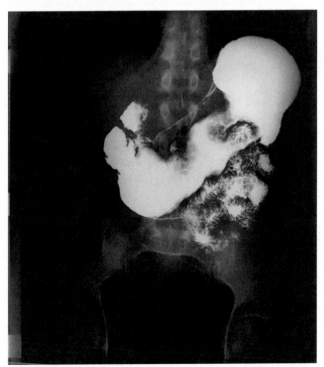

FIGURE 4-19 Positive contrast agents. Radiograph showing decreased density because of the increase in x-ray beam attenuation by use of a positive contrast agent.

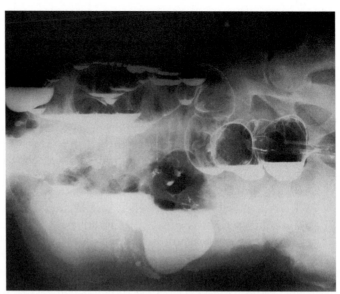

FIGURE 4-20 Negative contrast agents. Radiograph showing increased density because of the decrease in x-ray beam attenuation by use of a negative contrast agent.

TABLE 4-3	**Exposure Technique Mathematical Calculations**	
Exposure Technique Factor	**Relationship to Maintain Exposure to Image Receptor**	**Formula**
mAs	↑ mA and ↓ second	mA × second = mAs
kVp: 15% Rule	↑ kVp and ↓ mAs	kVp × 1.15 and mAs/2 kVp × .85 and mAs × 2
mAs/Distance Compensation Formula	↑ SID and ↑ mAs	$\dfrac{mAs_1}{mAs_2} = \dfrac{(SID_1)^2}{(SID_2)^2}$

Grid Conversion Factor:
    No grid = 1
    5:1 = 2
    6:1 = 3
    8:1 = 4
    12:1 = 5
    16:1 = 6
	↑ Grid ratio and ↑ mAs	$\dfrac{mAs_1}{mAs_2} = \dfrac{GCF_1}{GCF_2}$

Patient Thickness	↑ Thickness and ↑ mAs	Every 4-5 cm change in thickness change mAs by a factor of 2

The use of a contrast agent is an effective method of increasing the radiographic contrast when radiographing areas of low subject contrast.

The quality of the radiographic image depends on a multitude of variables. Knowledge of these variables and their radiographic effect assists the radiographer in producing quality radiographs. Table 4-3 summarizes common exposure technique mathematical calculations. Table 4-4 is a chart demonstrating how the variables discussed in this chapter affect IR exposure.

TABLE 4-4	**Exposure Factors and Their Effect on the Primary and Exit X-ray Beam**	
	Primary Beam Reaching Patient	**Exit Beam Reaching Image Receptor**
mAs		
Increasing mAs	↑ Quantity	↑ Quantity
Decreasing mAs	↓ Quantity	↓ Quantity
kVp		
Increasing kVp	↑ Quantity and quality	↑ Quantity and quality
Decreasing kVp	↓ Quantity and quality	↓ Quantity and quality
Focal Spot Size		
Smaller focal spot size	No effect	No effect
Larger focal spot size	No effect	No effect
SID		
Increasing SID	↓ Quantity	↓ Quantity
Decreasing SID	↑ Quantity	↑ Quantity
OID		
Increasing OID	No effect	↓ Quantity and scatter
Decreasing OID	No effect	↑ Quantity and scatter
Grid		
Increasing grid ratio	No effect	↓ Quantity and scatter
Decreasing grid ratio	No effect	↑ Quantity and scatter
Beam Restriction		
Increasing collimation	↓ Quantity	↓ Quantity and scatter
Decreasing collimation	↑ Quantity	↑ Quantity and scatter
Generator Output		
Single-phase generator	↓ Quantity and quality	↓ Quantity and quality
High-frequency generator	↑ Quantity and quality	↑ Quantity and quality
Compensating Filter		
Adding a compensating filter	↓ Quantity	↓ Quantity

CHAPTER SUMMARY

- The product of milliamperage and exposure time (mAs) has a direct proportional relationship with the quantity of x-rays produced and exposure to the IR.
- Milliamperage and exposure time have an inverse relationship to maintain exposure to the IR.
- The kVp changes the penetrating power of the x-ray beam and has a direct effect on exposure to the IR.
- Changing the kVp by 15% has the same effect on exposure to the IR as changing the mAs by a factor of 2.
- A numeric value or exposure indicator is displayed on the processed digital image that indicates the level of x-ray exposure received (incident exposure) to the IR.
- The kVp has an inverse relationship with radiographic contrast: A high kVp creates an image with low contrast, and a low kVp creates an image with high contrast.

- Radiation exposure to a film-screen IR affects the level of density and contrast, whereas brightness and contrast are primarily controlled by computer processing in digital imaging.
- Focal spot size affects only recorded detail or spatial resolution. A smaller focal spot size increases recorded detail or spatial resolution.
- SID has an inverse squared relationship with the intensity of radiation reaching the patient and the IR.
- Increasing OID decreases exposure to the IR.
- Decreasing SID and increasing OID increases size distortion (magnification) and decreases recorded detail or spatial resolution.
- Grids absorb scatter exiting the patient and increase radiographic contrast.
- Beam restriction affects the amount of tissue irradiated, scatter produced, and exposure to the IR.
- Changes in SID, grids, and patient thickness require a change in mAs to maintain the exposure to the IR.
- Generators with more efficient output, such as three-phase or high-frequency, require lower exposure techniques to produce the same exposure to the IR as a single-phase generator.
- Exposure factors may need to be modified for pediatric patients, varying projections and positions, casts and splints, body habitus, and pathologic conditions.

REVIEW QUESTIONS

1. Which of the following is accurate regarding the relationship between milliamperage (mA) and exposure time to maintain the exposure to the image receptor?
   A. Direct proportional
   B. Direct
   C. Inverse
   D. Inverse proportional

2. A radiographic film image has excessive density. Which of the following is best in order to correct the exposure error?
   A. Decrease kVp by 50%
   B. Increase mAs by 15%
   C. Decrease mAs by 50%
   D. Decrease mAs by 15%

3. What exposure factor affects both the quality and the quantity of the x-ray beam?
   A. kVp
   B. SID
   C. mA
   D. Focal spot size

4. Which of the following is *not* affected by kilovoltage?
   A. Compton interactions
   B. Spatial resolution
   C. Film density
   D. Radiation quantity

5. How is the quality of the image affected when more than needed radiation exposure reaches the digital image receptor?
   A. No effect
   B. Decreased brightness
   C. Increased brightness
   D. Higher contrast

6. Which of the following would maintain radiation exposure to the image receptor when the kilovoltage is decreased by 15%?
   A. Increase mAs 15%
   B. Increase mAs 50%
   C. Double the mAs
   D. Halve the mAs

7. A quality image is produced using 70 kVp and 25 mAs at a 40-inch SID. What calculated change in exposure technique is necessary to maintain radiation exposure to the image receptor when the SID is increased to 56 inches?
   A. 60 kVp at 25 mAs
   B. 70 kVp at 12.5 mAs
   C. 70 kVp at 50 mAs
   D. 60 kVp at 50 mAs

8. Without exposure technique compensation, increasing the OID by 4 inches for a knee film image would:
   (1) increase magnification
   (2) decrease density
   (3) increase contrast
   A. 1 and 2 only
   B. 1 and 3 only
   C. 2 and 3 only
   D. 1, 2, and 3

9. A quality image is produced using 80 kVp at 10 mAs with a 6:1 ratio grid. Calculate the change in exposure technique to maintain radiation exposure to the image receptor when changing to a 12:1 ratio grid.
   A. 80 kVp at 17 mAs
   B. 68 kVp at 20 mAs
   C. 80 kVp at 6 mAs
   D. 92 kVp at 5 mAs

10. Which of the following factors does *not* affect the radiation exposure to the image receptor?
A. Collimation
B. Focal spot size
C. Compensating filters
D. Body habitus

11. What exposure factor change is recommended to maintain radiation exposure to the image receptor when increasing patient thickness by 5 cm?
A. Double the kVp
B. Double the mAs
C. Decrease kVp by 15%
D. Increase mAs by 15%

12. Instilling a negative contrast agent in the gastrointestinal tract has what effect in the area of interest on the digital image?
A. Increased brightness
B. Decreased contrast
C. Decreased brightness
D. No effect

Scatter Control

OBJECTIVES

After completing this chapter, the reader will be able to perform the following:
1. Define all the key terms in this chapter.
2. State all the important relationships in this chapter.
3. Explain how scatter radiation affects digital and film-screen images.
4. State the purpose of beam-restricting devices.
5. Describe each of the types of beam-restricting devices.
6. State the purpose of automatic collimators or positive beam-limiting devices.
7. Describe the purpose of a radiographic grid.
8. Describe the construction of grids, including the different types of grid pattern, dimensions, and grid focus.
9. Calculate grid ratio.
10. List the various types of stationary grids, and describe the function and purpose of a moving grid.
11. Demonstrate use of the grid conversion formula.
12. Describe different types of grid cutoff that can occur and their radiographic appearance.
13. Identify the factors to be considered in using a grid.
14. Recognize how beam restriction and use of grids affect patient radiation exposure.
15. Explain the air gap technique and describe its use.

KEY TERMS

air gap technique
aperture diaphragm
automatic collimator
beam-restricting device
beam restriction
Bucky

Bucky factor
collimation
collimator
cone
convergent line
convergent point

crossed grid
cross-hatched grid
cylinder
focal distance
focal range
focused grid

KEY TERMS—cont'd

grid

grid cap

grid cassette

grid conversion factor

grid cutoff

grid focus

grid frequency

grid pattern

grid ratio

interspace material

linear grid

long dimension

moiré effect

nonfocused grid

parallel grid

positive beam-limiting device

short dimension

wafer grid

Controlling the amount of scatter radiation produced in a patient and ultimately reaching the image receptor (IR) is essential in creating a good-quality image. Scatter radiation is detrimental to radiographic quality because it adds unwanted exposure (fog) to the image without adding any patient information.

Digital IRs are more sensitive to lower-energy levels of radiation such as scatter, which results in increased fog in the image. Additionally, scatter radiation decreases radiographic contrast for both film-screen and digital images. Increased scatter radiation, either produced within the patient or higher-energy scatter exiting the patient, affects the exposure to the patient and anyone within close proximity. The radiographer must act to minimize the amount of scatter radiation reaching the IR.

Beam-restricting devices and radiographic grids are tools the radiographer can use to limit the amount of scatter radiation that affects the radiographic image and exposure to the patient or personnel. Beam-restricting devices decrease the x-ray beam field size and the amount of tissue irradiated, thereby reducing the amount of scatter radiation produced. Radiographic grids are used to improve radiographic image quality by absorbing scatter radiation that exits the patient, reducing the amount of scatter reaching the IR. It should be noted that grids do nothing to prevent scatter *production;* they merely reduce the amount of scatter reaching the IR.

SCATTER RADIATION

Scatter radiation, as described in Chapter 3, is primarily the result of the Compton interaction, in which the incoming x-ray photon loses energy and changes direction. Two major factors affect the amount and energy of scatter radiation exiting the patient: kilovoltage peak (kVp) and the volume of tissue irradiated. The volume of tissue depends on the thickness of the part and the x-ray beam field size. Increasing the volume of tissue irradiated results in increased scatter production. In addition, using a higher kVp increases x-ray transmission and reduces its overall absorption (photoelectric interactions); however, higher kVp increases the percentage of Compton interactions and the energy of scatter radiation exiting the patient. Using higher kVp or increasing the volume of tissue irradiated results in increased scatter radiation reaching the IR.

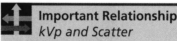

Important Relationship

kVp and Scatter

The amount and energy of scatter radiation exiting the patient depends, in part, on the kVp selected. Examinations using higher kVp produce a greater proportion of higher-energy scattered x-rays compared with examinations using low kVp.

Important Relationship
X-ray Beam Field Size, Thickness of the Part, and Scatter
The larger the x-ray beam field size, the greater the amount of scatter radiation produced.
The thicker the part being imaged, the greater the amount of scatter radiation produced.

 Important Relationship
Volume of Tissue Irradiated and Scatter
The volume of tissue irradiated is affected by both the part thickness and the x-ray beam field size. Therefore, the greater the volume of tissue irradiated, because of either or both factors, the greater the amount of scatter radiation produced.

BEAM RESTRICTION

It is the responsibility of the radiographer to limit the x-ray beam field size to the anatomic area of interest. **Beam restriction** serves two purposes: limiting patient exposure and reducing the amount of scatter radiation produced within the patient.

The unrestricted primary beam is cone-shaped and projects a round field on to the patient and IR (Figure 5-1). If not restricted in some way, the primary beam goes

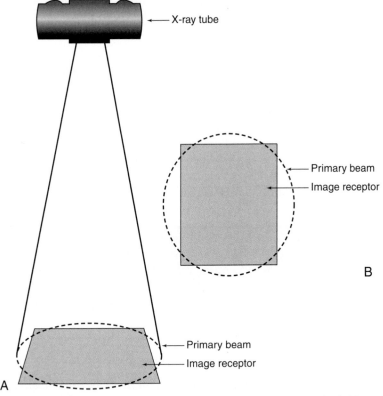

FIGURE 5-1 The unrestricted primary beam is cone-shaped, projecting a circular field. A, Side view. B, View from above.

beyond the boundaries of the IR, resulting in unnecessary patient exposure. Any time the x-ray field extends beyond the anatomic area of interest, the patient is receiving unnecessary exposure. Limiting the x-ray beam field size is accomplished with a **beam-restricting device.** Located just below the x-ray tube housing, the beam-restricting device changes the shape and size of the primary beam.

The terms **beam restriction** and **collimation** are used interchangeably; they refer to a decrease in the size of the projected radiation field. The term *collimation* is used more often than the term *beam restriction* because collimators are the most popular type of beam-restricting device. Increasing collimation means decreasing field size, and decreasing collimation means increasing field size.

Important Relationship
Beam Restriction and Patient Dose
As beam restriction or collimation increases, field size decreases, and patient dose decreases. As beam restriction or collimation decreases, field size increases, and patient dose increases.

Patient Protection Alert
Appropriate Beam Restriction
In performing a radiographic examination, the radiographer should be aware of the anatomic area of interest and limit the x-ray field size to just beyond this area. Collimating to the appropriate field size is a basic method for protecting the patient from unnecessary exposure.

BEAM RESTRICTION AND SCATTER RADIATION

In addition to decreasing patient dose, beam-restricting devices reduce the amount of scatter radiation that is produced within the patient, reducing the amount of scatter the IR is exposed to, and thereby increasing the radiographic contrast. The relationship between collimation (field size) and quantity of scatter radiation is illustrated in Figure 5-2. As stated previously, collimation means decreasing the size of the projected field, so increasing collimation means decreasing field size, and decreasing collimation means increasing field size.

Important Relationship
Collimation and Scatter Radiation
As collimation increases, the field size decreases, and the quantity of scatter radiation decreases; as collimation decreases, the field size increases, and the quantity of scatter radiation increases.

Collimation and Contrast

Because collimation decreases the x-ray beam field size, less scatter radiation is produced within the patient, and less scatter radiation reaches the IR. As described in Chapter 3, this affects the radiographic contrast.

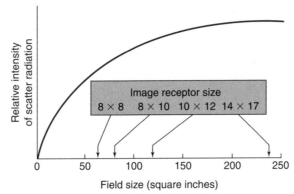

FIGURE 5-2 As field size increases, the relative quantity of scatter radiation increases.

> **Important Relationship**
> *Collimation and Radiographic Contrast*
> As collimation increases, the quantity of scatter radiation decreases, and radiographic contrast increases; as collimation decreases, the quantity of scatter radiation increases, and radiographic contrast decreases.

Compensating for Collimation

Increasing the collimation decreases the volume of tissue irradiated, the amount of scatter radiation produced, the number of photons that strike the patient, and the number of x-ray photons reaching the IR to produce the latent image. As a result, the exposure technique factors may need to be increased when increasing collimation to maintain exposure to the IR.

> **Important Relationship**
> *Collimation and Exposure to the Image Receptor*
> As collimation increases, exposure to the IR decreases; as collimation decreases, exposure to the IR increases.

It has been recommended that significant collimation requires an increase in 30% to 50% of the milliamperage/second (mAs) to compensate for the decrease in IR exposure.

Important relationships regarding the restriction of the primary beam are summarized in Table 5-1.

TYPES OF BEAM-RESTRICTING DEVICES

Several types of beam-restricting devices, which differ in sophistication and utility, are available. All beam-restricting devices are made of metal or a combination of metals that readily absorb x-rays.

TABLE 5-1	Restricting the Primary Beam
Increased Factor	**Result**
Collimation	Patient dose *decreases*
	Scatter radiation *decreases*
	Radiographic contrast *increases*
	Exposure to image receptor *decreases*
Field size	Patient dose *increases*
	Scatter radiation *increases*
	Radiographic contrast *decreases*
	Exposure to image receptor *increases*

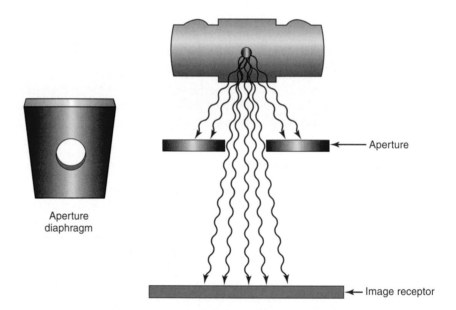

Aperture
diaphragm

Aperture

Image receptor

FIGURE 5-3 Commercially made aperture diaphragm.

Aperture Diaphragms

The simplest type of beam-restricting device is the aperture diaphragm. An **aperture diaphragm** is a flat piece of lead (diaphragm) that has a hole (aperture) in it. Commercially made aperture diaphragms are available (Figure 5-3), or hospitals make their own for purposes specific to a radiographic unit. Aperture diaphragms are easy to use. They are placed directly below the x-ray tube window. An aperture diaphragm can be made by cutting rubberized lead into the size needed to create the diaphragm and cutting the center to create the shape and size of the aperture.

Although the size and shape of the aperture can be changed, the aperture cannot be adjusted from the designed size, and therefore the projected field size is not

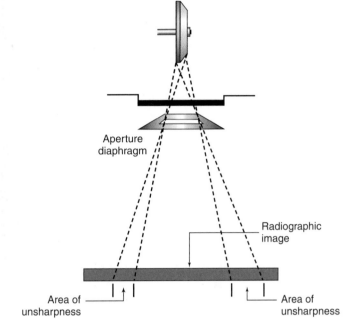

Aperture
diaphragm

Radiographic
image

Area of
unsharpness

Area of
unsharpness

FIGURE 5-4 Radiographic image unsharpness using an aperture diaphragm.

adjustable. In addition, because of the aperture's proximity to the radiation source (focal spot), a large area of unsharpness surrounds the radiographic image (Figure 5-4). Although aperture diaphragms are still used in some applications, their use is not as widespread as other types of beam-restricting devices.

Cones and Cylinders

Cones and cylinders are shaped differently (Figure 5-5), but they have many of the same attributes. A **cone** or **cylinder** is essentially an aperture diaphragm that has an extended flange attached to it. The flange can vary in length and can be shaped as either a cone or a cylinder. The flange can also be made to telescope, increasing its total length (Figure 5-6). Similar to aperture diaphragms, cones and cylinders are easy to use. They slide onto the tube, directly below the window. Cones and cylinders limit unsharpness surrounding the radiographic image more than aperture diaphragms do, with cylinders accomplishing this task slightly better than cones (Figure 5-7). However, they are limited in terms of available sizes, and they are not interchangeable among tube housings. Cones have a particular disadvantage compared with cylinders. If the angle of the flange of the cone is greater than the angle of divergence of the primary beam, the base plate or aperture diaphragm of the cone is the only metal actually restricting the primary beam. Therefore, cylinders generally are more useful than cones. Cones and cylinders are almost always made to produce a circular projected field, and they can be used to advantage for particular radiographic procedures (Figure 5-8).

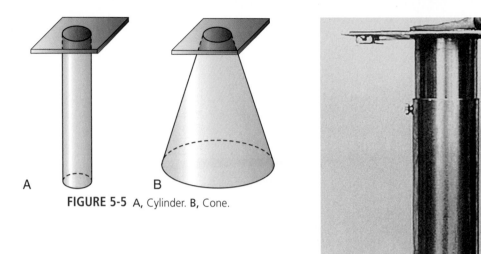

FIGURE 5-5 A, Cylinder. B, Cone.

FIGURE 5-6 Telescoping cylinder.

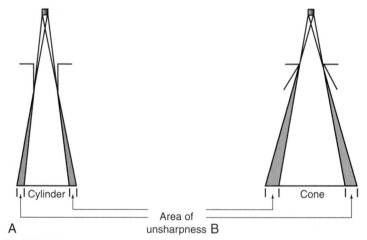

Cylinder

Cone

Area of
unsharpness

A   B

FIGURE 5-7 A cylinder (A) is better at limiting unsharpness than a cone (B).

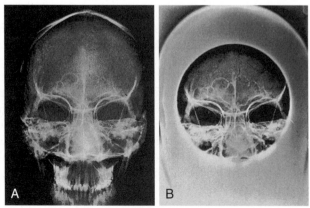

A   B

FIGURE 5-8 Radiograph of the frontal and maxillary sinuses not using a cone (A) and using a cone (B).

Collimators

The most sophisticated, useful, and accepted type of beam-restricting device is the **collimator.** Collimators are considered the best type of beam-restricting device available for radiography. Beam restriction accomplished with the use of a collimator is referred to as *collimation*. The terms *collimation* and *beam restriction* are used interchangeably.

A collimator has two or three sets of lead shutters (Figure 5-9). Located immediately below the tube window, the entrance shutters limit the x-ray beam much as the aperture diaphragm would. One or more sets of adjustable lead shutters are located 3 to 7 inches (8 to 18 cm) below the tube. These shutters consist of longitudinal and lateral leaves or blades, each with its own control. This design makes the collimator adjustable in terms of its ability to produce projected fields of varying sizes. The field shape produced by a collimator is always rectangular or square, unless an aperture diaphragm, cone, or cylinder is slid in below the collimator. Collimators are equipped with a white light source and a mirror to project a light field onto the patient. This light is intended to indicate accurately where the primary x-ray beam will be projected during exposure. In case of failure of this light, an x-ray field measurement guide (Figure 5-10) is present on the front of the collimator. This guide indicates the projected field size based on the adjusted size of the collimator opening at particular source-to-image receptor distances (SIDs). This guide helps ensure that

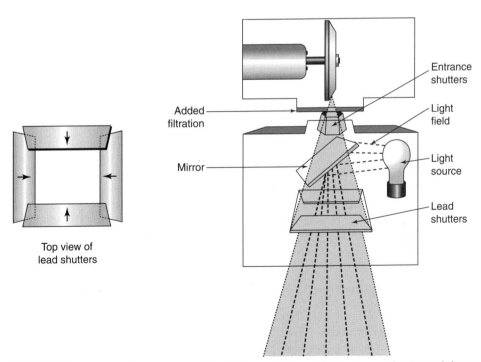

FIGURE 5-9 Collimators have two sets of lead shutters that are used to change the size and shape of the primary beam.

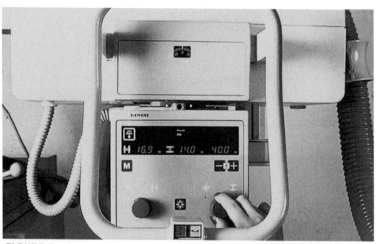

FIGURE 5-10 The x-ray field measurement guide on the front of a collimator.

BOX 5-1	Quality Control Check: Collimator and Beam Alignment

- Lack of congruence of the x-ray field light and the exposure field and misalignment of the light and Bucky tray may affect the quality of the radiograph. In addition, if the x-ray central ray is not perpendicular to the table and Bucky tray, radiographic quality may be compromised. A collimator and beam alignment test tool template and cylinder can be radiographed easily and evaluated for proper alignment.
- Collimator misalignment should be less than 2% of the SID used, and the perpendicularity of the x-ray central ray must be less than or equal to 1 degree misaligned.

the radiographer does not open the collimator to produce a field that is larger than the IR. Another problem that may occur is the lack of accuracy of the light field. The mirror that reflects the light down toward the patient or the light bulb itself could be slightly out of position, projecting a light field that inaccurately indicates where the primary beam will be projected. There is a means of testing the accuracy of this light field and the location of the center of projected beam (Box 5-1).

A plastic template with cross hairs is affixed to the bottom of the collimator to indicate where the center of the primary beam—the central ray—will be directed. This template is of great assistance to the radiographer in accurately centering the x-ray field to the patient.

Automatic Collimators

An **automatic collimator,** also called a **positive beam-limiting device,** automatically limits the size and shape of the primary beam to the size and shape of the IR. For many years, automatic collimators were required by U.S. federal law on all new radiographic installations. This law has since been rescinded, and automatic collimators are no longer a requirement on any radiographic equipment. They are still widely used, however. Automatic collimators mechanically adjust the primary beam size and shape to that of the IR when the IR is placed in the Bucky tray, just below the tabletop. Automatic collimation makes it difficult for the radiographer to increase the size of the primary beam to a field larger than the IR, which would result in increasing the patient's radiation exposure. Positive beam-limiting devices were seen as a way of protecting patients from overexposure to radiation. However, it should be noted that automatic collimators have an override mechanism that allows the radiographer to disengage this feature.

> **! Patient Protection Alert**
> *Limit Field Size to Image Receptor Size*
> Whether or not automatic collimation is being used, the radiographer should always be sure that the size of the x-ray field is the same as or less than the size of the IR except for digital flat panel detectors. When using a digital flat panel detector, the x-ray field size should be restricted to the anatomic area of interest. These digital IRs are typically one size and, in many instances, larger than the anatomic area of interest. Therefore, it is even more crucial for the radiographer to collimate appropriately for the imaging procedure so that the patient is not unnecessarily exposed to radiation.

RADIOGRAPHIC GRIDS

The radiographic grid was invented in 1913 by Gustave Bucky and continues to be the most effective means for limiting the amount of scatter radiation that reaches the IR. Approximately ¼-inch thick and ranging from 8 × 10 inches (20 × 25 cm) to 17 × 17 inches (43 × 43 cm), a **grid** is a device that has very thin lead strips with radiolucent interspaces, intended to absorb scatter radiation emitted from the patient. Placed between the patient and the IR, grids are invaluable in the practice of radiography. They work well to improve radiographic contrast but are not without drawbacks. As discussed later in this chapter, using a grid requires additional mAs, resulting in a higher patient dose. Therefore, grids are typically used only when the anatomic part is 10 cm (4 inches) or greater in thickness, and more than 60 kVp is needed for the examination.

As scatter radiation leaves the patient, a significant amount of it is directed at the IR. As stated previously, scatter radiation is detrimental to image quality because it adds unwanted exposure to the IR without adding any radiographic information. Scatter radiation decreases radiographic contrast. Ideally, grids would absorb, or clean up, all scattered photons directed toward the IR and would allow all transmitted photons emitted from the patient to pass from the patient to the IR. Unfortunately, this does not happen (Figure 5-11). When used properly, however, grids can greatly increase the contrast of the radiographic image.

> **Important Relationship**
> *Scatter Radiation and Image Quality*
> Scatter radiation adds unwanted exposure to the IR and decreases image quality.

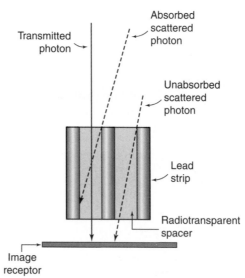

FIGURE 5-11 Ideally, grids would absorb all scattered radiation and allow all transmitted photons to reach the film. In reality, however, some scattered photons pass through to the film, and some transmitted photons are absorbed.

Grid Construction

Grids contain thin lead strips or lines that have a precise height, thickness, and space between them. Radiolucent **interspace material** separates the lead lines. Interspace material typically is made of aluminum. The lead lines and interspace material of the grid are covered by an aluminum front and back panel.

Grid construction can be described by grid frequency and grid ratio. **Grid frequency** expresses the number of lead lines per unit length, in inches, centimeters, or both. Grid frequencies can range in value from 25 to 80 lines/cm (63 to 200 lines/inch). A typical value for grid frequency might be 40 lines/cm (100 lines/inch). Another way of describing grid construction is by its grid ratio. **Grid ratio** is defined as the ratio of the height of the lead strips to the distance between them (Figure 5-12). Grid ratio can also be expressed mathematically as follows:

$$\text{Grid ratio} = h / D$$

where h is the height of the lead strips and D is the distance between them.

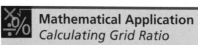

Mathematical Application
Calculating Grid Ratio
What is the grid ratio when the lead strips are 2.4 mm high and separated by 0.2 mm?

$$\text{Grid ratio} = h / D$$
$$\text{Grid ratio} = \frac{2.4}{0.2} = 12 \text{ or } 12:1$$

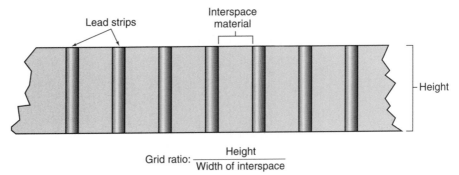

$$\text{Grid ratio: } \frac{\text{Height}}{\text{Width of interspace}}$$

FIGURE 5-12 Grid ratio is the ratio of the height of the lead strips to the distance between them.

Grid ratios range from 4:1 to 16:1. High-ratio grids remove, or clean up, more scatter radiation than lower-ratio grids having the same grid frequency and thus increase radiographic contrast further.

There is a relationship among grid ratio, grid frequency, and the amount of lead content (measured in mass per unit area). Increasing grid ratio for the same grid frequency increases the amount of lead content and therefore increases scatter absorption.

> **Important Relationship**
> *Grid Ratio and Radiographic Contrast*
> As grid ratio increases for the same grid frequency, scatter cleanup improves, and radiographic contrast increases; as grid ratio decreases for the same grid frequency, scatter cleanup is less effective, and radiographic contrast decreases.

Information about a grid's construction is contained on a label placed on the tube side of the grid. This label usually states the type of interspace material used, grid frequency, grid ratio, grid size, and information about the range of SIDs that can be used with the grid. The radiographer should read this information before using the grid because these factors influence grid performance, exposure technique selection, grid alignment, and image quality.

Grid Pattern

Grid pattern refers to the linear pattern of the lead lines of a grid. Two types of grid pattern exist: linear and crossed or cross-hatched. A **linear grid** has lead lines that run in only one direction (Figure 5-13). Linear grids are the most popular in terms of grid pattern because they allow angulation of the x-ray tube along the length of the lead lines. A **crossed grid** or **cross-hatched grid** has lead lines that run at a right angle to one another (Figure 5-14). Crossed grids remove more scattered photons than linear grids because they contain more lead strips, oriented in two directions. However, applications are limited with a crossed grid because the x-ray tube cannot be angled in any direction without producing grid cutoff (i.e., absorption of the transmitted x-rays). Grid cutoff is undesirable and is discussed later in this chapter.

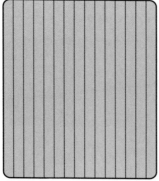

FIGURE 5-13 Linear grid pattern.

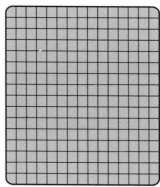

FIGURE 5-14 Crossed or cross-hatched grid pattern.

Grid Focus

Grid focus refers to the orientation of the lead lines to one another. Two types of grid focus exist: parallel (nonfocused) and focused. A **parallel grid** or **nonfocused grid** has lead lines that run parallel to one another (Figure 5-15). Parallel grids are used primarily in fluoroscopy and mobile imaging. A **focused grid** has lead lines that are angled, or canted, to match approximately the angle of divergence of the primary beam (Figure 5-16). The advantage of focused grids compared with parallel grids is that focused grids allow more transmitted photons to reach the IR. As seen in Figure 5-17, transmitted photons are more likely to pass through a focused grid to reach the IR than they are to pass through a parallel grid.

> **Important Relationship**
> *Focused versus Parallel Grids*
> Focused grids have lead lines that are angled to match approximately the divergence of the primary beam. Thus, focused grids allow more transmitted photons to reach the IR than parallel grids.

As seen in Figure 5-18, if imaginary lines were drawn from each of the lead lines in a linear focused grid, these lines would meet to form an imaginary point, called the **convergent point**. If points were connected along the length of the grid, they would form an imaginary line, called the **convergent line**. Both the convergent line and the convergent point are important because they determine the focal distance of a focused grid. The **focal distance** (sometimes referred to as *grid radius*) is the distance between the grid and the convergent line or point. The focal distance is important because it is used to determine the focal range of a focused grid. The **focal range** is the recommended range of SIDs that can be used with a focused grid. The convergent line or point always falls within the focal range (Figure 5-19). For example, a common focal range is 36 to 42 inches (90 to 105 cm), with a focal distance of 40 inches (100 cm). Another common focal range is 66 to 74 inches (165 to 185 cm), with a focal distance of 72 inches (180 cm). Because the lead lines in a parallel grid are not angled, they have a focal range extending from a minimum SID to infinity.

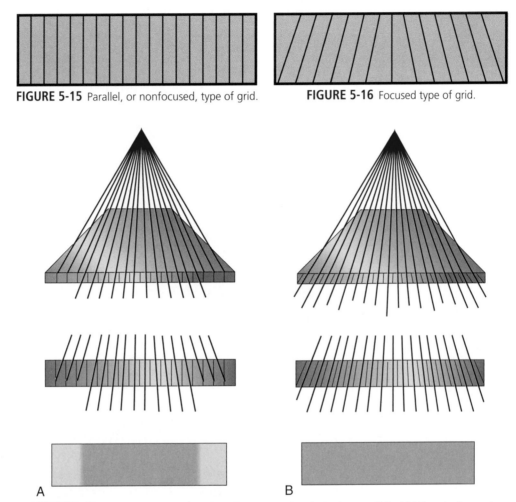

FIGURE 5-15 Parallel, or nonfocused, type of grid.

FIGURE 5-16 Focused type of grid.

FIGURE 5-17 Comparison of transmitted photons passing through a parallel grid **(A)** and a focused grid **(B)**.

Types of Grids

Grids are available for use by the radiographer in several forms and can be stationary or moving. Stationary, nonmoving grids include the wafer grid, grid cassette, and grid cap. A **wafer grid** matches the size of the cassette and is used by placing it on top of the IR. Wafer grids typically are taped to the IR to prevent them from sliding during the radiographic procedure. A **grid cassette** is an IR that has a grid permanently mounted to its front surface. A **grid cap** contains a permanently mounted grid and allows the IR to slide in behind it; this is useful because the grid is secure, and many IRs can be interchanged behind the grid before processing the image.

Stationary and Reciprocating Grids. When grids are stationary, it is possible to examine closely and see the grid lines on the radiographic image. Slightly moving the grid during the x-ray exposure blurs the grid lines (motion unsharpness), rendering them less visible.

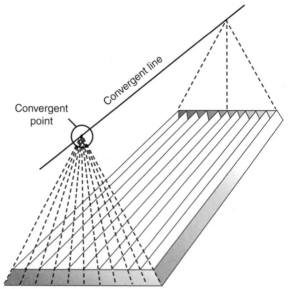

FIGURE 5-18 Imaginary lines drawn above a linear focused grid from each lead strip meet to form a convergent point; the points form a convergent line.

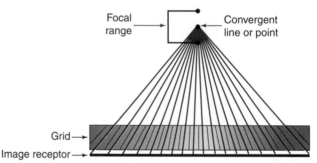

FIGURE 5-19 The convergent line or point of a focused grid falls within a focal range.

Moving or reciprocating grids are part of the **Bucky,** more accurately called the *Potter-Bucky diaphragm.* Located directly below the radiographic tabletop, the grid is found just above the tray that holds the IR. Grid motion is controlled electrically by the x-ray exposure switch. The grid moves slightly back and forth in a lateral direction over the IR during the entire exposure. These grids typically have dimensions of 17 × 17 inches (43 × 43 cm) so that a 14 × 17 inch (35 × 43 cm) IR can be positioned under the grid either lengthwise or crosswise, depending on the examination requirements.

Long Dimension versus Short Dimension Grids. Linear grids can be constructed as either long dimension or short dimension. A **long dimension** linear grid has lead strips running parallel to the long axis of the grid. A **short dimension** linear grid has lead strips running perpendicular to the long axis of the grid (Figure 5-20). For example, a 14 × 17 inch (35 × 43 cm) long dimension grid has lead strips 17 inches (43 cm) long, whereas a short dimension grid has lead strips 14 inches (35 cm) long.

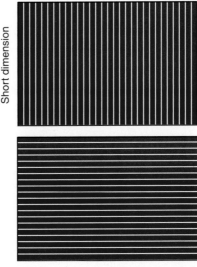

FIGURE 5-20 A long dimension grid has lead strips running parallel to the long axis of the grid. A short dimension grid has lead strips running perpendicular to the long axis of the grid.

A short dimension grid may be useful for examinations where it is difficult to center the central ray correctly for the long dimension grid.

Grid Performance

The purpose of using grids in radiography is to increase radiographic contrast. In addition to improving contrast by cleaning up scatter, grids reduce the total amount of x-rays reaching the IR. The better the grid is at absorbing scattered photons, such as with a higher-ratio grid, the fewer the photons reaching the IR. To compensate for this reduction, additional mAs must be used to maintain exposure to the IR. The **grid conversion factor** (GCF), or **Bucky factor,** can be used to determine the adjustment in mAs needed when changing from using a grid to nongrid (or vice versa) or for changing to grids with different grid ratios.

The GCF can be expressed mathematically as follows:

$$GCF = \frac{mAs\ with\ the\ grid}{mAs\ without\ the\ grid}$$

Important Relationship
Grid Ratio and Exposure to Image Receptor

As grid ratio increases, exposure to IR decreases; as grid ratio decreases, exposure to IR increases.

Table 5-2 presents specific grid ratios and grid conversion factors. When a grid is added to the IR, mAs must be increased by the factor indicated to maintain the same number of x-ray photons reaching the IR. This calculation requires multiplication by the GCF for the particular grid ratio.

TABLE 5-2	Bucky Factor/Grid Conversion Factor (GCF)
Grid Ratio	**Bucky Factor/GCF**
No grid	1
5:1	2
6:1	3
8:1	4
12:1	5
16:1	6

 Mathematical Application
Adding a Grid

If a radiographer produced a shoulder radiograph with a nongrid exposure using 3 mAs and next wanted to use a 12:1 ratio grid, what mAs should be used to produce the same exposure to the IR?

Nongrid exposure = 3 mAs
GCF (for 12:1 grid) = 5 (from Table 5-2)

$$GCF = \frac{\text{mAs with the grid}}{\text{mAs without the grid}}$$

$$3 = \frac{\text{mAs with the grid}}{5}$$

$$15 = \text{mAs with the grid}$$

When adding a 12:1 ratio grid, the mAs must be increased by a factor of 5, in this case to 15 mAs.

Likewise, if a radiographer chooses not to use a grid during a procedure, but knows the appropriate mAs only for when a grid is used, the mAs must be decreased by the GCF. This calculation requires division by the GCF for the particular grid ratio.

 Mathematical Application
Removing a Grid

If a radiographer produced a knee radiograph using a 8:1 ratio grid and 10 mAs and on the next exposure wanted to use a nongrid exposure, what mAs should be used to produce the same exposure to the IR?

Grid exposure = 10 mAs
GCF (for 8:1 grid) = 4 (from Table 5-2)

$$GCF = \frac{\text{mAs with the grid}}{\text{mAs without the grid}}$$

$$4 = \frac{10 \text{ mAs}}{\text{mAs without the grid}}$$

$$2.5 = \text{mAs without the grid}$$

When removing an 8:1 ratio grid, the mAs must be decreased by a factor of 4, in this case to 2.5 mAs.

The GCF is also useful when changing between grids with different grid ratios. When changing from one grid ratio to another, the following formula should be used to adjust the mAs:

$$\frac{mAs_1}{mAs_2} = \frac{GCF_1}{GCF_2}$$

Mathematical Application
Decreasing the Grid Ratio

If a radiographer used 40 mAs with a 12:1 ratio grid, what mAs should be used with a 6:1 ratio grid to produce the same exposure to the IR?

Exposure 1: 40 mAs, 12:1 grid, GCF = 5
Exposure 2: _____ mAs, 6:1 grid, GCF = 3

$$\frac{mAs_1}{mAs_2} = \frac{GCF_1}{GCF_2}$$

$$\frac{40}{mAs_2} = \frac{5}{3}$$

$$mAs_2 = 24$$

Decreasing the grid ratio requires less mAs.

Mathematical Application
Increasing the Grid Ratio

If a radiographer performed a routine portable pelvic examination using 40 mAs with an 8:1 ratio grid, what mAs should be used if a 12:1 ratio grid is substituted?

Exposure 1: 40 mAs, 8:1 grid, GCF = 4
Exposure 2: _____ mAs, 12:1 grid, GCF = 5

$$\frac{mAs_1}{mAs_2} = \frac{GCF_1}{GCF_2}$$

$$\frac{40}{mAs_2} = \frac{4}{5}$$

$$mAs_2 = 50$$

Increasing the grid ratio requires additional mAs.

The increase in mAs required to maintain the exposure to the IR results in an increase in patient dose. This increase in patient dose is significant, as the numbers for the GCF indicate. It is important to remember that patient dose is increased because of the following:

1. Using a grid compared with not using a grid
2. Using a higher-ratio grid

Important Relationship
Grid Ratio and Patient Dose

As grid ratio increases, patient dose increases; as grid ratio decreases, patient dose decreases.

> **! Patient Protection Alert**
> *Grid Selection*
> Decisions regarding the use of a grid and grid ratio should be made by balancing image quality and patient protection. In order to keep patient exposure as low as possible, grids should be used only when appropriate, and the grid ratio should be the lowest that would provide sufficient contrast improvement.

Grid Cutoff

In addition to the disadvantage of increased patient dose associated with grid use, another disadvantage is the possibility of grid cutoff. **Grid cutoff** refers to a decrease in the number of transmitted photons that reach the IR because of some misalignment of the grid. The primary radiographic effect of grid cutoff is a further reduction in the number of photons reaching the IR. Grid cutoff often requires that the radiographer repeat the radiograph, increasing patient dose yet again. Grid ratio has a significant impact on grid cutoff, with higher grid ratios resulting in more potential cutoff.

Types of Grid Cutoff Errors. Grid cutoff can occur as a result of four types of errors in grid use. To reduce or eliminate grid cutoff, the radiographer must have a thorough understanding of the importance of proper grid alignment in relation to the IR and x-ray tube.

Upside-Down Focused. Upside-down focused grid cutoff occurs when a focused grid is placed upside-down on the IR, resulting in the grid lines going opposite the angle of divergence of the x-ray beam. Radiographically, there is significant loss of exposure along the edges of the image (Figure 5-21). Photons easily pass through the

FIGURE 5-21 Radiograph produced with an upside-down focused grid.

center of the grid because the lead lines are perpendicular to the IR surface. Lead lines that are more peripheral to the center are angled more and absorb the transmitted photons. Upside-down focused grid error is easily avoided because every focused grid should have a label indicating "Tube Side." This side of the grid should always face the tube, away from the IR.

 Important Relationship
Upside-Down Focused Grids and Grid Cutoff
Placing a focused grid upside-down on the IR causes the lateral edges of the radiograph to be very underexposed.

Off-Level. Off-level grid cutoff results when the x-ray beam is angled across the lead strips. It is the most common type of cutoff and can occur from either the tube or the grid being angled (Figure 5-22). Off-level grid cutoff can often be seen with mobile radiographic studies or horizontal beam examinations and appears as a loss of exposure across the entire image. This type of grid cutoff is the only type that occurs with both focused and parallel grids.

Important Relationship
Off-Level Error and Grid Cutoff
Angling the x-ray tube across the grid lines or angling the grid itself during exposure produces an overall decrease in exposure on the radiograph.

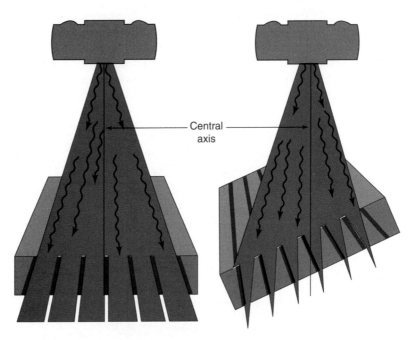

Central axis

Proper position   Off-level
FIGURE 5-22 An off-level grid can cause grid cutoff.

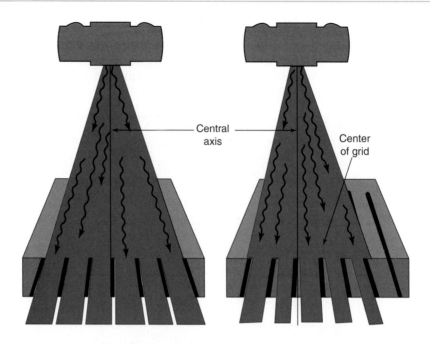

Proper position   Off-center

FIGURE 5-23 Centering to one side of a focused grid can cause off-center grid cutoff.

Off-Center. Also called *lateral decentering*, off-center grid cutoff occurs when the central ray of the x-ray beam is not aligned from side to side with the center of a focused grid. Because of the arrangement of the lead lines of the focused grid, the divergence of the primary beam does not match the angle of these lead strips when not centered (Figure 5-23). Off-center grid cutoff appears as an overall loss of density on radiographic film (Figure 5-24).

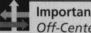
Important Relationship
Off-Center Error and Grid Cutoff
If the center of the x-ray beam is not aligned from side to side with the center of a focused grid, grid cutoff occurs.

Off-Focus. Off-focus grid cutoff occurs when using an SID outside of the recommended focal range. Grid cutoff occurs if the SID is less than or greater than the focal range. Both appear the same radiographically as a loss of density at the periphery of the film (Figure 5-25).

Important Relationship
Off-Focus Error and Grid Cutoff
Using an SID outside of the focal range creates a loss of exposure at the periphery of the radiograph.

FIGURE 5-24 Radiograph demonstrating off-center grid cutoff.

FIGURE 5-25 Radiograph demonstrating off-focus grid cutoff.

! Patient Protection Alert
Grid Errors

A radiographic image that has suboptimal exposure can be the result of many factors, one of which is grid cutoff. Before assuming that an underexposed image is due to technique factors and then reexposing the patient, the radiographer should evaluate grid alignment. If misalignment is the cause of the underexposure, the patient can be protected from reexposure with a technique factor adjustment.

Table 5-3 summarizes important relationships regarding the use of radiographic grids.

Moiré Effect

The **moiré effect** or zebra pattern is an artifact that can occur when a stationary grid is used during computed radiography (CR) imaging (Figure 5-26). If the grid frequency is similar to the laser scanning frequency during CR image processing, a zebra pattern can result on the digital image. Use of a higher grid frequency or a moving grid with CR digital imaging eliminates this type of grid error. In addition, if a grid cassette is placed in a Bucky, imaging the double grids creates a zebra pattern on the radiograph.

TABLE 5-3	Radiographic Grids
Increased Factor	**Result**
Grid ratio*	Contrast *increases*
	Patient dose *increases*
	The likelihood of grid cutoff *increases*

*mAs adjusted to maintain exposure to IR.

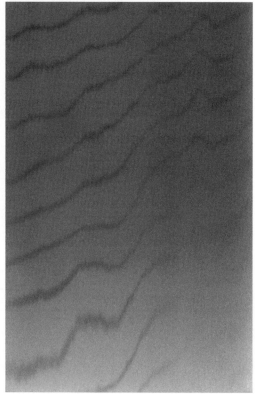

FIGURE 5-26 Moiré effect. Radiograph demonstrating the zebra pattern as a result of the moiré effect.

Grid Usage

The radiographer needs to consider numerous factors when deciding on the type of grid, if any, to be used for an examination. Although quite efficient at preventing scatter radiation from reaching the IR, grids are not appropriate for all examinations. When appropriate, selection of a grid involves consideration of contrast improvement, patient dose, and the likelihood of grid cutoff. Radiographers typically choose between parallel and focused grids, high-ratio and low-ratio grids, grids with different focal ranges, and whether or not to use a grid at all.

As indicated earlier, the choice of whether or not to use a grid is based on the kVp necessary for the examination and the thickness of the part. Parts 10 cm (4 inches) or larger, together with kVp greater than 60, produce enough scatter to necessitate the use of a grid. The next question is which grid to use. There is no single best grid for all situations. A 16:1 focused grid provides excellent contrast improvement, but the patient's dose is high, and the radiographer must ensure that the grid and x-ray tube are perfectly aligned to prevent grid cutoff. The 5:1 parallel grid does a mediocre job of scatter cleanup, especially at kVp greater than 80. However, the patient dose is significantly lower, and the radiographer need not be concerned with cutoff caused by being off-center, SID used, or having the grid upside-down. Selection between grids with different focal ranges depends on the radiographic examination. Supine abdomen studies should use a grid that includes 40 inches (100 cm) in the focal range; upright chest studies should have grids that include 72 inches (180 cm). In general, most radiographic rooms use a 10:1 or 12:1 focused grid, which provides a compromise between contrast improvement and patient dose. Stationary grids, for mobile examinations in particular, may be lower ratio, parallel, or both to allow the radiographer greater positioning latitude.

Box 5-2 lists attributes of the grid typically used in radiography. Box 5-3 provides information on quality control checks for grid uniformity and alignment.

BOX 5-2 | Typical Grid

- Is linear instead of crossed
- Is focused instead of parallel
- Is of mid-ratio (8:1 to 12:1)
- Has a focal range that includes an SID of 40 (100 cm) or 72 (180 cm) inches

---

BOX 5-3 | Quality Control Check: Grid Uniformity and Alignment

- Nonuniformity of a grid (lack of uniform lead strips) may create artifacts on the image. Grid uniformity can be easily evaluated by imaging a grid and measuring optical densities throughout the image. Optical density readings should be within ± 0.10 for proper uniformity.
- Misalignment of a focused grid (off-center) can reduce exposure to the IR as a result of grid cutoff. A grid alignment tool made of radiopaque material with cut-out holes in a line can be imaged to evaluate correct alignment of the grid with the x-ray field. A properly aligned grid would produce a greater center hole optical density than the optical densities of the side holes.

AIR GAP TECHNIQUE

Although the radiographer may use the grid most often to prevent scatter from reaching the IR, the grid is not the only available tool. The air gap technique, although limited in its usefulness, provides another method for limiting the scatter reaching the IR. The **air gap technique** is based on the simple concept that much of the scatter will miss the IR if there is increased distance between the patient and IR (increased object-to-image receptor distance [OID]) (Figure 5-27). The greater the gap, the greater the reduction in scatter reaching the IR. Similar to a grid, contrast is increased, the number of photons reaching the IR is reduced because less scatter reaches the IR, and the mAs must be increased to compensate. Exposure may be slightly less because a grid absorbs some of the transmitted photons (grid cutoff), whereas the air gap technique does not.

The air gap technique is limited in its usefulness because the necessary OID results in decreased recorded detail. To overcome this increase in unsharpness, an increase in SID is required, which may not always be feasible.

> **Important Relationship**
> *Air Gap Technique and Scatter Control*
> The air gap technique is an alternative to using a grid to control scatter reaching the IR. By moving the IR away from the patient, more of the scatter radiation will miss the IR. The greater the gap, the less scatter reaches the IR.

Scatter control is important when using digital or film-screen imaging systems. Reducing the amount of scatter produced through beam restriction, reducing the amount of scatter reaching the IR by using a grid, avoiding grid cutoff errors, and making appropriate exposure adjustments as needed all help to produce quality radiographic images.

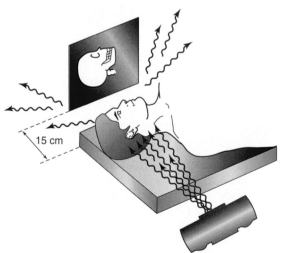

FIGURE 5-27 The air gap technique used in magnification radiography of the lateral skull.

CHAPTER SUMMARY

- Scatter radiation, the result of Compton interactions, is detrimental to radiographic image quality. Excessive scatter results in additional unwanted exposure and reduced contrast.
- The effect of scatter radiation can be reduced by limiting the amount produced and by absorbing the scatter before it reaches the IR.
- The amount of scatter produced increases as the volume of irradiated tissue increases, and the proportion and energy of scatter exiting the patient increase as the kVp increases.
- Beam restriction limits the area exposed to radiation, the patient dose, and the amount of scatter produced in the patient. Aperture diaphragms, cones and cylinders, and collimators are types of beam restrictors.
- Radiographic grids are devices placed between the patient and the IR to absorb scatter radiation. Consisting of a series of lead strips and radiolucent interspaces, grids allow transmitted radiation to pass through while scatter radiation is absorbed.
- Grid designs include linear parallel, focused parallel, crossed, short dimension, and long dimension, each with advantages and disadvantages.
- The use of a grid in a radiographic examination results in fewer photons reaching the IR. The grid conversion, or Bucky, factor is used to calculate the exposure needed when grids are used.
- Grid errors, producing grid cutoff, include using a focused grid upside-down and errors caused by off-level, off-center, and off-focus equipment alignment.
- The use and type of grid depend on the thickness of the part, kVp, patient dose, contrast improvement, and likelihood of grid errors.
- The air gap technique is another method, although seldom used, for reducing the amount of scatter reaching the IR.
- Scatter control is of the same, or greater, importance with digital imaging, owing to the increased sensitivity to low-energy radiation.

REVIEW QUESTIONS

1. The projected shape of the unrestricted primary beam is _____.
   A. square
   B. rectangular
   C. circular
   D. elliptical

2. A purpose of beam-restricting devices is to _____ by changing the size and shape of the primary beam.
   A. increase patient dose
   B. decrease scatter radiation produced
   C. increase exposure to the image receptor
   D. decrease image contrast

3. The most effective type of beam-restricting device is the _____.
   A. cone
   B. aperture diaphragm
   C. cylinder
   D. collimator

4. Of the beam-restricting devices listed in question 3, which two are most similar to one another?
   A. A and B
   B. A and C
   C. B and C
   D. B and D

5. The purpose of automatic collimation is to ensure that _____.
   A. the quantity of scatter production is minimal
   B. the field size does not exceed the image receptor size
   C. maximal recorded detail and contrast are achieved
   D. exposure to the image receptor is maintained

6. When making a significant increase in collimation, _____.
   A. mAs should be increased
   B. kVp should be increased
   C. mAs should be decreased
   D. kVp should be decreased

7. Which one of the following increases as collimation increases?
   A. Patient exposure
   B. Scatter production
   C. Fog
   D. Contrast

8. Which of the following statements is true of positive beam-limiting devices?
   A. They are required on all radiographic installations.
   B. They are required on all new radiographic installations.
   C. They have never been required on radiographic installations.
   D. They were once required on new radiographic installations.

9. The purpose of a grid in radiography is to _____.
   A. increase exposure to the image receptor
   B. increase image contrast
   C. decrease patient dose
   D. increase recorded detail

10. Grid ratio is defined as the ratio of the _____.
    A. height of the lead strips to the distance between them
    B. width of the lead strips to their height
    C. number of lead strips to their width
    D. width of the lead strips to the width of the interspace material

11. Compared with parallel grids, focused grids _____.
    A. have a greater grid frequency and lead content
    B. can be used with either side facing the tube
    C. have a wider range of grid ratios and frequencies
    D. allow more transmitted photons to reach the image receptor

12. With which one of the following grids would a convergent line be formed if imaginary lines from its grid lines were drawn in space above it?
    A. Linear focused
    B. Crossed focused
    C. Linear parallel
    D. Crossed parallel

13. If 15 mAs is used to produce a particular level of exposure to the image receptor without a grid, what mAs would be needed to produce that same level of exposure using a 16:1 grid?
    A. 45
    B. 60
    C. 90
    D. 105

14. Grid cutoff, regardless of the cause, is most recognizable on a film radiograph as reduced _____.
    A. contrast
    B. recorded detail
    C. density
    D. positioning

15. Off-focus grid cutoff occurs by using an SID that is not _____.
    A. within the focal range of the grid
    B. equal to the focal distance of the grid
    C. at the level of the convergent line of the grid
    D. at the level of the convergent point of the grid

16. The type of motion most used for moving grids today is _____.
    A. longitudinal
    B. reciprocating
    C. circular
    D. single stroke

17. A grid should be used whenever the anatomic part size exceeds _____.
    A. 3 cm
    B. 6 cm
    C. 10 cm
    D. 12 cm

18. The air gap technique uses an increased _____ instead of a grid.
A. kVp
B. mAs
C. SID
D. OID

Image Receptors and Image Acquisition

OBJECTIVES

After completing this chapter, the reader will be able to perform the following:

1. Define all the key terms in this chapter.
2. State all the important relationships in this chapter.
3. Differentiate among the types of image receptors (IRs) used in radiography.
4. Compare and contrast the construction of digital and film-screen IRs in order to acquire the latent image.
5. Differentiate between computed radiography (CR) and direct digital radiography (DR) IRs.
6. Explain the relationship between sampling frequency and spatial resolution.
7. Describe how the size of a CR imaging plate can affect spatial resolution.
8. Recognize the differences between indirect and direct conversion digital IRs.
9. Compare film-screen and digital IRs in terms of their dynamic range and explain the importance of dynamic range in exposure technique selection and image quality.
10. Define signal-to-noise ratio (SNR), and explain its importance to digital image quality.
11. Define sensitometry, and discuss film speed, contrast, latitude, and spectral sensitivity.
12. Explain the use of intensifying screens in film-screen imaging.
13. Recognize the effect intensifying screens have on image quality and patient radiation exposure.

KEY TERMS

cassette
double-emulsion film
dynamic range
emulsion layer
film speed
flat panel detectors
fluorescence
imaging plate
intensifying screen

latent image centers
luminescence
phosphor layer
photostimulable luminescence
photostimulable phosphor
pixel pitch
rare earth elements
relative speed
sampling frequency

sampling pitch
screen film
screen speed
signal-to-noise ratio
silver halide
spectral emission
spectral matching
spectral sensitivity

During radiographic imaging, the radiation exiting the patient is composed of a range of intensities that reflect the absorption characteristics of the anatomic tissues. The image receptor (IR) receives the exit radiation and creates the latent or invisible image. The latent image is acquired differently depending on the type of IR. This chapter describes the common types of IRs used in radiography and how the latent image is formed. Latent image processing and display of the visible image are discussed in Chapter 7.

DIGITAL IMAGE RECEPTORS

Two types of digital IRs are typically used in radiography: computed radiography (CR) and direct digital radiography (DR) IRs. These IRs differ in their construction and how they acquire the latent image. Once the latent image is acquired and the raw data are digitized, image processing and display are essentially the same, regardless of the type of IR.

Computed Radiography

CR IRs can be portable or fixed in a table or upright x-ray unit. The CR IR includes a cassette that houses the **imaging plate** (IP) (Figure 6-1). The radiation exiting the patient interacts with the IP, where the photon intensities are absorbed by the phosphor. Although some of the absorbed energy is released as visible light (luminescence), a sufficient amount of energy is stored in the phosphor to produce a latent image. **Luminescence** is the emission of light when stimulated by radiation.

The IP primarily consists of a support layer, phosphor layer, and protective layer (Figure 6-2). The phosphor layer is composed of barium fluorohalide crystals doped with europium, referred to as the **photostimulable phosphor** (PSP). This type of phosphor emits visible light when stimulated by a high-intensity laser beam, a phenomenon termed **photostimulable luminescence**.

CR imaging requires a two-step process for image acquisition: image capture in the IP and image readout. The latent image is formed in the PSP when the exit x-ray

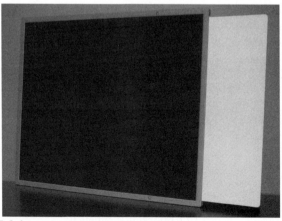

FIGURE 6-1 Typical CR cassette showing the imaging plate housed within.

intensities are absorbed by the phosphor and the europium atoms become ionized by the photoelectric effect. The absorbed energy excites the electrons, and they are elevated to a higher energy state where they become stored or trapped (Figure 6-3). The number and distribution of these trapped electrons are proportional to the tissue's differential x-ray absorption and form the latent image. These electrons remain in this higher energy state until released during the laser beam scanning of the read-out stage. The acquired image data (released energy) are extracted from the digital receptor, converted to digital data, and computer processed for image display. Exposed IPs should be processed within a relatively short amount of time (within 1 hour) because the latent image dissipates over time.

Important Relationship
Computed Radiography Digital Image Receptors
The CR latent image is acquired in the PSP layer of the IP. Most energy from the exit radiation intensities is stored in the PSP for extraction in the reader unit.

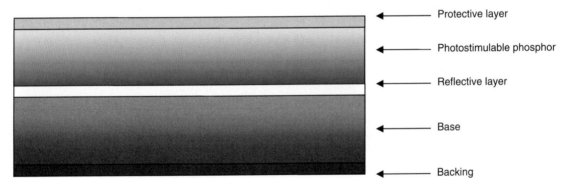

— Protective layer

— Photostimulable phosphor

— Reflective layer

— Base

— Backing

FIGURE 6-2 Cross-section of CR imaging plate.

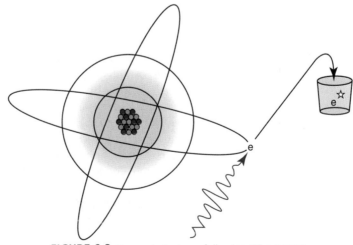

FIGURE 6-3 Trapped electrons following CR exposure.

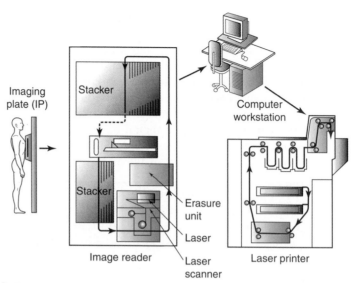

FIGURE 6-4 The exposed CR imaging plate is placed in a reader unit to release the stored image, convert the analog image to a digital image, and send the data to a computer monitor, laser printer for a hard copy or both. The reader unit also erases the exposed imaging plate in preparation for the next exposure.

The exposed IP is placed in or sent to a reader unit that converts the analog data into digital data for computer processing (Figure 6-4). Reader units are available in single-plate or multiplate configurations. The major components of a typical reader unit are a drive mechanism to move the IP through the scanning process; an optical system, which includes the laser, beam-shaping optics, collecting optics, and optical filters; a photodetector, such as a photomultiplier tube (PMT); and the analog-to-digital converter (ADC). Manufacturers differ in the CR reader mechanics. Some devices move the IP, and some move the optical components. There are three important stages in digitizing the latent image: scanning, sampling, and quantization.

The purpose of scanning is to convert the latent image into an electrical signal (voltage) that can be subsequently digitized and displayed as a manifest digital image. Once in the reader unit, the IP is removed from the cassette and scanned with a helium-neon laser beam or a solid-state laser diode to release the stored energy as visible light (Figure 6-5). Absorption of the laser beam energy releases the trapped electrons, and they return to a lower energy state. During this process, the excess energy is emitted as visible light (photostimulable luminescence). The scanning of the plate results in a continuous pattern of light intensities being sent to the PMT, whose output is directed to the ADC for sampling and quantization.

A PMT collects, amplifies, and converts the visible light to an electrical signal proportional to the range of energies stored in the IP. The signal output from the PMT is digitized by an ADC in order to produce the digital image. To digitize the analog signal from the PMT, it must first be sampled. An important performance characteristic of an ADC is the **sampling frequency,** which determines how often the analog signal is reproduced in its discrete digitized form. Increasing the sampling frequency of the

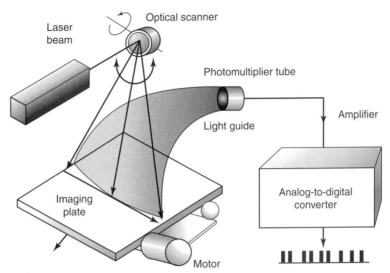

FIGURE 6-5 A neon-helium laser beam scans the exposed CR imaging plate to release the stored energy as visible light. The photomultiplier tube collects, amplifies, and converts the light to an electrical signal. The analog-to-digital converter converts the analog data to digital data.

analog signal increases the pixel density of the digital data and improves the spatial resolution of the digital image (Figure 6-6). The closer the samples are to each other (increased sampling frequency), the smaller the **sampling pitch,** or distance between the sampling points (Figure 6-7). Increased sampling frequency decreases the sampling pitch and results in smaller-sized pixels. The distance between the midpoint of one pixel to the midpoint of an adjacent pixel describes the **pixel pitch.** Spatial resolution is improved with an increased number of smaller pixels resulting in a more faithful digital representation of the acquired analog image.

> **Important Relationship**
> *Sampling Frequency and Spatial Resolution*
> Increasing the sampling frequency results in a smaller sampling and pixel pitch, which improves the spatial resolution of the digital image. Decreasing the sampling frequency results in a larger sampling and pixel pitch and decreased spatial resolution.

Manufacturers of CR equipment vary in the method of sampling IPs of different sizes. Some manufacturers fix the sampling frequency to maintain a fixed spatial resolution, whereas others vary the sampling frequency to maintain a fixed matrix size. If the spatial resolution is fixed, the image matrix size is simply proportional to the IP size. A larger IP has a larger matrix to maintain spatial resolution (Figure 6-8). If the matrix size is fixed, changing the size of the IP would affect the spatial resolution of the digital image. For example, with a fixed matrix size system, changing from a 14 × 17 inch (35 × 43 cm) to a 10 × 12 inch (25 × 30 cm) IP size, for the same field of view (FOV), would result in improved spatial resolution (Figure 6-9). Spatial resolution is improved because in order to maintain the same matrix size and

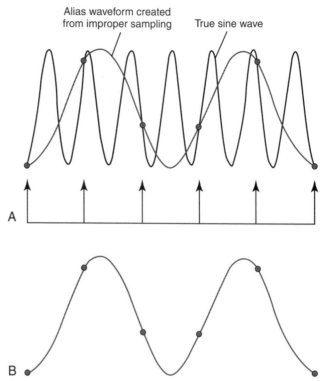

FIGURE 6-6 CR sampling and its effect on the digital data. **A** represents the sampling points of the analog waveform. **B** shows the improper digital waveform that results from low sampling frequency.

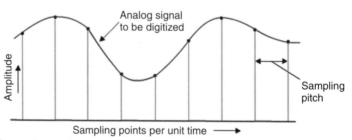

FIGURE 6-7 Sampling and pixel pitch. The sampling frequency determines the distance between the midpoint of one pixel to the midpoint of an adjacent pixel.

number of pixels, the pixels must be smaller in size. It is recommended to use the smallest IP size reasonable for the anatomic area of interest.

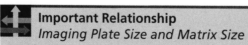

Important Relationship
Imaging Plate Size and Matrix Size

For a fixed matrix size CR system, using a smaller IP for a given field of view (FOV) results in improved spatial resolution of the digital image. Increasing the size of the IP for a given FOV results in decreased spatial resolution.

FIXED SAMPLING FREQUENCY

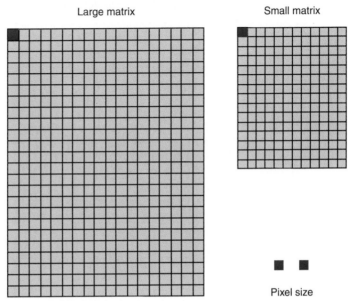

FIGURE 6-8 Fixed sampling frequency. A fixed sampling frequency will maintain a fixed spatial resolution. A larger IP size will have a larger matrix to maintain the same pixel size. Note: Pixel size not to scale and used for illustration only.

FIXED MATRIX SIZE

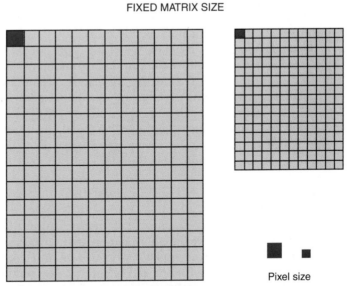

FIGURE 6-9 Fixed matrix size. A fixed matrix size will vary the sampling frequency for a different IP size. A larger IP size will result in a larger pixel size and decrease spatial resolution. Note: Pixel size not to scale and used for illustration only.

BOX 6-1 | **Quality Control Check: Computed Radiography**

- Manufacturers of CR equipment have developed quality control activities specific to their equipment; however, there are basic universal procedures.
- The sensitivity of individual IPs should be checked routinely to ensure the consistency of optical densities. Expose selected IPs to varying amounts of x-ray intensities, print the images, and measure the optical density to verify it does not vary more than ±0.20.
- Linearity of the system can be evaluated by proportionally increasing and decreasing the radiation exposure to the IP and validating that the exposure indicator responds accordingly and within ±20%.
- Reproducibility of optical densities within an individual IP and uniformity among multiple IPs should be within ±0.25 optical density.
- Spatial resolution can be monitored by imaging a line-pair resolution test tool; the resolution should be within 10% of the resolution specified by the manufacturer.
- The laser beam performance can be evaluated by imaging an opaque straight-edge object and visually checking for any jitter along the edges of the object.
- Contrast resolution can be measured by imaging a phantom or step wedge device and measuring density differences. Optical density differences should remain stable over time.
- The thoroughness of the IP erasure function can be evaluated by performing a secondary erasure on the IP and checking for any residual optical density (ghosting).

Another important ADC performance characteristic is degree of quantization or pixel bit depth, which controls the number of gray shades or contrast resolution of the image. During the process of quantization, each pixel, representing a brightness value, is assigned a numeric value. Quantization reflects the precision with which each sampled point is recorded. Chapter 3 discussed the characteristics of a digital image in terms of matrix size, pixel, and pixel bit depth. As previously discussed, the pixel size and pitch determine the spatial resolution, and the pixel bit depth determines the system's ability to display a range of shades of gray to represent the anatomic tissues. Pixel bit depth is fixed by the choice of ADC, and CR systems manufactured with a greater pixel bit depth (i.e., 14-bit [2^{14} can display 16,384 shades of gray]) improve the contrast resolution of the digital image.

Before the IP is returned to service, the plate is exposed to an intense white light to release any residual energy that could affect future exposures. PSPs can be reused and are estimated to have a life of 10,000 readings before they need to be replaced. Advancements in the PSP material, laser beam technology, and dual-sided IP scanning will continue to improve the process of CR image acquisition. (Box 6-1 describes quality control methods for evaluating CR equipment.)

Direct Digital Radiography

DR IRs have a self-scanning readout mechanism that employs an array of x-ray detectors that receive the exit radiation and convert the varying x-ray intensities into proportional electronic signals for digitization. In contrast to CR, which requires a two-step image acquisition process, DR imaging combines image capture and image readout. As a result, DR images are available almost instantly after exposure. However, DR receptors are more fragile and much more expensive than CR IRs. Several types of electronic detectors are available for DR.

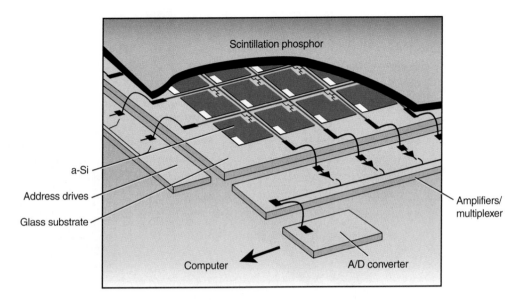

FIGURE 6-10 Flat panel detector array.

Flat Panel Detectors. **Flat panel detectors** are solid-state IRs employing a large area active matrix array of electronic components ranging in size from 43 × 35 cm to 43 × 43 cm (17 × 14 inches to 17 × 17 inches). Flat panel detectors are constructed with layers in order to receive the x-ray photons and convert them to electrical charges for storage and readout (Figure 6-10). Signal storage, signal readout, and digitizing electronics are integrated into the flat panel device. The first layer is composed of the x-ray converter, the second layer houses the thin-film transistor (TFT) array, and the third layer is a glass substrate. The TFT array is divided into square detector elements (DEL), each having a capacitor to store electrical charges and a switching transistor for readout. Electrical charges are read out separately from each detector element. The electronic signal is then sent to the ADC for digitization.

The detector system is usually dedicated to a single room and is permanently mounted in the table or upright Bucky system. Flat panel digital detectors are also available as mobile IRs and can be removed from the Bucky and used on the tabletop or a stretcher. After exposure, the digital image is available within a few seconds on a viewing monitor, and no separate reader unit is involved (Figure 6-11). Flat panel systems are highly dose-efficient and provide quicker access to images compared with CR and film-screen. The spatial resolution of flat panel receptors is generally superior to the spatial resolution of CR. Because the pixel detector is built into the DR flat panel IR, the size and pitch of the pixel are determined by the DEL and fixed. Therefore, spatial resolution for flat panel detector IRs is limited to the DEL. A system that uses a smaller DEL size has improved spatial resolution. Flat panel detectors are manufactured in two different ways to create the electrical charges that are proportional to the x-ray exposure: indirect and direct conversion methods.

Indirect Conversion Detectors. Indirect conversion detectors use a scintillator such as cesium iodide (CsI) or gadolinium oxysulfide (Gd_2O_2S) to convert the exit

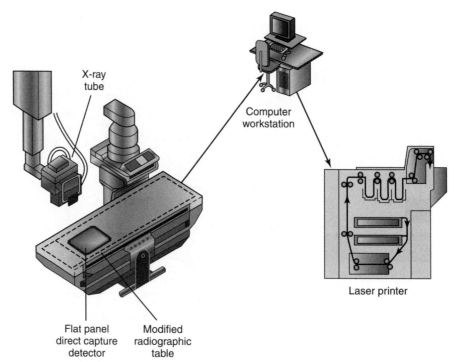

FIGURE 6-11 Flat panel digital detector fixed in a modified x-ray table.

radiation into visible light. The visible light, in proportion to the x-ray exposure, is then converted to electrical charges by the photodetectors (layer of amorphous silicon in the TFT array). The electrical charges are temporarily stored by capacitors in the TFT array before being digitized and processed in the computer (Figure 6-12).

The design of the scintillator used to convert the x-ray intensities into visible light can be structured or unstructured. Structured scintillators, usually crystalline CsI, reduce the spread of visible light and therefore yield images with higher spatial resolution compared with unstructured scintillators. *Indirect conversion detectors* are so named because they involve a two-stage process of converting x-ray intensities first to visible light and then to electrical charges during image acquisition. The electrical signals are then directed to amplifiers and the ADC to produce the raw digital image.

Direct Conversion Detectors. Direct conversion detectors use an amorphous selenium-coated (a-Se) detector to convert the exit radiation directly into electrical charges (Figure 6-13). To compensate for the moderately low atomic number of selenium ($Z = 34$), the thickness of the amorphous selenium is relatively high (approximately 1 mm). An electrical field is applied across the selenium layer to limit lateral diffusion of electrons as they migrate toward the thin-film transistor array. By this means, excellent spatial resolution is maintained. Similar to indirect conversion detectors, the electronic charge is stored in a TFT array before it is amplified, digitized, and processed in the computer.

Regardless of the type of digital imaging system, the varying electrical signals are sent to the ADC for conversion into digital data. The digitized pixel intensities are

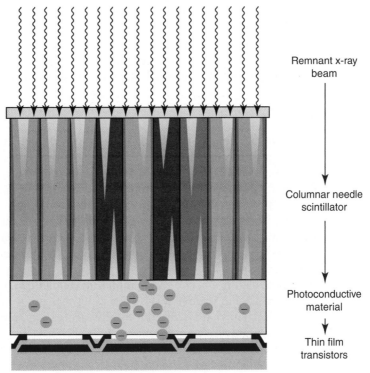

FIGURE 6-12 Flat panel detector—indirect conversion.

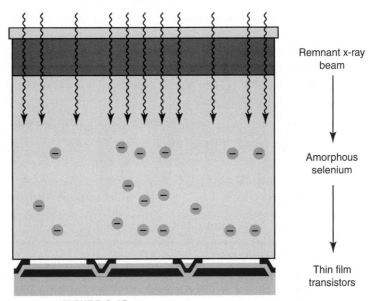

FIGURE 6-13 Flat panel detector—direct conversion.

patterned in the computer to form the image matrix. The image matrix is a digital composite of the varying x-ray intensities exiting the patient. Each pixel has a brightness level representing the attenuation characteristic of the volume of tissue imaged. Once the varying x-ray intensities are converted to numeric data, the digital image can be processed, manipulated, transported, or stored electronically.

Dynamic Range

The **dynamic range** of the digital imaging system refers to the ability of the detector to capture accurately the range of photon intensities that exit the patient. Compared with film-screen detectors, digital IRs have much larger exposure latitude (wide dynamic range). In practical terms, this wide dynamic range means that a small degree of underexposure or overexposure would still result in acceptable image quality. This characteristic of digital receptors is advantageous in situations where automatic exposure control (AEC) is not normally available, such as in portable radiography. During ADC, a numeric value (digital data) is assigned to the pixel that represents the attenuation characteristics of that volume of tissue. Processing the digital data provides a radiographic image that can be viewed on a display monitor and altered in various ways. Even if optimal exposure techniques were not used, image rescaling that occurs during this processing step can produce images with appropriate grayscale appearance.

The ability of the IR to capture a wide range of exit photon intensities does not mean a quality image is always created. Although lower than necessary x-ray exposures can be detected and processed, image quality suffers because there is insufficient exposure to the IR and quantum noise results. The computer can process the data resulting from an IR exposed to higher than necessary radiation and produce a quality image but at the expense of patient overexposure. It is the responsibility of the radiographer to determine the amount of exposure necessary to produce a quality digital image within the *as low as reasonably achievable* (ALARA) principle.

Important Relationship
Digital Detectors and Dynamic Range
Digital IRs have a large dynamic range; that is, they can capture accurately a wide range of x-ray intensities exiting the patient. The computer then processes the raw pixel data to compensate for exposure errors and create a radiographic image. However, lower or higher than necessary exposure techniques do not guarantee a quality digital image with reasonable radiation exposure to the patient.

Signal-to-Noise Ratio

Signal-to-noise ratio (SNR) is a method of describing the strength of the radiation exposure compared with the amount of noise apparent in a digital image. Image noise is a concern with any electronic digital image. Because the photon intensities are converted to an electronic signal that is digitized by the ADC, the term *signal* refers to the strength or amount of radiation exposure captured by the IR to create the image. Increasing the SNR improves the quality of the digital image. Increasing the SNR means that the strength of the signal is high compared with the amount of noise, and therefore image quality is improved. Decreasing the SNR means there is increased noise compared with the strength of the signal, and therefore the quality of the radiographic image is degraded. Quantum noise results when there are too few x-ray photons captured by the IR to create the latent image. In addition to quantum noise, sources of noise include the electronics that capture, process, and display the digital image.

The ability to visualize anatomic tissues is affected by the SNR. Noise interferes with the signal strength just as background static would interfere with the clarity of music heard. When the digital image displays increased noise, regardless of the source, anatomic details have decreased visibility.

Important Relationship
Signal-to-Noise Ratio and Image Quality
Increasing the SNR increases the visibility of anatomic details, whereas decreasing the SNR decreases the visibility of anatomic details.

FILM-SCREEN IMAGE RECEPTORS

Before the development of digital IRs, radiographic images were acquired, processed, and displayed on film. Film is placed in a cassette housing two intensifying screens for the purpose of reducing patient exposure. Although film-screen images are being replaced with digital IRs, knowledge of these IRs is useful.

Radiographic Film

Radiographic film acquires the latent image and must be chemically processed before it is visible. As a result, film serves as the medium for image acquisition, processing, and display. Several types of radiographic film are still used in medical imaging departments. Depending on the specific application, film manufacturers produce film in a variety of sizes ranging from 20 × 25 cm (8 × 10 inches) to 35 × 43 cm (14 × 17 inches). The composition of film can be described in layers (Box 6-2). The most important layer for creating the image is the emulsion layer. The **emulsion layer** is the radiation-sensitive and light-sensitive layer of the film. The emulsion of film consists of silver halide crystals suspended in gelatin. **Silver halide** is the material that is sensitive to radiation and light. The emulsion layer is fragile and must have a layer composed of a polyester base so that the film can be handled and processed, yet remain physically strong after processing. Most film used in radiographic procedures has a dye or tint added to the base layer to decrease eye strain when viewed on a view (illuminator) box.

Screen film is the most widely used radiographic film. As its name implies, it is intended to be used with one or two intensifying screens. Screen film is more sensitive to light and less sensitive to x-rays. Screen film can have either a single-emulsion or double-emulsion coating. **Double-emulsion film** has an emulsion coating on both sides of the base. Film-screen imaging typically uses double-emulsion film with two intensifying screens.

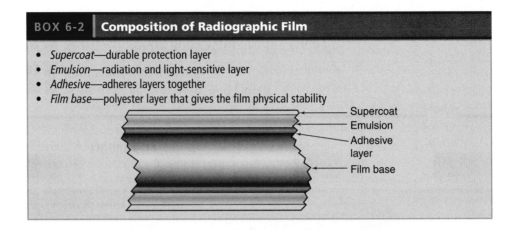

- *Supercoat*—durable protection layer
- *Emulsion*—radiation and light-sensitive layer
- *Adhesive*—adheres layers together
- *Film base*—polyester layer that gives the film physical stability

Latent Image Formation. The specific way in which the latent image is formed is unknown, but the Gurney-Mott theory of latent image formation is most widely believed to explain best the manner in which this process occurs. To explain latent image formation, it is necessary to describe what happens at the molecular level in the emulsion layer of film—specifically what happens to silver halide crystals when exposed to x-rays and light.

Physical imperfections, known as *sensitivity specks*, in the silver halide crystals are the site of the latent image formation. Exposure to x-rays and light ionizes the silver halide crystals, and the freed electrons become trapped at the sensitivity specks. The negatively charged sensitivity specks attract the freed silver ions. Every silver ion that combines with an electron is neutralized by that electron, thereby becoming metallic silver. Several sensitivity specks with many silver ions attracted to them become **latent image centers.** These latent image centers appear as radiographic density on the manifest image after processing. It is believed that for a latent image center to appear, it must contain at least three sensitivity specks that have at least three silver atoms each. With more exposure to the film, more metallic silver is visualized as radiographic density.

Important Relationship
Sensitivity Specks and Latent Image Centers

Sensitivity specks serve as the focal point for the development of latent image centers. After exposure, these specks trap the free electrons and then attract and neutralize the positive silver ions. After enough silver is neutralized, the specks become a latent image center and are converted to metallic silver after chemical processing.

Film Characteristics. Current manufacturers of radiographic film offer a wide variety of films. These differ not only in size and general type, but also in film speed, film contrast, exposure latitude, and spectral sensitivity. Film speed, contrast, and latitude are graphically demonstrated in a film's characteristic (sensitometric) curve. Sensitometry is the study of the relationship between radiation exposure and the amount of density produced after processing. This information is displayed as a

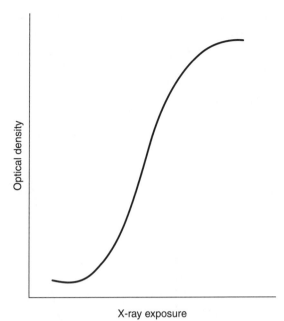

X-ray exposure

FIGURE 6-14 The characteristic (sensitometric) curve graphically represents the relationship between varying x-ray exposure and image density.

curve on a graph (Figure 6-14), and films manufactured differently display a unique curve. In contrast to digital IRs, where the response of the detector to radiation exposure is linear, film can be manufactured to yield a particular speed or contrast response to radiation exposure. Figure 6-15 shows the response of different types of radiographic film to radiation exposure.

Film Speed. **Film speed** is the degree to which the emulsion is sensitive to x-rays or light. The greater the speed of a film, the more sensitive it is. Because sensitivity increases, less exposure is necessary to produce a specific density. Two primary factors, both relating to the silver halide crystals found in the emulsion layers, affect the speed of radiographic film. The first factor is the number of silver halide crystals present, and the second factor is the size of the silver halide crystals. Radiographic film manufacturers control film speed by manipulating both of these factors in the production of specific speeds of radiographic film.

Important Relationship
Silver Halide and Film Sensitivity

As the number of silver halide crystals increases, film sensitivity or speed increases; as the size of the silver halide crystals increases, film sensitivity or speed increases. A faster film speed requires less radiation exposure to produce a specific density.

Film Contrast and Latitude. *Film contrast* refers to the ability of radiographic film to provide a certain level of image contrast (density differences). High-contrast film accentuates more black and white areas, whereas low-contrast film primarily shows shades of gray. The latitude of film affects the range of radiation exposures that can provide diagnostic densities. Radiographic films that are capable of responding to a wide range of exposures to produce diagnostic densities are considered *wide-latitude film*. Films manufactured to display higher contrast have narrow exposure latitude compared with low-contrast films having wider exposure latitude. Although film can be manufactured to respond to a range of radiation exposures (dynamic

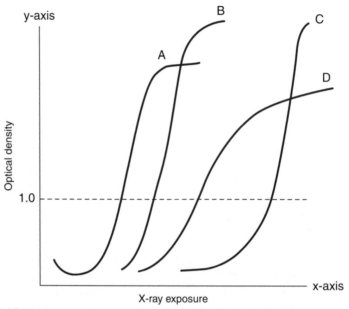

FIGURE 6-15 Film types and sensitometric graphs *(A-D)*. The shape and position of the graph along the x-axis, displays the differing characteristics of fim speed, contrast, and latitude.

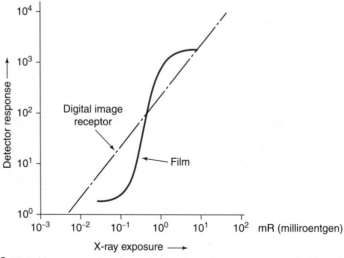

FIGURE 6-16 Digital image receptors have a wider dynamic range compared with radiographic film.

range), this range is more limited than digital image detectors. Radiographic film has a limited dynamic range compared with digital IRs (Figure 6-16).

Spectral Sensitivity. **Spectral sensitivity** refers to the color of light to which a particular film is most sensitive. In radiography, there are generally two categories of spectral sensitivity films: blue-sensitive and green-sensitive (orthochromatic). When radiographic film is used with intensifying screens, it is important to match the spectral sensitivity of the film with the spectral emission of the screens. **Spectral emission** refers to the color of light produced by a particular intensifying screen. In radiography, two categories of spectral emission generally exist: blue light–emitting screens and green light–emitting screens. It is critical to use blue-sensitive film with blue light–emitting screens and green-sensitive film with green light–emitting screens. **Spectral matching** refers to correctly matching the color sensitivity of the film to the color emission of the intensifying screen. An incorrect match of film and screens based on spectral emission and sensitivity results in radiographs that display inappropriate levels of radiographic density.

Intensifying Screens

An **intensifying screen** is a device found in radiographic cassettes that contains phosphors that convert x-ray energy into light, which then exposes the radiographic film. The purpose of this device is to intensify the action of the x-rays and permit much lower x-ray exposures compared with film alone.

As with radiographic film, the construction of screens can be described in layers (Box 6-3). The **phosphor layer,** or active layer, is the most important screen component because it contains the phosphor material that absorbs the transmitted x-rays and converts them to visible light. The most common phosphor materials consist of chemical compounds of elements from the rare earth group of elements. **Rare earth elements** are elements that range in atomic number from 57 to 71 on the periodic table; they are referred to as *rare earth elements* because they are relatively difficult and expensive to extract from the earth.

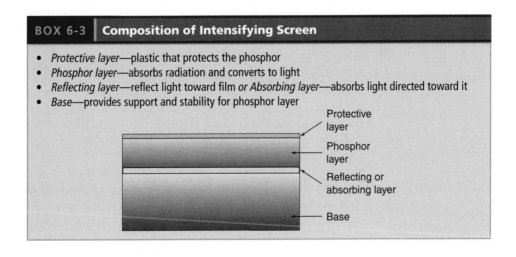

| BOX 6-3 | **Composition of Intensifying Screen** |

- *Protective layer*—plastic that protects the phosphor
- *Phosphor layer*—absorbs radiation and converts to light
- *Reflecting layer*—reflect light toward film or *Absorbing layer*—absorbs light directed toward it
- *Base*—provides support and stability for phosphor layer

Protective layer
Phosphor layer
Reflecting or absorbing layer
Base

Intensifying screen systems used in cassettes generally include two screens. The screen that is mounted in the side of the cassette facing the x-ray tube is called the *front screen,* and the screen that is mounted in the opposite side is called the *back screen.* With two screens, the film (double-emulsion) is exposed to approximately twice as much light as a single-screen system because the film is exposed to light from both sides. Some screen systems use only a single screen and are used with single-emulsion film. When a single screen is used, it is mounted as a back screen on the side of the cassette that is opposite from the tube side. When loading a single-emulsion film into the appropriate cassette with a single screen, the emulsion side of the film must be placed against the intensifying screen.

Film is much more sensitive to visible light than to x-rays. By converting each absorbed high-energy x-ray photon into thousands of visible light photons, intensifying screens amplify film optical density. Without screens, the total amount of energy to which the film is exposed consists of only x-rays. With screens, the total amount of energy to which the film is exposed is divided between x-rays and light. When intensifying screens are used, approximately 90% to 99% of the total energy to which the film is exposed is light. X-rays account for the remaining 1% to 10% of the energy.

Intensifying screens operate by a process known as *luminescence.* **Luminescence** is the emission of light from the screen when stimulated by radiation. The desired type of luminescence in imaging is *fluorescence.* **Fluorescence** refers to the ability of phosphors to emit visible light only while exposed to x-rays (with little or no afterglow). An undesired type of luminescence is phosphorescence. *Phosphorescence* is the emission of light after the x-ray exposure has terminated. Phosphorescence or afterglow causes unwanted exposure to the film.

Screen Speed.   The purpose of intensifying screens is to decrease the radiation dose to the patient. Because screen phosphors can intensify the action of the x-rays by converting them to visible light, the use of screens allows the radiographer to use considerably lower mAs values. The disadvantage of using screens is the reduction in recorded detail. The reason for decreased recorded detail is that visible light photons created within the screen tend to disperse before reaching the film emulsion; this blurs the image.

Important Relationship
Screen Speed and Recorded Detail

As screen speed is increased, recorded detail is decreased; as screen speed decreases, recorded detail increases.

Screen manufacturers produce a variety of intensifying screens, which differ in how well they intensify the action of the x-rays and therefore differ in their capacity to produce accurate recorded detail.

The capability of a screen to produce visible light is called **screen speed.** A faster screen produces more light than a slower screen given the same exposure. Although very fast screens reduce patient exposure, they also degrade image resolution (recorded detail) and increase quantum mottle (noise), so a balance must be chosen.

> **Important Relationship**
> *Screen Speed, Light Emission, and Patient Dose*
> The faster an intensifying screen, the more light is emitted for the same intensity of x-ray exposure. As screen speed increases, less radiation is necessary, and radiation dose to the patient is decreased; as screen speed decreases, more radiation is necessary, and radiation dose to the patient is increased.

Several factors affect how fast or slow an intensifying screen is, including absorption efficiency, conversion efficiency, thickness of the phosphor layer, and size of the phosphor crystal (Table 6-1). The presence of a reflecting layer, an absorbing layer, or dye in the phosphor layer also affects screen speed.

Absorption efficiency refers to the ability of the screen to absorb the incident x-ray photons. A rare earth phosphor screen absorbs approximately 60% of the incident photons. *Conversion efficiency* describes how well the screen phosphor takes these x-ray photons and converts them to visible light. Increased absorption and conversion efficiency mean that rare earth phosphors have increased speed compared with a previously used screen phosphor, calcium tungstate. This increased speed allows the radiographer to reduce substantially the x-ray exposure needed to produce images with the appropriate amount of density.

The thickness of the phosphor layer and the size of the crystal also have an effect on screen speed. A thicker phosphor layer contains more phosphor material than a thinner phosphor layer. The phosphor is the material that converts x-rays into light, so if more phosphor material is present in a screen, more light is produced, increasing the screen speed. The size of the phosphor material crystals also affects screen speed. Larger phosphor crystals produce more light than smaller phosphor crystals. Again, more light being produced means that the screen is faster.

The final factors that affect screen speed are the presence or absence of a reflecting layer, a light-absorbing layer, or light-absorbing dyes in the phosphor layer. When present, a reflecting layer increases screen speed (at the expense of decreased recorded detail) by redirecting retrograde light back toward the film emulsion. Conversely, a light-absorbing layer or light-absorbing dyes present in the phosphor layer are used to decrease screen speed (and increase recorded detail) by absorbing light that would otherwise reach and expose the film.

TABLE 6-1	Summary of Effect of Screen Factors on Screen Speed, Recorded Detail, and Patient Dose		
Screen Factor	**Screen Speed**	**Recorded Detail**	**Patient Dose**
Thicker phosphor layer	↑	↓	↓
Larger phosphor crystal size	↑	↓	↓
Reflective layer	↑	↓	↓
Absorbing layer	↓	↑	↑
Dye in phosphor layer	↓	↑	↑

The ability of the screen to produce visible light can also be described in terms of its **relative speed** (RS). RS results from comparing screen-film systems based on the amount of light produced for a given exposure. Film-screen relative speeds range from 50 RS to 800 RS. Most radiology departments that use film-screen technology have at least two different speeds of intensifying screen systems. A fast system usually is available with an RS of about 400. A 400-speed system is a good compromise between the beneficial effect of decreasing the patient dose and the detrimental effect of decreasing the recorded detail. A slower system is usually available, and it is sometimes labeled on the outside of the cassette as *detail* or *extremity*. The RS of this system typically is 100. Detail or extremity screen systems are relatively slow and require greater exposure and result in higher patient doses. However, the anatomic parts imaged with detail or extremity screen systems generally are small; therefore, they do not require large exposures. Detail or extremity screen systems produce excellent recorded detail. The radiographer must be careful in selecting the appropriate screen system for the examination ordered. Cassettes with extremity and detail screens should be used only for tabletop examinations. They should never be used in the Bucky tray because of the excessive amount of exposure needed. (Box 6-4 describes quality control methods for evaluating intensifying screens.)

Because the film-screen system speed affects radiographic density, the mAs should be adjusted if the film-screen speed is changed. Increasing the film-screen system speed requires a decrease in the mAs to maintain radiographic density. A decrease in the film-screen system speed requires an increase in the mAs to maintain density.

Important Relationship
Film-Screen System Speed and mAs

Increasing the film-screen speed requires a decrease in the mAs to maintain density. Decreasing the film-screen speed requires an increase in the mAs to maintain density.

The RS classification for film-screen systems provides a method whereby exposure techniques can be adjusted for changes in film-screen speed. The relative film-screen

---

BOX 6-4 | **Quality Control Check: Intensifying Screens**

- Intensifying screens should produce an image with uniform density, provide uniform resolution, and not create image artifacts. Several simple quality control procedures can be performed to monitor the performance of intensifying screens.
- A step wedge or homogeneous phantom can be imaged to evaluate the uniformity of optical densities within one screen and compare optical densities for screens of the same speed. Optical densities should be within ±0.05 throughout each image and within ±0.20 among screens of the same speed.
- A resolution test tool can be imaged to measure spatial resolution of each screen. Intensifying screens with the same speed should visualize the same number of line pairs per millimeter.
- An ultraviolet (UV) lamp can be used to evaluate the condition of the surface of the screen. The surface should be free of dirt, stains, and defects.

speed conversion formula is a mathematical formula for adjusting the mAs for changes in the film-screen system speed:

$$\frac{mAs_1}{mAs_2} = \frac{RS_2}{RS_1}$$

The correct relative film-screen speed factors must be used to calculate the new mAs required to compensate for the change in density. The new mAs then produces an exposure comparable with that of the original exposure technique.

Mathematical Application
Adjusting mAs for Changes in Film-Screen System Speed

A quality radiograph is obtained using 10 mAs at 65 kVp and 100 speed film-screen system. What new mAs is used to maintain radiographic density when changing to a 400 speed film-screen system?

$$\frac{10 \text{ mAs}}{X} = \frac{400 \text{ speed}}{100 \text{ speed}}$$

$$10 \text{ mAs} \times 100 \,;\, 1000 = 400X \,;\, \frac{1000}{400} = 2.5 \text{ mAs} = X$$

The remaining component in the film-screen IR is the cassette. Serving as a container for both the intensifying screens and the film, the **cassette** must be light-proof, lightweight for portability, and rigid enough not to bend under a patient's weight, all while allowing the maximum amount of radiation to pass through and reach the screens. Low x-ray–absorbing materials, such as thermoset plastic, magnesium, or even graphite carbon fiber, can be found in the front of cassettes. Inside the back of cassettes may be a thin sheet of lead foil designed to absorb backscatter before it exposes the film.

CHAPTER SUMMARY

- CR and DR IRs differ in their construction and how they acquire the latent image. Once the latent image is acquired and the raw data are digitized, image processing and display are essentially the same, regardless of the type.
- In CR, the imaging plate has a photostimulable phosphor layer that absorbs the exit radiation and excites electrons, which become elevated to a higher energy state and trapped.
- The exposed imaging plate is placed in a reader unit where the trapped electrons are released during the laser beam scanning, and the excess energy is emitted as visible light. A PMT collects, amplifies, and converts the visible light to an electrical signal proportional to the range of energies stored in the imaging plate.
- The signal output from the PMT is digitized by an ADC converter in order to produce the digital image.
- The sampling frequency determines how often the analog signal is reproduced in its discrete digitized form. Increasing the sampling frequency increases the pixel density of the digital data and improves the spatial resolution of the digital image.
- Following data extraction, CR imaging plates must be erased by exposure to an intense white light to release any residual energy before reuse.
- In contrast to CR, DR IRs combine image capture and readout.

- Signal storage, signal readout, and digitizing electronics are integrated into a solid-state flat panel detector.
- Flat panel detectors use both indirect and direct conversion methods to create the proportional electrical charges to send to the ADC for conversion into digital data.
- Indirect conversion detectors use a scintillator to convert the exit radiation into visible light, and then the visible light is converted to electrical charges for storage in the TFTs.
- Direct conversion detectors convert the exit radiation directly into electrical charges.
- Once the varying x-ray energies are converted to numeric data, the digital image can be processed, manipulated, transported, or stored electronically.
- Digital IRs have a wide dynamic range, which means they can accurately capture the wide range of photon energies that exit the patient. However, lower or higher than necessary exposure techniques do not guarantee a quality digital image with reasonable radiation exposure to the patient.
- SNR is a method of describing the strength of the radiation exposure compared with the amount of noise apparent in a digital image. When the digital image displays increased noise, regardless of the source, anatomic details have decreased visibility.
- In film-screen radiography, film serves as the medium for image acquisition, processing, and display.
- Silver halide crystals suspended in the film's emulsion layer absorb the radiant energy (x-rays and visible light) and form the latent image.
- Sensitometry is the study of the relationship between radiation exposure and the amount of density produced after the film is chemically processed.
- Radiographic film can be manufactured to differ in terms of speed, contrast, latitude, and spectral sensitivity.
- The greater the speed of the film, the more sensitive it is to radiant energy.
- Film is placed in a cassette between two intensifying screens and permits lower x-ray exposures compared with film alone.
- The intensifying screen phosphors emit visible light (fluoresce) in proportion to the exit radiation to expose the film.
- Intensifying screens can be manufactured to vary in speed. Increasing intensifying screen speed reduces the required radiation exposure but also decreases the recorded detail in the image.

REVIEW QUESTIONS

1. The type of image receptor that uses a photostimulable phosphor to acquire the latent image is _____.
   A. an intensifying screen
   B. a flat panel detector
   C. computed radiography
   D. radiographic film

2. Which of the following is used to extract the latent image from an imaging plate?
   A. Laser beam
   B. Photomultiplier tube
   C. Analog-to-digital converter
   D. Thin-film transistor

3. Which of the following will improve the quality of the digital image?
   A. Decreased sampling frequency and increased sampling pitch
   B. Decreased sampling frequency and decreased sampling pitch
   C. Increased sampling frequency and increased sampling pitch
   D. Increased sampling frequency and decreased sampling pitch

4. Which of the following would improve the quality of the digital image for a given field of view (FOV)?
   A. A fixed matrix size and larger imaging plate
   B. A decreased sampling frequency and larger imaging plate
   C. A small matrix size and larger pixel size
   D. A fixed matrix size and small imaging plate

5. What is the process of assigning a numeric value to represent a brightness value?
   A. Dynamic range
   B. Signal-to-noise ratio
   C. Quantization
   D. Spectral sensitivity

6. Which of the following pixel bit depths would display a greater range of shades of gray to represent the anatomic tissues?
   A. 8-bit
   B. 10-bit
   C. 14-bit
   D. 16-bit

7. Digital imaging systems have a wider dynamic range than film-screen image receptors.
   A. True
   B. False

8. A lower signal-to-noise ratio improves the quality of a digital image.
   A. True
   B. False

9. Which of the following is the latent image center for radiographic film?
   A. Phosphor layer
   B. Polyester base
   C. Detector element
   D. Sensitivity speck

10. Which of the following describes a film's sensitivity to x-rays or light?
A. Gamma
B. Speed
C. Contrast
D. Latitude

11. Intensifying screens are used to _____.
A. decrease patient exposure
B. increase recorded detail
C. increase film latitude
D. decrease contrast

12. The ability to emit light only when stimulated by x-rays is known as _____.
A. phosphorescence
B. sensitometry
C. conversion efficiency
D. fluorescence

Image Processing and Display

OBJECTIVES

After completing this chapter, the reader will be able to perform the following:

1. Define all the key terms in this chapter.
2. State all the important relationships in this chapter.
3. Explain histogram analysis, automatic rescaling, and lookup tables and their role during computer processing to create a quality digital image.
4. Differentiate among the vendor-specific types of exposure indicators.
5. Compare and contrast the types of display monitors used for diagnostic interpretation and image reviewing.
6. Identify the important features of monitors that may affect the quality of the displayed image.
7. Explain the difference between luminance and luminance ratio.
8. Recognize postprocessing functions, including electronic collimation, window level and width, subtraction, contrast enhancement, edge enhancement, and smoothing.
9. Define the acronyms PACS, DICOM, and HL7.
10. Explain how the latent image is converted to a manifest image during automatic film processing.
11. State the developing and fixing agents used in chemical processing.
12. List the sequential stages and systems needed to process a quality radiographic film image.
13. State methods to maintain the archival quality of film radiographs.
14. Discuss the role of chemical replenishment, temperature control, and silver recovery during film processing.
15. State the requirements for darkroom safelights, temperature, and humidity control.

KEY TERMS

ambient lighting
automatic film processor
automatic rescaling
contrast resolution

developing agents
Digital Imaging and
  Communications in
  Medicine (DICOM)

electronic collimation
exposure indicator
feed tray
fixing agent

After a latent image is created, it must be processed to produce the manifest or visible image. Processing differs significantly between digital and film-screen imaging. This chapter discusses computer processing and display for a digital image and chemical processing and display for a film image. In addition, unique features of digital imaging in display and postprocessing are presented.

DIGITAL IMAGE PROCESSING

The previous chapter described how digital image receptors (IRs) (computed radiography [CR] and digital radiography [DR]) capture the intensity pattern of exit radiation in order to create radiographic images. After the raw image data are extracted from the digital receptor and converted to digital data, the image must be computer processed before its display and diagnostic interpretation. The term *digital image processing* refers to various computer manipulations applied to digital images for the purpose of optimizing their appearance. Although many of the possible digital image processing operations are outside the scope of this textbook, several of the most important and commonly used processing steps are described.

Histogram Analysis

Histogram analysis is an image processing technique commonly used to identify the edges of the image and assess the raw data prior to image display. In this method, the computer first creates a histogram of the image (Figure 7-1). A histogram is a graphic representation of a data set. A data set includes all the pixel values that represent the image before edge detection and rescaling. This graph represents the number of digital pixel values versus the relative prevalence of the pixel values in the image. The *x*-axis represents the amount of exposure, and the *y*-axis represents the incidence of pixels for each exposure level. The computer analyzes the histogram using processing algorithms and compares it with a preestablished histogram specific to the anatomic part being imaged. This process is called **histogram analysis**. The computer software has stored histogram models, each having a shape characteristic of the selected anatomic region and projection. These stored histogram models have **values of interest (VOI)**, which determine the range of the histogram data set that should be included in the displayed image.

In CR imaging, the entire imaging plate is scanned to extract the image from the photostimulable phosphor. The computer identifies the exposure field and the edges of the image, and all exposure data outside this field are excluded from the

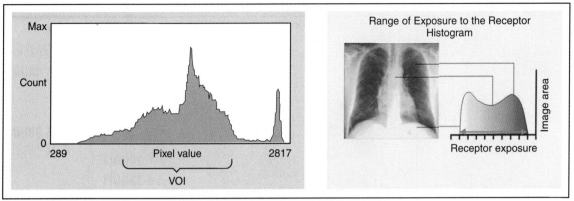

FIGURE 7-1 The histogram represents the number of digital pixel values versus the relative prevalence of those values in the latent image. The *x*-axis represents the amount of exposure and the *y*-axis the incidence of pixels for each exposure level. Each image has its own histogram.

histogram. Ideally, all four edges of a collimated field are recognized. If at least three edges are not identified, all data, including raw exposure or scatter outside the field, may be included in the histogram, resulting in a histogram analysis error. Histogram analysis errors are less likely to occur with DR IRs compared with CR IRs because the image data are extracted from the exposed detectors only.

Important Relationship
Histogram Analysis
With digital systems, the computer creates a histogram of the data set. The histogram is a graph of the exposure received to the pixel elements and the prevalence of the exposures within the image. This created histogram is compared with a stored histogram model for that anatomic part; VOIs are identified, and the image is displayed.

Histogram analysis is also employed to maintain consistent image brightness despite overexposure or underexposure of the IR. This procedure is known as **automatic rescaling.** The computer rescales the image based on the comparison of the histograms, which is actually a process of mapping the grayscale to the VOI to present a specific display of brightness (Figure 7-2). Although automatic rescaling is a convenient feature, radiographers should be aware that rescaling errors occur for a variety of reasons and can result in poor-quality digital images.

Exposure Indicator. An important feature of digital image processing is its ability to create an image with the appropriate amount of brightness regardless of the exposure to the IR. As a result of the histogram analysis, valuable information is provided to the radiographer regarding the exposure to the digital IR. The **exposure indicator** provides a numeric value indicating the level of radiation exposure to the digital IR. Currently, exposure indicators are not standardized among various digital imaging equipment in use today; however, the industry is working toward standardization of the exposure indicator. See Table 7-1 for a list of CR vendor-specific exposure indicators.

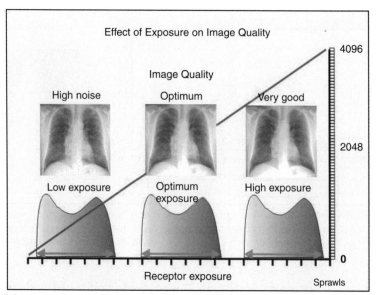

FIGURE 7-2 Automatic rescaling is employed during histogram analysis to maintain consistent image brightness despite overexposure or underexposure of the IR.

TABLE 7-1	**Computed Radiography Vendor-Specific Exposure Indicators**			
		Value = 1 mR		
Vendor	Exposure Indicator	exposure	**2× Exposure**	**½ Exposure**
Fuji and Konica	Sensitivity (S)	200	100	400
Carestream (Kodak)	Exposure index (EI)	2000	2300	1700
Agfa	Log median value (lgM)	2.5	2.8	2.2

In CR, the exposure indicator value represents the exposure level to the imaging plate, and the values are vendor specific. Fuji and Konica use sensitivity (S) numbers, and the value is inversely related to the exposure to the plate. A 200 S number is equal to 1 mR of exposure to the plate. If the S number increases from 200 to 400, this would indicate a decrease in exposure to the IR by half. Conversely, a decrease in the S number from 200 to 100 would indicate an increase in exposure to the IR by a factor of 2, or doubling of the exposure. Carestream (Kodak) uses exposure index (EI) numbers; the value is directly related to the exposure to the plate, and the changes are logarithmic expressions. For example, a change in EI from 2000 to 2300, a difference of 300, is equal to a factor of 2 and represents twice as much exposure to the plate. Agfa uses log median (lgM) numbers; the value is directly related to exposure to the plate, and changes are also logarithmic expressions. For example, a change in lgM from 2.5 to 2.8, a change of 0.3, is equal to a factor of 2 and represents twice as much exposure to the IR. Optimal ranges of the exposure indicator values are vendor specific and vary among the types of procedures, such as abdomen and chest imaging versus extremity imaging.

DR imaging systems may also display an exposure indicator that varies according to the manufacturer's specifications. The radiographer should monitor the exposure indicator values as a guide for proper exposure techniques. If the exposure indicator value is within the acceptable range, adjustments can be made for contrast and brightness with postprocessing functions, and this will not degrade the image. However, if the exposure is outside of the acceptable range, attempting to adjust the image data with postprocessing functions would not correct for improper receptor exposure and may result in noisy or suboptimal images that should not be submitted for interpretation.

The radiographer has a role in the selection of the appropriate anatomic part and projection before computer processing. This step indicates to the computer which histogram to use. If the radiographer selects a part other than the one imaged, a histogram analysis error may occur. In addition, any errors that occur, such as during data extraction from the IR or rescaling during computer processing, could affect the exposure indicator and provide a false value. It is important for radiographers not only to consider the exposure indicator value carefully but also to recognize its limitations.

Important Relationship
Exposure Indicators

The radiographer should strive to select techniques that result in exposure indicator values within the indicated optimum range for that digital imaging system. However, the radiographer also needs to recognize the limitations of exposure indicators in providing accurate information.

Lookup Tables

Following histogram analysis, **lookup tables** provide a method of altering the image to change the display of the digital image in various ways. Because digital IRs have a linear exposure response and a very large dynamic range, raw data images exhibit low contrast and must be altered to improve visibility of anatomic structures. Lookup tables provide the means to alter the brightness and grayscale of the digital image using computer algorithms. They are also sometimes used to reverse or invert image grayscale. Figure 7-3 visually compares pixel values of the original image with a processed image. If the image is not altered, the graph would be a straight line. If the original image is altered, the original pixel values would be different in the processed image and the graph would no longer be a straight line but might resemble a characteristic curve for radiographic film (Figure 7-4).

For example, each pixel value could be altered to display the digital image with a change in contrast. New pixel intensities would be calculated that result in the image being displayed with higher contrast (Figure 7-5). Figure 7-6 shows the original image, the graph following changes in the pixel values, and the processed higher contrast image. Lookup tables provide a method of processing digital images in order to change the brightness and contrast displayed (Figure 7-7).

Important Relationship
Lookup Tables

Lookup tables provide the means to alter the original pixel values to improve the brightness and contrast of the image.

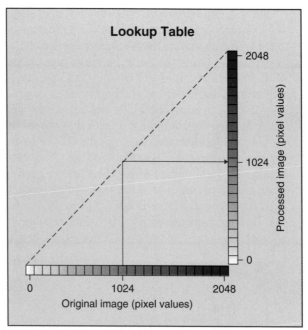

FIGURE 7-3 Straight line graph demonstrating no change in the pixel values from the original to the processed image.

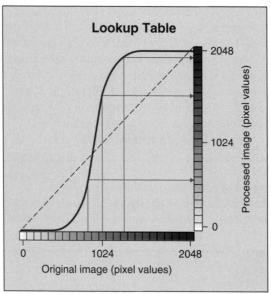

FIGURE 7-4 Graph demonstrating a change in pixel values from the original image to the processed image. The shape of the graph is similar to the characteristic curve for radiographic film.

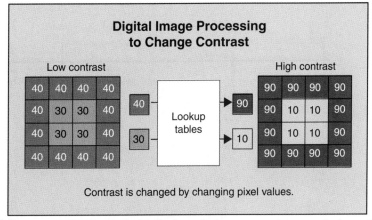

FIGURE 7-5 Lookup table altering the pixel values of a low-contrast image to display an image with higher contrast.

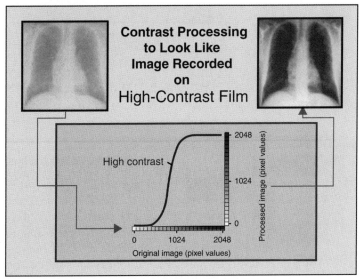

FIGURE 7-6 The original low-contrast chest image is altered to display a higher-contrast chest image. The graph shows a change in the pixel values from the original image.

IMAGE DISPLAY

Following computer processing, the digital image is ready to be displayed for viewing. *Soft copy viewing* refers to the display of the digital image at a computer workstation, as opposed to viewing images on film or another physical medium (hard copy). The quality of the digital image is also affected by important features of the display monitor, such as its luminance, resolution, and viewing conditions such as ambient lighting and monitor placement. Specialized postprocessing software is used at the display workstation to aid the radiologist in image interpretation. In

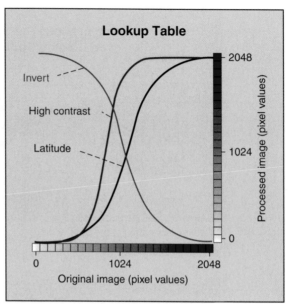

FIGURE 7-7 Similar to radiographic film sensitometry, the shape and location of the curve vary for changes in the processed image.

addition to soft copy viewing, the digital image can be printed on specialized film by a laser printer.

Display Monitors

As discussed previously, the quality of the digital image is affected by its acquisition parameters and subsequent computer processing. In addition, the quality of the digital image is affected by the performance of the display monitor. The quality of display monitors may not be equal among all those used for viewing of digital images. Monitors used by radiologists for diagnostic interpretation, referred to as *primary,* must be of higher quality than the monitors used only for routine image review. However, the radiographer's monitor should be of sufficiently high quality in order to discern all the image quality characteristics accurately before sending the image to the radiologist for diagnostic interpretation. Display monitors used for diagnostic interpretation are typically monochrome high-resolution monitors and can be formatted as portrait or landscape and configured with one, two, or four monitors (Figure 7-8). A display monitor having diagonal dimensions of 54 cm (21 inches) is adequate to view images sized 35 × 43 cm (14 × 17 inches).

Types of Monitors. Cathode ray tubes (CRTs) and liquid crystal displays (LCDs) are types of monitors typically used for viewing digital images. LCDs are replacing CRTs, and newer technology, such as plasma-type monitors, continue to be developed.

A CRT monitor creates an image by accelerating and focusing electrons to strike the faceplate composed of a fluorescent screen (Figure 7-9). Because the image is scanned on the screen in lines, the number of lines affects the quality of

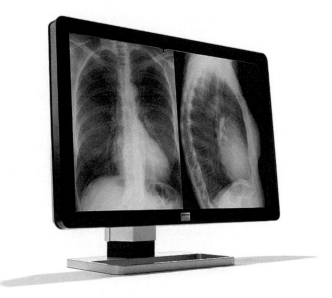

FIGURE 7-8 A set of portrait display monitors used for soft-copy viewing.

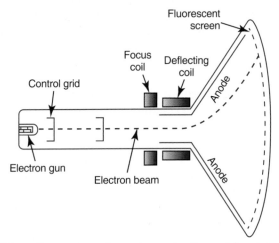

FIGURE 7-9 The CRT monitor creates an image by accelerating and focusing electrons to stike the faceplate composed of a fluorescent screen.

the image displayed. It is recommended that CRT monitors scan at least 525 lines per $\frac{1}{30}$ of a second. The major components of the CRT monitor are the electron gun encasing a cathode, focusing coils and deflecting coils, and the anode. This type of display monitor typically has a curved faceplate, and its dimensions are deeper.

The LCD monitor passes light through liquid crystals to display the image on the glass faceplate. Additional components include a source for the electrical signal and light waveforms and polarizing filters (Figure 7-10). The electrical signals can vary

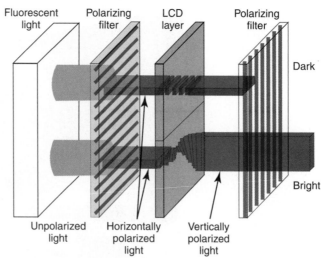

Fluorescent light • Polarizing filter • LCD layer • Polarizing filter • Dark • Bright • Unpolarized light • Horizontally polarized light • Vertically polarized light

FIGURE 7-10 The LCD monitor passes light through liquid crystals to display the image on the glass faceplate.

the light waveforms that pass through the crystals for viewing on the faceplate. The LCD monitor has a flat faceplate, and its dimensions are thinner.

Several important features of monitors can affect the quality of the displayed image. Spatial resolution (as determined by screen size and matrix size), luminance, and contrast resolution are just some of the important characteristics of display monitors.

Viewing Conditions. Placement of the display monitors and the level of light in the room, referred to as **ambient lighting,** can affect soft copy viewing of digital images. Positioning the monitor away from any direct light sources reduces the amount of reflection on the faceplate of the monitor. In addition, maintaining a low level of ambient lighting can help to enhance the viewer's perception of image brightness and contrast displayed on the monitor. Display monitors that have a thicker faceplate such as a CRT have a tendency to reflect more of the ambient lighting than monitors with thinner faceplates such as an LCD.

Performance Criteria. Several important features of display monitors affect their performance. Digital images are captured and processed to display a specific matrix size. As previously discussed, an image created with a large matrix having many smaller-sized pixels improves the spatial resolution of the digital image (pixel image). If the monitor used for viewing the digital image cannot display a matrix of that size (because it has too few display pixels), image quality is decreased. Therefore, the monitor matrix size should be at least as large as the image matrix size. It is recommended that a high-resolution 5-megapixel (2048 × 2560 pixels) display monitor be used for diagnostic interpretation.

Because anatomic tissue is visualized as brightness levels, the amount of light emitted from the monitor (luminance) affects the quality of the displayed image. **Luminance** is a measurement of the light intensity emitted from the surface of the monitor and is expressed in units of candela per square meter (cd/m^2). Primary display monitors should exhibit an average luminance between 300-500 cd/m^2. A ratio of the maximum to minimum luminance is evaluated as a part of display monitor quality control and is recommended to be at least 250/100.

The contrast resolution of a digital image is determined by the pixel bit depth. A digital imaging system capable of displaying 16,384 shades of gray (14-bit) requires a monitor capable of displaying a large grayscale range. Monitors that have a higher luminance ratio are capable of displaying a greater grayscale range. The DICOM Grayscale Standard Display Function (GSDF) as recommended by the American Association of Physicists in Medicine (AAPM) Task Group 18 should not vary more than 10%.

Additional concerns of display monitors are geometric distortions, such as concavity and convexity; veiling glare, which adversely affects image contrast; and display noise, which is typically a result of statistical fluctuations or luminance differences in the image.

Postprocessing. Postprocessing functions are computer software operations available to the radiographer and radiologist that allow manual manipulation of the displayed image. These functions allow the operator to adjust manually many presentation features of the image to enhance the diagnostic value.

Electronic Collimation. Collimating or restricting the radiation field size to the area of interest is an important tool used to reduce patient exposure and improve the quality of the radiographic image. In order to process and display the image correctly, it is important that only the area of interest be included within the radiation exposure area. Once the image is processed, regions viewed on the image can be altered further by **electronic collimation**, also known as *masking* or *shuttering*. For example, when the area of interest is properly collimated, the image may display increased brightness surrounding the radiation-exposed field. This region of brightness provides no useful information and can be removed from the displayed image. In addition, electronic collimation can remove regions within the radiation-exposed field that provide no useful information. Electronic collimation has no effect on overall image quality or patient exposure.

Brightness. Because the image is composed of numeric data, the brightness level displayed on the computer monitor can be easily altered to visualize the range of anatomic structures recorded. This adjustment is accomplished using the windowing function. The **window level** (or center) sets the midpoint of the range of brightness visible in the image. Changing the window level on the display monitor allows the image brightness to be increased or decreased throughout the entire range. When the range of brightness displayed is less than the maximum, the processed image presents only a subset of the total information contained within the computer (Figure 7-11).

Assume that pixel values from 0 to 2048 are used to represent the full range of digital image brightness levels. A high pixel value could represent a volume of tissue that attenuated fewer x-ray photons and is displayed as a decreased brightness level. Therefore, a low pixel value represents a volume of tissue that attenuates more x-ray photons and is displayed as increased brightness.

Moving the window level up to a high pixel value increases visibility of the darker anatomic regions (e.g., lung fields) by increasing overall brightness on the display monitor. Conversely, to visualize better an anatomic region represented by a low pixel value, one would decrease the window level to decrease the brightness on the display monitor.

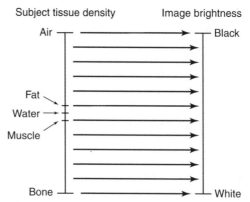

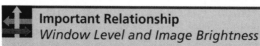

FIGURE 7-11 Changing the window level increases or decreases the image brightness throughout the range of densities recorded in the image.

Important Relationship
Window Level and Image Brightness

A direct relationship exists between window level and image brightness on the display monitor. Increasing the window level increases the image brightness; decreasing the window level decreases the image brightness.

Contrast. The number of different shades of gray that can be stored and displayed by a computer system is termed **grayscale**. **Contrast resolution** is another term associated with digital imaging and is used to describe the ability of the imaging system to distinguish between objects that exhibit similar densities because they attenuate the x-ray beam similarly. An important distinguishing characteristic of a digital image is its improved contrast resolution compared with a film-screen image. As mentioned previously, the contrast resolution of a pixel is determined by the bit depth or number of bits (i.e., 12, 14, or 16), which affects the number of shades of gray available for image display. Increasing the number of shades of gray increases the contrast resolution within the image. An image with increased contrast resolution, when windowed optimally, increases the visibility of very subtle anatomic features.

Once the digital image is processed, radiographic contrast can be adjusted to vary visualization of the area of interest; this is necessary because the contrast resolution of the human eye is limited. The **window width** is a control that adjusts the radiographic contrast. Because the digital image can display shades of gray ranging from black to white, the display monitor can vary the range or number of shades of gray visible on the image to show the desired anatomy. Adjusting the range of shades of gray visible varies the image contrast. When the entire number of shades of gray are displayed (wide window width), the image has lower contrast; when a smaller number of shades of gray are displayed (narrow window width), the image has higher contrast (Figure 7-12).

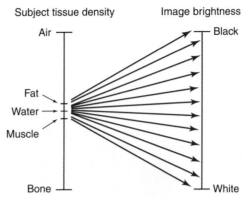

FIGURE 7-12 Changing the window width increases or decreases the range of brightness levels visible. A narrow window width decreases the range of brightness levels and increases contrast. Wider window width increases the range of brightness levels and reduces contrast.

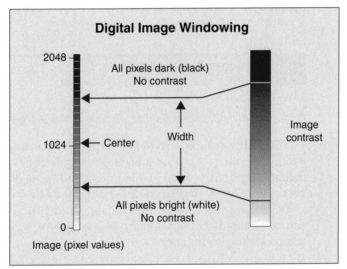

FIGURE 7-13 The level or center of the window and the window width change the visual display of the digital image.

In digital imaging, an inverse relationship exists between window width and image contrast. A wide window width displays an image with lower contrast than the same area of interest displayed with a narrow window width.

The center or midpoint of the window level and the width of the window determine the brightness and contrast of the displayed image (Figure 7-13). Figure 7-14 demonstrates how the image is altered when the window level is changed for a given window width.

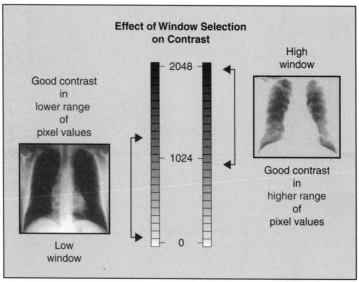

FIGURE 7-14 Changing the window level for a chest x-ray varies the visibility of the anatomic detail or contrast for both low-density and high-density areas.

Important Relationship
Window Width and Image Contrast
A narrow (decreased) window width displays higher radiographic contrast, whereas a wider (increased) window width displays lower radiographic contrast.

The ability to optimize image display in real time using the window level and width controls is a major advantage of soft copy (versus hard copy) viewing of digital images. Also, keep in mind that windowing does not alter the original stored pixel values of an image, but rather alters only how they are displayed.

Depending on the software available during soft copy viewing, the digital image can be manipulated additionally in a variety of ways. Following are five common postprocessing techniques:

1. *Subtraction* (Figure 7-15) is a technique that can remove superimposed structures so that the anatomic area of interest is more visible. Because the image is in a digital format, the computer can subtract selected brightness values to create an image without superimposed structures.
2. *Contrast enhancement* (Figure 7-16) is a postprocessing technique that alters the pixel values to increase image contrast.
3. *Edge enhancement* (Figure 7-17) is a postprocessing technique that improves the visibility of small, high-contrast structures. Image noise may be slightly increased, however.
4. *Black/white reversal* (Figure 7-18) is a postprocessing technique that reverses the grayscale from the original radiograph.
5. *Smoothing* is a postprocessing technique that suppresses image noise (quantum noise). Spatial resolution is degraded, however.

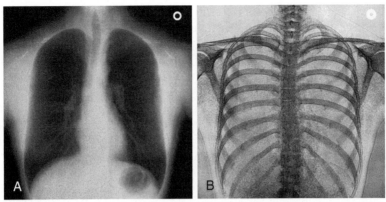

FIGURE 7-15 Subtraction postprocessing techniques. **A,** Skeletal areas are removed. **B,** Lungs and soft tissue are removed.

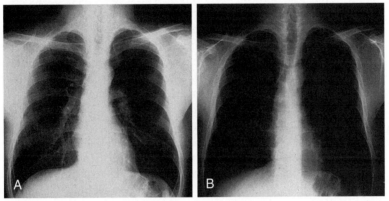

FIGURE 7-16 Postprocessing adjustment in radiographic contrast. **A,** Longer-scale contrast typical of chest radiography. **B,** Contrast has been adjusted to present a higher scale.

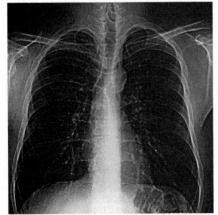

FIGURE 7-17 Radiographic image demonstrates an edge enhancement postprocessing technique.

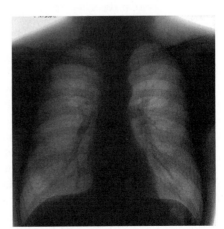

FIGURE 7-18 Radiographic image demonstrates a black/white reversal postprocessing technique.

A word of caution is warranted regarding postprocessing: Overuse of these functions can drastically and negatively alter the data set that is the digital image. Overwriting the original image with a postprocessed replica may reduce the diagnostic and archival quality of the data. One should also keep in mind that in many facilities the radiographer's workstations use monitors of significantly lower quality and viewing conditions that are very different compared with the radiologist's workstations. How an image looks on the radiographer's workstation in a brightly lit work area may be very different from the way it looks on the radiologist's high-resolution monitor in a darkened reading room. Therefore, care should be taken in the postprocessing of an image before forwarding it for interpretation.

Laser Printers

Although not commonly needed for interpretation, hard copy records of digital images may still occasionally be desired. Digital images can be windowed while being viewed on a display monitor and then printed onto film by a laser camera. Multiple images can be printed on a single sheet, and multiple copies of images can be printed that were processed differently. Laser printers are available that use either wet or dry printing methods. Wet laser printers use liquid chemicals (developer and fixer) to process the image. In dry processing, the chemicals are part of the film. The image is created by use of heat instead of liquid chemicals.

DIGITAL COMMUNICATION NETWORKS

Modern radiologic practice requires efficient and facile acquisition, storage, retrieval, transmission, and display of digital image data from multiple imaging modalities. Digital communication needs in radiology also include the processing and delivery of patient data and subsequent interpretation of radiologic procedures. The ability to integrate image, voice, and medical information simultaneously involves a more complex system. **Picture archival and communication system (PACS)** is a computer system designed for digital imaging that can receive, store, distribute, and display digital images; radiology information systems (RIS) and hospital information systems (HIS) are computer systems that provide medical information.

The ability to integrate these systems can be accomplished by networks. A network system links all of these computer systems so that images, patient data, and interpretations can be viewed simultaneously by people at different workstations (Figure 7-19). An important goal of a radiology network system is to provide the referring physician with the radiology report, patient data, and radiographic images at a convenient location and in a timely manner.

Digital Imaging and Communications in Medicine (DICOM) is a communication standard for information sharing between PACS and imaging modalities. **Health Level Seven standard (HL7)** is a communication standard for medical information. Connectivity and communication among these systems are necessary for radiology to realize the full potential of digital communication. Network systems are currently being marketed to meet the demands in the radiation sciences. A well-integrated system would improve patient care through cost-effective, reliable, secure, and timely delivery of diagnostic information.

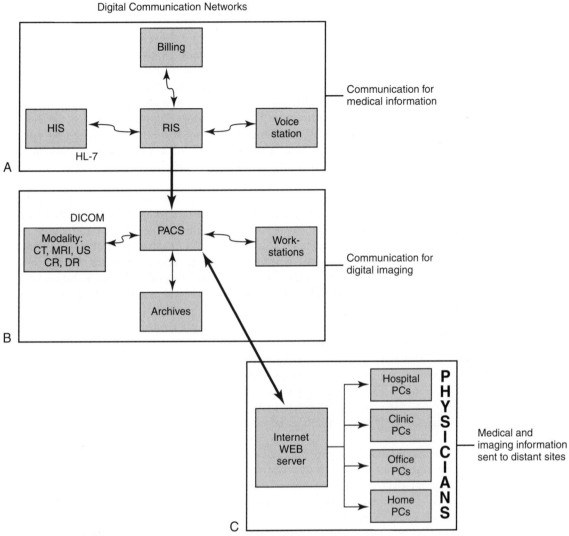

FIGURE 7-19 A, Communication among the computer systems for medical information. **B,** Communication among the computer systems for imaging. **C,** Referring physicians can receive radiology reports, patient data, and radiographic images through the Internet.

Although digital imaging has replaced most of film-screen imaging, knowledge of film processing and film display is important.

RADIOGRAPHIC FILM PROCESSING

Following exposure of the film to radiant energy from x-rays and the light from the intensifying screens, the film must be chemically processed in order to view the radiographic image. Automatic film processing is the method used to produce a visible permanent image.

Automatic Film Processing

The purpose of radiographic film processing is to convert the latent image into a manifest image. According to the Gurney-Mott theory, exposure of the silver bromide crystals in the film emulsion by light or x-ray photons creates the latent image and initiates the conversion process. Chemical processing of the exposed film completes the conversion process and transforms the image into a permanent visible image.

Processing Stages. An **automatic film processor** (Figure 7-20) is a device that encompasses chemical tanks, a roller transport system, and a dryer system for the processing of radiographic film. The processing of a radiograph occurs in four stages: developing, fixing, washing, and drying. Each stage has its specific function and implementation method (Table 7-2).

Developing. The primary function of developing is to convert the latent image into a manifest, or visible, image. The purpose of the **developing agents,** or **reducing agents,** is to reduce exposed silver halide to metallic silver and to add electrons to exposed silver halide. Two chemicals are used to accomplish this purpose: phenidone and hydroquinone. *Phenidone* is said to be a fast reducer, producing gray (lower) densities. *Hydroquinone* is said to be a slow reducer, producing black (higher) densities. The developer solution needs an alkaline pH environment for the chemicals to function properly.

> **Important Relationship**
> *Developing or Reducing Agents*
> The developing agents are responsible for reducing the exposed silver halide crystals to metallic silver, visualized as radiographic densities. Phenidone is responsible for creating the lower densities, and hydroquinone is responsible for creating the higher densities. Their combined effect results in the range of visible densities on the radiograph.

During the development process, developer solution donates additional electrons to the sensitivity specks, or electron traps, in the emulsion layers of the film. These additional electrons attract more silver to these areas, amplifying the amount of atomic silver at each latent image center. Exposed silver halide is reduced to metallic silver when bromide and iodide ions are removed from the emulsion. The atomic silver that was exposed to radiant energy (light and x-rays) is converted to metallic silver and presented as radiographic densities. Unexposed silver halide does not react immediately to the developer because it has not been ionized and does not accept electrons from the developer. Given extended exposure to developing solution or exposure to excessively heated developing solution, however, even unexposed areas of film can react to developing solution.

Fixing. The primary functions of the fixing stage are to remove unexposed silver halide from the film and to make the remaining image permanent. There are also two secondary functions of fixing. One is to stop the development process; the other is to harden the emulsion further. Fixing solution must function to remove all undeveloped silver halide, while not affecting the metallic silver image.

The purpose of the **fixing agent** is to clear undeveloped silver halide from the film. A thiosulfate (sometimes also called *hypo*), such as ammonium thiosulfate, is the chemical used as this agent. The fixer solution needs an acidic pH environment for the chemicals to function properly.

>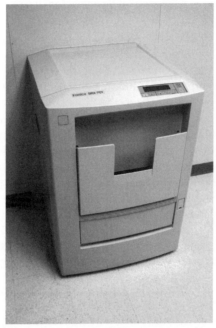
>
> **↕ Important Relationship**
> *Clearing the Unexposed Crystals*
> The fixing agent, ammonium thiosulfate, is responsible for removing the unexposed crystals from the emulsion.

Washing. The purpose of the washing process is to remove fixing solution from the surface of the film. This is a further step in making the manifest image permanent. If not properly washed, the resulting radiograph shows a brown staining of the

FIGURE 7-20 Type of automatic film processor used in radiography.

TABLE 7-2	**Automatic Film Processing Stages**

Developing
Converts latent image to a manifest or visible image
    Developing or Reducing Agents
      • Phenidone—faster and produces gray densities
      • Hydroquinone—slower and produces black densities

Fixing
Removes unexposed silver halide from film; stops the development process; hardens the emulsion
    Fixing Agent
      • Ammonium thiosulfate

Washing
Removes fixing solution from surface of film

Drying
Removes 85%-90% of moisture from film

image, resulting in image loss and a decrease in its diagnostic value. This staining is caused by thiosulfate (fixing agent) that remains in the emulsion layers. Some thiosulfate always remains within the film, but the goal of washing is to remove enough so that the radiograph can be used for an extended period.

Important Relationship
Archival Quality of Radiographs
Maintaining the archival (long-term) quality of radiographs requires that most of the fixing agent be removed (washed) from the film. Staining or fading of the permanent image results when too much thiosulfate remains on the film.

The process by which washing works is referred to as *diffusion*. Diffusion exposes the film to water that contains less thiosulfate than the film. Because the film contains more fixing agent than the water, the fixing agent diffuses into the water.

Eventually, thiosulfate concentrations in the wash water can become greater than the concentrations in the films being processed; therefore, the wash water must be replaced frequently. Water flows freely from the input water supply through the wash tank and down the drain while the roller transport system is operating. This type of system provides a constant supply of fresh wash water to aid in the diffusion process. The moving water also causes agitation and increases diffusion.

Drying. The final process in automatic processing is drying. The purpose of drying films is to remove 85% to 90% of the moisture from the film so that it can be handled easily and stored while maintaining the quality of the diagnostic image. As a result, finished radiographs should retain 10% to 15% of their moisture when processing is complete. If films are dried excessively, the emulsion layers can crack, which decreases the diagnostic quality of the radiograph.

Important Relationship
Archival Quality of Radiographs
Permanent radiographs must retain moisture of 10% to 15% to maintain archival quality. Excessive drying can cause the emulsion layers to crack.

Increased relative humidity decreases the efficiency of dryers in processors, so an increased drying temperature is necessary. Processors are equipped with thermostatic controls to allow selection of a wide range of dryer temperatures.

To process a radiographic image chemically, specialized equipment and systems must perform concurrently to move the film through the processing stages according to the manufacturer's specifications.

Processor Systems. Automatic processors use a vertical transport system of rollers that advance the film through the various stages of film processing (Figure 7-21). A film is introduced into the processor on the feed tray. The **feed tray** is a flat metal surface with an edge on either side that permits the film to enter the processor easily while remaining correctly aligned. Automatic processors use different types of rollers to move the film through the processor. Transport and crossover rollers ensure the film is moved into and through the tanks at a constant speed.

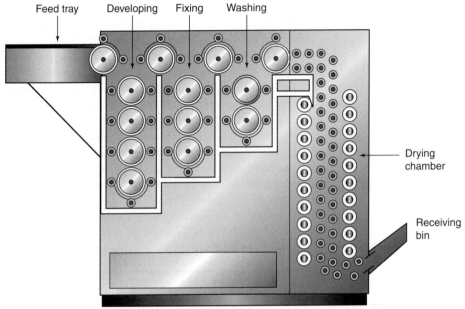

FIGURE 7-21 Cross-section of an automatic processor showing the vertical transport system of rollers.

An electric motor provides power for the roller assemblies to transport the film through the processor. The on-off switch that provides electrical power to the processor activates this motor. Most processors are also equipped with a standby control. The **standby control** is an electrical circuit that shuts off power to the roller assemblies when the processor is not being used. Pushing the standby control switch when one is ready to process a film can reactivate the roller assemblies and water intake.

Replenishment refers to the replacement of fresh chemicals after the loss of chemicals during processing, specifically developer solution and fixer solution. The replenishment of chemicals used in the automatic processor is necessary because these chemicals eventually become exhausted or inactive, and their ability to perform their functions decreases. Developing solution becomes exhausted from both use and exposure to air, which reduces its chemical strength.

Fixer solution becomes exhausted for several reasons: It becomes weakened from use as a result of accumulations of silver halide that are removed from the film during the fixing process and because developer solution remains in the film, which decreases the strength and activity of the fixer solution.

Important Relationship
Replenishment and Solution Performance
The replenishment system provides fresh chemicals to the developing and fixing solutions to maintain their chemical activity and volume when they become depleted during processing.

The amount of solution that is replenished is preset and based on the size of the film or occurs at timed intervals. Replenishment systems usually are adjusted so that more fixer solution is replenished per film compared with developer solution.

Automatic processors have a recirculation system for the developer and fixer tanks. Each tank has a separate system that consists of a pump and connecting tubing. The **recirculation system** acts to circulate the solutions in each of these tanks by pumping solution out of one portion of the tank and returning it to a different location within the same tank from which it was removed. The recirculation system keeps the chemicals mixed, which helps maintain solution activity and provides agitation of the chemicals around the film to facilitate fast processing.

Recirculation also helps maintain the proper temperature of the developer solution. The developer recirculation system includes an in-line filter that removes impurities as the developer solution is being recirculated.

Temperature control of the developer solution is important because the activity of this solution depends directly on its temperature. An increase or decrease in developer temperature can adversely affect the quality of the radiographic image.

In most 90-second automatic processors, developer temperature must be maintained at 93° F to 95° F (33.8° C to 35° C). An **immersion heater** is a heating coil that is immersed in the bottom of the developer and fixer tank. Most automatic pro-

> **Important Relationship**
> *Developer Temperature and Radiographic Quality*
> Variations in developer temperature can adversely affect the quality of the radiographic image. Increasing developer temperature increases the density, and decreasing developer temperature decreases the density. Radiographic contrast also may be adversely affected by changes in the developer temperature.

cessors are thermostatically controlled to heat the developer solution to its proper temperature and maintain that temperature as long as the processor is turned on.

Radiographs must be properly dried to be viewed and stored. The film is dried by hot air that is blown onto both surfaces of the film as it moves through the dryer. This air is forced through the dryer by a blower and is directed onto the film by air tubes. The temperature of the air that is used to dry films is thermostatically monitored to control moisture removal from the film accurately.

Inadequate processing is evidenced by certain appearances of the finished radiograph. Particular problems can be pinpointed by analyzing the radiographs. These problems and the radiographic appearances that indicate them are summarized in Table 7-3.

Quality Control

Unexposed film should be stored in its original packaging so that important information about the film can be maintained, such as expiration date and lot number. Film boxes should be stored vertically, not horizontally, to prevent pressure artifacts on the film. Film should be stored away from heat sources and ionizing radiation. Both heat and radiation can cause the silver halide in film emulsion to break down, which results in fogged film. The shelf life of film, as expressed by its expiration date, must be observed. Film should not be used beyond the expiration date.

How film is handled in the darkroom can have a profound effect on the radiographs. Common hazards to radiographic quality that can be found in the darkroom

TABLE 7-3	Indicators of Inadequate Processing
Radiographic Appearance	**Processing Problem**
Decrease in density	Developer exhausted
	Developer underreplenishment
	Processor running too fast
	Low developer temperature
	Developer improperly mixed
Increase in density	Developer overreplenishment
	High developer temperature
	Light leak in processor
	Developer improperly mixed
Pinkish stain (dichroic fog)	Contamination of developer by fixer
	Developer or fixer underreplenishment
Brown stain (thiosulfate stain)	Inadequate washing
Emulsion removed by developer	Insufficient hardener in developer
Milky appearance	Fixer exhausted
	Inadequate washing
Streaks	Dirty processor rollers
	Inadequate washing
	Inadequate drying
Water spots	Inadequate drying
Minus-density scratches	Scratches from guide plates caused by roller or plate misalignment

are white-light exposure, safelight exposure, ionizing radiation exposure, and other potential hazards.

Darkrooms must be free from all outside white-light exposure. A white-light source may be located inside the darkroom, but it should be connected to an interlock system whereby the film bin may not be opened as long as the darkroom white-light source is on. In addition, the temperature and humidity can adversely affect the film. Film should be stored and handled at temperatures ranging from 55° F to 75° F (14° C to 24° C) with a relative humidity of 30% to 60%. Without moisture in the air (low humidity), any buildup of static charges can expose the film.

Countertops must be clean and static free to avoid the formation of radiographic artifacts on the films. Several brands of commercial cleaning fluids contain an antistatic component ideal for cleaning darkroom countertops and processor feed trays.

Other potential hazards to film in the darkroom include heat and chemical exposure. Film stored within the darkroom should not be near any heat source. Processing chemicals must be kept away from film and film-handling areas to prevent exposure and contamination of these areas.

Ionizing radiation exposure to film in the darkroom is a potential hazard because many darkrooms share common walls with radiographic rooms. The walls that are

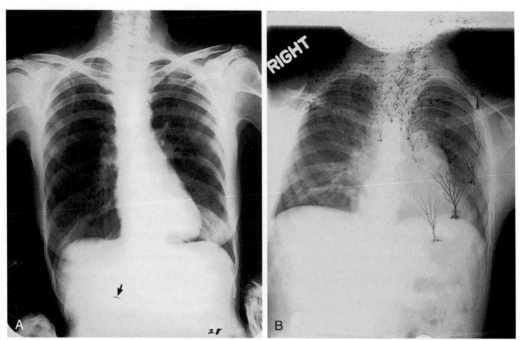

FIGURE 7-22 Film artifacts. **A,** Plus-density half-moon artifacts can be caused by bending or kinking the film *(arrow)*. **B,** Plus-density static discharge artifact can be caused by sliding a film over a flat surface.

common with the darkroom and a radiographic room must be lined with lead as required by law for standard protection from radiographic exposures. The film bin where film is stored and available for immediate use should also be lined with lead to prevent fog that may result from radiation exposure.

Safelights used in the darkroom must be equipped with a safelight filter appropriate for the type of film being handled in the darkroom. Commonly used filters include Kodak Wratten 6B for blue-sensitive film and Kodak GBX for orthochromatic film, which is sensitive to both blue-violet and green visible light. Safelight filters must be free of cracks because white light that leaks from the safelight could expose the film. The power rating of the light bulbs used in safelights should be no greater than that recommended by film manufacturers (generally 7.5 to 15 W), which is indicated on the outside of the box of radiographic film.

Good radiographic quality cannot be achieved when film is improperly stored, mishandled before or after exposure, or incorrectly processed. Common film artifacts resulting from improper storage, darkroom handling, or improper processing are shown in Figure 7-22. A quality control program also must be implemented and systematically followed to ensure proper processing of radiographic film. Box 7-1 describes quality control methods for evaluating the darkroom and film processor.

Silver Recovery

Because fixer solution is used to remove unexposed silver halide from the film, used fixer solution contains a high concentration of accumulated silver. Some type of silver recovery must be used when radiographic processing accumulates high

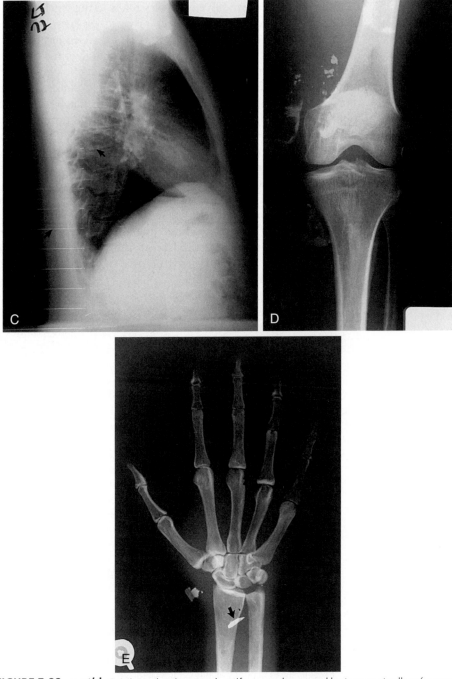

FIGURE 7-22, cont'd C, Minus-density scratch artifacts can be caused by transport rollers *(arrows).*
D, Minus-density caused by moisture on finger. **E,** Dirty screens or cassettes can cause nonspecific
minus-density artifacts.

concentrations of silver. **Silver recovery** refers to the removal of silver from used fixer solution. For some facilities that regularly process large volumes of radiographs, the financial rewards of silver recovery may be an added incentive.

Silver-recovery units are available for on-site silver recovery and generally require servicing by an outside contractor familiar with the equipment and its method of removing silver. These silver-recovery units are connected directly to the drain system of the fixer tank to remove silver as used fixer solution passes through the unit. After the silver has been recovered, the used fixer is drained.

Silver-recovery units work by one of two methods. One method of silver recovery is called *metallic replacement*. There are two types of metallic replacement silver-recovery units. One uses steel wool, and the other uses a silver-extraction filter. A steel wool metallic replacement unit uses steel wool to filter the used fixer solution. Silver replaces the iron in the steel wool and can then be removed easily after significant accumulation in a canister or replacement cartridge occurs. A silver-extraction unit uses a foam filter that is impregnated with steel wool. Again, the silver from used fixer solution replaces the iron in the steel wool. A silver-extraction filter is more efficient at removing silver from used fixer and lasts longer than a simple steel wool metallic replacement unit.

BOX 7-1 | Quality Control: Darkroom and Film Processor

A quality control program must be implemented and systematically followed to ensure proper processing of radiographic film. A good quality control program should include steps for monitoring all of the equipment and activities required for the production of quality radiographic images, to include but not limited to the following:

- Sensitometric monitoring of the film processor provides valuable information on the daily functioning of the processor.
  - Following the establishment of baseline measurements, expose and process a sensitometric strip daily, measure the appropriate optical density points with a densitometer, and plot on a control chart with predetermined upper and lower acceptable limits. The graph provides a visual indicator of any acute or evolving processor malfunction.
- Typically, a processor control chart monitors base + fog, medium optical density or speed, and upper and lower density differences to evaluate contrast.
  - Speed and contrast indicators should not vary more than ±0.15 optical density from baseline measurements.
  - Base + fog should not be greater than +0.05 optical density from the baseline measurement.
  - Developer temperature should be measured daily with a digital thermometer and should not vary ±0.5°F (0.3° C).
- The darkroom environment should be well ventilated, clean, organized, and safe.
- A safelight fog test should be performed semiannually and result in less than +0.05 optical density of added fog.
- Replenishment rates should be checked weekly and fall within ±5% of manufacturer's specification.
- Recommended quarterly quality control checks include:
  - Developer solution pH should be maintained between 10 and 11.5.
  - Fixer pH should be maintained between 4 and 4.5.
  - Developer specific gravity should not vary more than ±0.004 from manufacturer's specifications.

Another method of silver recovery is the *electrolytic method*. It is the most efficient method, but the units needed for this process are also more expensive than metallic replacement units. Electrolytic units have an electrically charged drum or disk that attracts silver. The silver plates onto the drum or disk and can be removed when a substantial amount of silver has been collected.

Silver is considered a heavy metal, and its disposal is regulated by local and state agencies. In many locales, strict limits are placed on the concentrations of silver in used fixer that can be disposed of via the sewer system. Silver recovery is an important process in radiology because silver is a natural resource, can be toxic to the environment, and has monetary value.

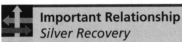

Important Relationship
Silver Recovery
Silver is a natural resource, is a heavy metal that can be toxic to the environment, and needs to be removed from the used fixer.

Image Display

In order to view a processed film image, it must be displayed on an illuminator. **Illuminators** or viewboxes are devices that provide light illumination so that the anatomy, displayed as various shades of optical densities, can be visualized.

Illuminators. The dimensions of an illuminator are typically 14 × 17 inches (35 × 43 cm) and can be arranged individually or combined in rows as a bank of illuminators (Figure 7-23). The most important performance criterion of film illuminators is the uniformity of light intensity within and among viewboxes. Variations in the light emission can affect visibility of anatomic detail, and therefore maintaining clean and damage-free viewboxes along with the proper bulb wattage are essential to quality control.

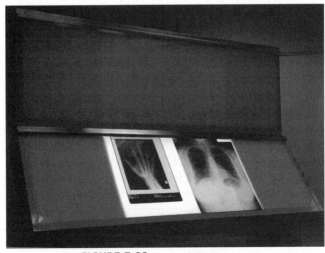

FIGURE 7-23 Bank of illuminators.

CHAPTER SUMMARY

- With digital systems, the computer creates a histogram or graph of the exposure received to the pixel elements and the prevalence of those exposures within the image.
- Histogram analysis is an image processing technique used to identify the edges of the image and to compensate for image overexposure and underexposure.
- The computer analyzes the histogram using processing algorithms and compares it with a preestablished histogram specific to the anatomic part imaged.
- Automatic rescaling is a process employed to maintain consistent image brightness despite overexposure and underexposure.
- During histogram analysis, the exposure indicator provides a numeric value indicating the level of radiation exposure to the digital IR.
- Following histogram analysis, lookup tables provide the means to alter the original pixel values to improve the brightness and contrast of the image.
- Display monitors provide soft copy viewing of digital radiographs. Primary monitors are high-quality monitors used for diagnostic interpretation.
- Two commonly used display monitors are CRT and LCD. CRT monitors create an image by accelerating and focusing electrons to strike the faceplate composed of a fluorescent screen. LCD monitors pass light through liquid crystals to display the image on a glass plate.
- Important features regarding display monitors are viewing conditions, matrix size, luminance, luminance ratio, and contrast resolution.
- Postprocessing functions, such as electronic collimation, window level and width, subtraction, contrast enhancement, edge enhancement, and smoothing, allow manipulation of the displayed image.
- Laser printers are available that use either wet or dry methods to print hard copy images.
- PACS is the communication system for the digital imaging modalities and can receive, store, distribute, and display digital images.
- DICOM is a communication standard for information sharing between PACS and imaging modalities, and HL7 is a communication standard for medical information.
- Automatic film processing incorporates several chemical stages and systems to convert the latent image into a manifest image.
- Hydroquinone and phenidone are chemical reducing agents used during the developing stage to convert the exposed silver halide crystals to black metallic silver.
- Ammonium thiosulfate is the chemical fixing agent to clear undeveloped crystals from the film's emulsion.
- Maintaining the archival quality of radiographs requires that most of the fixing agent be washed from the film.
- During the drying stage, 85% to 90% of the moisture needs to be removed from the film for long-term storage.
- Important systems to processing films include replenishment, chemical recirculation, temperature control, and the transport system to move the film through the tanks at a constant speed.

- Film should be stored and handled in a darkroom at temperatures ranging from 55° F to 75° F (14° C to 24° C) and with relative humidity of 30% to 60%. Without moisture in the air (low humidity), any buildup of static charges can expose the film.
- Safelights used in the darkroom must be equipped with a safelight filter appropriate for the type of film handled.
- Silver recovery can be accomplished by the electrolytic method or metallic replacement and is an important process because silver is a natural resource, is a heavy metal that can be toxic to the environment, and needs to be removed from the used fixer.
- Radiographic films are displayed on illuminators that emit uniform light intensity.

REVIEW QUESTIONS

1. Which of the following is defined as a graphic representation of the pixel values?
   A. Automatic rescaling
   B. Values of interest
   C. Histogram
   D. Exposure indicator

2. What process is employed to maintain consistent digital image brightness for overexposure or underexposure?
   A. Automatic rescaling
   B. Histogram
   C. Exposure indicator
   D. Lookup tables

3. Which of the following is *not* a numeric value indicating the level of radiation exposure to the digital image receptor?
   A. Sensitivity number
   B. Exposure indicator
   C. Window level
   D. Exposure index

4. What digital process alters image brightness and grayscale to improve the visibility of anatomic structures?
   A. Automatic rescaling
   B. Histogram analysis
   C. Exposure indicator
   D. Lookup tables

5. What type of monitor passes light through liquid crystals to display the digital image?
   A. TFT
   B. LCD
   C. CRT
   D. PACS

6. Maintaining a low level of ambient lighting can improve soft copy viewing of digital images.
A. True
B. False

7. Display monitors used for soft copy viewing of digital images should have _____.
A. increased ambient lighting
B. decreased matrix size
C. low spatial resolution
D. high luminance

8. Which of the following is *not* a function during postprocessing of the displayed digital image?
A. Automatic rescaling
B. Electronic collimation
C. Windowing
D. Edge enhancement

9. A wider window width _____.
A. increases brightness
B. decreases brightness
C. increases contrast
D. decreases contrast

10. What reducing agent acts slowly to produce the higher densities on a film radiograph?
A. Ammonium thiosulfate
B. Hydroquinone
C. Phenidone
D. Cesium iodide

11. What chemical agent is responsible for clearing the unexposed silver halide crystals during film processing?
A. Ammonium thiosulfate
B. Hydroquinone
C. Phenidone
D. Cesium iodide

12. How is the archival quality of radiographic film maintained?
A. Remove most of the fixing agent from the film
B. Retain at least 10% of moisture in the film
C. Store film in an area of high humidity
D. A and B only

13. Which automatic processing system primarily maintains the activity level of the chemistry?
    A. Replenishment
    B. Standby control
    C. Recirculation
    D. Quality control

14. Why is silver recovery necessary during film processing?
    A. It is a natural resource.
    B. It is toxic to the environment.
    C. It has monetary value.
    D. All of the above

15. Film radiographs are best viewed on illuminators having variability of light intensity.
    A. True
    B. False

Exposure Technique Selection

OBJECTIVES

After completing this chapter, the reader will be able to perform the following:

1. Define all the key terms in this chapter.
2. State all the important relationships in this chapter.
3. State the purpose of automatic exposure control (AEC) in radiography.
4. Differentiate among the types of radiation detectors used in AEC systems.
5. Recognize how the detector size and configuration affect the response of the AEC device.
6. Explain how alignment and positioning affect the response of the AEC device.
7. Discuss patient and exposure technique factors and their effect on the response of the AEC device.
8. Analyze unacceptable images produced using AEC, and identify possible causes.
9. Recognize the effect of the type of image receptor on AEC calibration, its use, and image quality.
10. Describe patient protection issues associated with AEC.
11. State the importance of calibration of the AEC system to the type of image receptor used.
12. Define anatomically programmed radiography (APR).
13. Differentiate between the types of exposure technique charts.

KEY TERMS

anatomically programmed
  radiography (APR)
anatomic programming
automatic exposure control
  (AEC)
backup time
calipers
comparative anatomy

density controls
detectors
exposure technique charts
extrapolated
fixed kVp/variable mAs
  technique chart
ionization chamber
ion chamber

mAs readout
minimum response time
optimal kVp
photomultiplier tube
phototimer
variable kVp/fixed mAs
  technique chart

The radiographer is responsible for selecting exposure factor techniques to produce quality radiographs for a wide variety of equipment and patients. There are many thousands of possible combinations of kVp, mA, SID, exposure time, image receptors (IRs), and grid ratios. When combined with patients of various sizes and with various pathologic conditions, the selection of proper exposure factors becomes a formidable task. Tools are available to assist the radiographer in selecting appropriate exposure techniques: automatic exposure control (AEC) devices, anatomically programmed radiography, and exposure technique charts. Knowledge about the performance of these tools and their operation assists the radiographer in producing quality radiographic images.

AUTOMATIC EXPOSURE CONTROL

An AEC system is a tool available on most modern radiographic units to assist the radiographer in determining the amount of radiation exposure to produce a quality image. **Automatic exposure control (AEC)** is a system used to control consistently the amount of radiation reaching the IR by terminating the length of exposure. AEC systems also are called *automatic exposure devices,* and sometimes they are erroneously referred to as *phototiming.* When using AEC systems, the radiographer must still use individual discretion to select an appropriate kVp, mA, IR, and grid. However, the AEC device determines the exposure time (and total exposure) that is used.

> **Important Relationship**
> *Principle of Automatic Exposure Control Operation*
> Once a predetermined amount of radiation is transmitted through a patient, the x-ray exposure is terminated. This determines the exposure time and therefore the total amount of radiation exposure to the IR.

AEC systems are excellent at producing consistent levels of exposure when used properly, but the radiographer must also be aware of the limitations of using an AEC system in patient positioning and centering, detector size and selection, collimation, and IR variation.

Radiation Detectors

All AEC devices work by the same principle of operation: Radiation is transmitted through the patient and converted into an electrical signal, terminating the exposure time; this occurs when a predetermined amount of radiation has been detected, as indicated by the level of electrical signal that has been produced. The predetermined level of radiation that must be reached before exposure termination is calibrated by service personnel to meet the departmental standards of image quality.

The difference in AEC systems lies in the type of device that is used to convert radiation into electricity. Two types of AEC systems have been used: phototimers and ionization chambers. Phototimers represent the first generation of AEC systems used in radiography, and it is from this type of system that the term *phototiming* has evolved. *Phototiming* specifically refers to the use of an AEC device that uses photomultiplier tubes or photodiodes, even though these systems are uncommon today. Therefore, the use of the term *phototiming* is usually incorrect. The more common type of AEC system uses ionization chambers. Regardless of the specific type of AEC system used, almost all systems use a set of three radiation-measuring detectors, arranged in some specific manner (Figure 8-1). The radiographer selects the configuration of these devices, determining which one (or more) of the three actually measures radiation exposure reaching the IR. These devices are variously referred to as *sensors, chambers, cells,* or *detectors*. These radiation-measuring devices are referred to here for the remainder of the discussion as **detectors**.

> **Important Relationship**
> *Radiation-Measuring Devices*
> Detectors are the AEC devices that measure the amount of radiation transmitted. The radiographer selects the combination of the three detectors to use.

Phototimers. **Phototimers** use a fluorescent (light-producing) screen and a device that converts the light to electricity. A **photomultiplier tube** is an electronic device that converts visible light energy into electrical energy. A photodiode is a solid-state device that performs the same function. Phototimer AEC devices are considered exit-type devices because the detectors are positioned behind the IR (Figure 8-2) so that radiation must exit the IR before it is measured by the detectors. Light paddles, coated with a fluorescent material, serve as the detectors, and the radiation interacts with the paddles, producing visible light. This light is transmitted to remote photomultiplier tubes or photodiodes that convert this light into electricity. The timer is tripped, and the radiographic exposure is terminated when a sufficiently large charge has been received. This electrical charge is in proportion to the radiation to which the light paddles have been exposed. Phototimers have largely been replaced with ionization chamber systems.

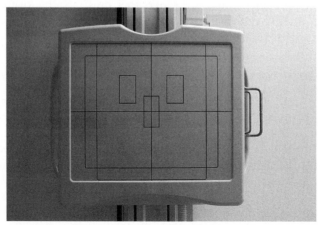

FIGURE 8-1 The size and arrangement of the three AEC detectors are clear on this upright chest unit.

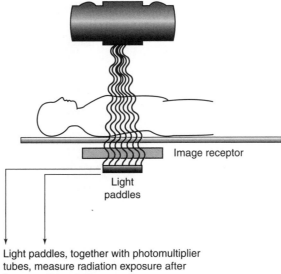

Image receptor

Light
paddles

Light paddles, together with photomultiplier
tubes, measure radiation exposure after
it passes through the cassette.

FIGURE 8-2 The phototimer AEC system has the light paddles (detectors) located directly below the IR. This is an exit-type device in that the x-rays must exit the IR before they are measured by the detectors.

Ionization Chamber Systems. An **ionization chamber,** or **ion chamber,** is a hollow cell that contains air and is connected to the timer circuit via an electrical wire. Ionization chamber AEC devices are considered entrance-type devices because the detectors are positioned in front of the IR (Figure 8-3) so that radiation interacts with the detectors just before interacting with the IR. When the ionization chamber is exposed to radiation from a radiographic exposure, the air inside the chamber becomes ionized, creating an electrical charge. This charge travels along the wire to the timer circuit. The timer is tripped, and the radiographic exposure is terminated when a sufficiently large charge has been received. This electrical charge is in proportion to the radiation to which the ionization chamber has been exposed. Compared with phototimers, ion chambers are less sophisticated and less accurate, but they are less prone to failure. Most AEC systems today use ionization chambers.

> **Important Relationship**
> *Function of the Ionization Chamber*
> The ionization chamber interacts with exit radiation before it reaches the IR. Air in the chamber is ionized, and an electrical charge that is proportional to the amount of radiation is created.

mAs Readout

When a radiographic study is performed using an AEC device, the total amount of radiation (mAs) required to produce the appropriate exposure to the IR is determined by the system. Many radiographic units include an **mAs readout** display, where

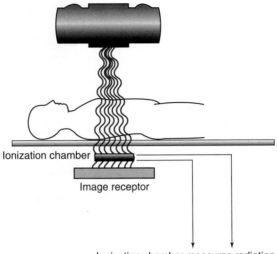

Ionization chamber measures radiation
exposure before it reaches the image receptor.

FIGURE 8-3 The ionization chamber AEC system has the detectors located directly in front of the IR. This system is termed *entrance-type* because the x-ray exposure is measured just before entering the IR.

the actual amount of mAs used for that image is displayed immediately after the exposure, sometimes for only a few seconds. It is critical for the radiographer to take note of this information when it is available. Knowledge of the mAs readout has numerous advantages. It allows the radiographer to become more familiar with manual exposure technique factors. If the image is suboptimal, knowing the mAs readout provides a basis from which the radiographer can make exposure adjustments by switching to manual technique. There may be studies with different positions where AEC and manual technique are combined because of difficulty with accurate centering. For example, knowing the mAs readout for the anteroposterior (AP) lumbar spine gives the radiographer an option to switch to manual technique for the oblique exposures, making technique adjustments based on reliable mAs information.

> **Important Relationship**
> *Automatic Exposure Control and mAs Readout*
> If the radiographic unit has an mAs readout display, the radiographer should take note of the reading after the exposure is made. This information can be invaluable.

kVp and mA Selections

AEC controls only the quantity of radiation reaching the IR and has no effect on other image characteristics, such as contrast. The kVp for a particular examination should be selected as it would be for that examination, regardless of whether an AEC device is used. The radiographer must select the kVp level that provides an appropriate level of contrast and is at least the minimum kVp to penetrate the part. Although in digital imaging contrast can be computer manipulated, the kVp should still be selected to visualize best the area of interest. In addition, the higher the kVp value used, the shorter the exposure time needed by the AEC device. Because high kVp radiation is more penetrating (reducing the total amount of x-ray exposure to the patient because more x-ray photons exit the patient) and the detectors are measuring quantity of radiation, the preset amount of radiation exposure is reached sooner with a high kVp.

Important Relationship
kVp Levels and Automatic Exposure Control Response
The radiographer must set the kVp value as needed to ensure adequate penetration and to produce the appropriate level of contrast. The kVp selected determines the length of exposure time when using AEC. A low kVp requires more exposure time to reach the pre-determined amount of exposure. A high kVp decreases the exposure time to reach the pre-determined amount of exposure and reduces the overall radiation exposure to the patient.

Patient Protection Alert
Kilovoltage Selection
Using higher kVp with AEC decreases the exposure time and overall mAs needed to produce a diagnostic image, significantly reducing the patient's exposure. The kVp selected for an examination should produce the desired image contrast for the part examined and be as high as possible to minimize the patient's radiation exposure.

When the radiographer uses a control panel that allows the mA and time to be set independently, he or she should select the mA value as it would be for that particular examination, regardless of whether an AEC device is used. The mA value selected will affect the exposure time needed by the AEC device. Therefore, if the radiographer wants to decrease exposure time for a particular examination, he or she may easily do so by increasing the mA value. For a given procedure, increasing the mA on the control panel decreases the exposure time, and decreasing the mA selected on the control panel increases the exposure time.

Important Relationship
mA Level and Automatic Exposure Control Response
If the radiographer can set the mA level when using AEC, it will affect the time of exposure for a given procedure. Increasing the mA decreases the exposure time to reach the pre-determined amount of exposure. Decreasing the mA increases the exposure time to reach the predetermined amount of exposure.

Minimum Response Time

The term **minimum response time** refers to the shortest exposure time that the system can produce. Minimum response time (1 ms with modern AEC systems) usually is longer with AEC systems than with other types of radiographic timers (i.e., other types of radiographic timers usually are able to produce shorter exposure times than

AEC devices). This can be a problem with some segments of the patient population, such as pediatric patients and uncooperative patients. Typically, the radiographer increases the mA so that the time of exposure terminates more quickly. If the minimum response time is longer than the amount of time needed to terminate the preset exposure, it results in an increased amount of radiation reaching the IR. With pediatric patients and other patients who cannot or will not cooperate with the radiographer by holding still or holding their breath during the exposure, AEC devices may not be the technology of choice.

Backup Time

Backup time refers to the maximum length of time the x-ray exposure will continue when using an AEC system. The backup time may be set by the radiographer or controlled automatically by the radiographic unit. It may be set as backup exposure time or as backup mAs (the product of mA and exposure time). The backup time acts as a safety mechanism when an AEC system fails or the equipment is not used properly. In either case, the backup time protects the patient from receiving unnecessary exposure and protects the x-ray tube from reaching or exceeding its heat-loading capacity. If the backup time is controlled automatically, it should terminate at a maximum of 600 mAs.

Important Relationship
Function of Backup Time
Backup time, the maximum exposure time allowed during an AEC examination, serves as a safety mechanism when AEC is not used properly or is not functioning properly.

The backup time might be reached as the result of operator oversight when an AEC examination, such as a chest x-ray, is done at the upright Bucky and the radiographer has set the control panel for table Bucky. The table detectors are forced to wait an excessively long time to measure enough radiation to terminate the exposure. The backup time is reached and the exposure is terminated, limiting the patient's exposure and keeping the tube from overloading. However, newer x-ray units with AEC include a sensor in the Bucky tray for the IR and do not allow an exposure to activate if the table Bucky detectors were selected but the x-ray tube centered to the upright Bucky.

When controlled by the radiographer, the backup time should be set high enough to be greater than the exposure needed but low enough to protect the patient from excessive exposure in case of a problem. Setting the backup time at 150% of the expected exposure time is appropriate. If the backup timer periodically or routinely terminates the exposure, higher mA values should be used to shorten the exposure time.

Important Relationship
Setting Backup Time
Backup time should be set at 150% to 200% of the expected exposure time. This allows the properly used AEC system to terminate the exposure appropriately but protects the patient and tube from excessive exposure if a problem occurs.

> **! Patient Protection Alert**
> *Monitoring Backup Time*
> To minimize patient exposure, the backup time should be neither too long nor too short. Backup time that is too short results in the exposure being stopped prematurely, and the image may need to be repeated because of poor image quality. Backup time that is too long results in the patient receiving unnecessary radiation if a problem occurs and the exposure does not end until the backup time is reached. In addition, the image may have to be repeated because of poor image quality.

Density Adjustment

AEC devices are equipped with **density controls** that allow the radiographer to adjust the amount of preset radiation detection values. These generally are in the form of buttons on the control panel that are numbered –2, –1, +1, and +2. The actual numbers presented on density controls vary, but each of these buttons changes exposure time by some predetermined amount or increment expressed as a percentage. A common increment is 25%, meaning that the predetermined exposure level needed to terminate the timer can be either increased or decreased from normal in one increment (+25% or –25%) or two increments (+50% or –50%). Manufacturers usually provide information for their equipment on how these density controls should be used. Common sense and practical experience should also serve as guidelines for the radiographer. Routinely using plus or minus density settings to produce an acceptable radiograph indicates that a problem exists, possibly a problem with the AEC device.

Alignment and Positioning Considerations

Detector Selection. Selection of the detectors to be used for a particular examination is critical when using an AEC system. AEC systems with multiple detectors typically allow the radiographer to select any combination of one, two, or all three detectors. The selected detectors actively measure radiation during exposure, and the electrical signals are averaged. Typically, the detector that receives the greatest amount of exposure has a greater impact on the total exposure.

Measuring radiation that passes through the anatomic area of interest is important. The general guideline is to select the detectors that would be superimposed by the anatomic structures that are of greatest interest and need to be visualized on the radiograph. Failure to use the proper detectors could result in either underexposure or overexposure to the IR. In the case of a posteroanterior (PA) chest radiograph, the area of radiographic interest includes the lungs and heart; therefore, one or two outside detectors should be selected to place the detectors directly beneath the critical anatomic area. If the center detector were mistakenly selected, the anatomy superimposing this detector includes the thoracic spine. If the exposure is made, the resultant image shows sufficient exposure in the spine, with the lungs overexposed (Figure 8-4). In the manual that accompanies a radiographic unit, the AEC device manufacturer provides recommendations for which detectors to use for specific examinations. Recommendations for detector combination also can be found in many radiographic procedures textbooks.

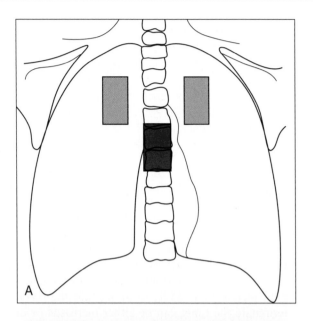

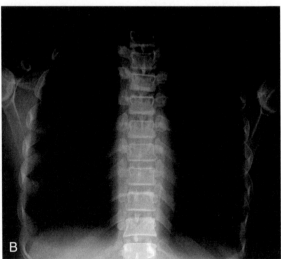

FIGURE 8-4 Selecting the detectors to be located directly under the critical anatomic area may make the difference between a diagnostic image and an unacceptable image. The PA chest should be imaged using both outside detectors to locate them directly under the lung tissue. **A,** This diagram shows that the center detector was inappropriately selected for the PA chest image, placing the thoracic spine directly over the detector. **B,** The resulting chest radiograph demonstrates diagnostic density in the area of the spine, but the lungs are notably overexposed.

Many radiographic units have AEC devices in both the table Bucky and an upright Bucky. If more than one Bucky per radiographic unit uses AEC, the radiographer must be certain to select the correct Bucky before making an exposure. Failure to do so may result in the patient and IR being exposed to excessive radiation. The backup time is reached, the exposure is terminated prematurely, and a repeat radiographic study may need to be done, increasing the patient's dose.

A similar problem can occur in some systems when not using a Bucky, such as with cross-table, tabletop, or stretcher or wheelchair studies. If the AEC system is activated with these types of examinations, an unusually long exposure results because the detectors are not being exposed to radiation. Again, the backup time will likely be reached, and the patient's dose will be excessive. Some radiographic units are designed so that an exposure does not occur if the AEC device has been selected and there is no IR detected in the Bucky.

Important Relationship
Detector Selection

The combination of detectors affects the amount of exposure reaching the IR. If the area of radiographic interest is not directly over the selected detectors, that area likely will be overexposed or underexposed. When performing any radiographic study where the IR is located outside of the Bucky, the AEC system should be deactivated, and a manual technique should be used.

Patient Centering. Proper centering of the part being examined is crucial when using an AEC system. The anatomic area of interest must be centered properly over the detectors that the radiographer has selected. Improper centering of the part over the selected detectors may underexpose or overexpose the IR. For example, when an AEC device is used for a lateral lumbar spine image, if the central ray is too far posterior and the center detector is selected (as appropriate), the soft tissue superimposes the detector rather than the spine. In this case, the soft tissue behind the spine demonstrates sufficient exposure, but the spine itself is underexposed (Figure 8-5).

Important Relationship
Patient Centering

Accurate centering of the area of interest over the detectors is critical to ensure proper exposure to the IR. If the area of interest is not properly centered to the detectors, overexposure or underexposure may occur.

Inaccurate centering is probably the most common cause of suboptimal film-screen images when AEC is used. When the anatomy of interest is not centered directly over the detector, the image is underexposed or overexposed, possibly requiring the image to be repeated and the patient to receive more radiation than necessary.

If a digital IR is underexposed or overexposed, the computer adjusts for the exposure error, but the image quality or patient exposure, or both, is compromised. Underexposure may result in the visibility of quantum noise, and overexposure increases patient exposure and may decrease contrast.

Detector Size. The size of the detectors manufactured within an AEC system is fixed and cannot be adjusted. Therefore, it is important for the radiographer to determine whether AEC should be used during the radiographic procedure. The radiographer must first determine whether the patient's anatomic area of interest can adequately cover the detector combination. For example, if the patient for a procedure is very small, such as a toddler, his or her chest may not adequately cover the outer two detectors. In this case, the patient's chest is smaller than the dimensions of the selected detectors. If a portion of the detector is exposed directly to the primary beam, the radiation exposure level necessary to terminate the exposure is reached almost immediately, resulting in underexposure of the area of interest.

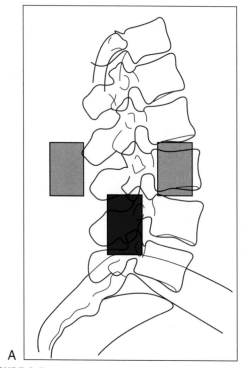

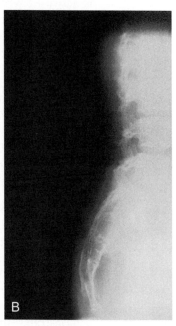

FIGURE 8-5 Centering the key anatomic area directly over the AEC detector is critical in producing diagnostic radiographs. Whatever anatomic area is located over the detector has diagnostic exposure. **A,** With the center detector selected, the centering for this lateral lumbar spine image is posterior to the lumbar vertebral bodies. The lamina, spinous processes, and soft tissue cover the detector. **B,** The resulting radiograph demonstrates appropriate density just posterior to the vertebral bodies, but the bodies themselves are underexposed. This radiograph is unacceptable because of inaccurate centering resulting in underexposure of the anatomy of interest.

It is critical that the radiographer determine whether the anatomic area of interest can adequately superimpose the dimension of the detector combination. If the detector combination is larger in size than the area of interest, it would necessitate the use of a manual exposure technique.

Compensating Issues

Patient Considerations. The AEC system is designed to compensate for changes in patient thickness. If the area of interest is thicker because of an increase in the patient's size, the exposure time will lengthen in order to reach the preset exposure to the detectors. AEC systems that do not adequately compensate for changes in patient thickness may need to be calibrated.

Some patients may require greater technical consideration when AEC is used for radiographic procedures. Abdominal examinations using AEC can be compromised if a patient has an excessive amount of bowel gas. If a detector is superimposed by an area of the abdomen with excessive gas, the timer will terminate the exposure prematurely, resulting in underexposure to the IR. Likewise, destructive pathologic conditions can cause underexposure of the area of radiographic interest. The presence of positive contrast media, an additive pathologic condition, or a prosthetic device that superimposes the detector can cause excessive exposure.

If the anatomic area directly over the detector does not represent the anatomic area of interest, inappropriate exposure to the IR may result. This can happen when the anatomic area over the detector contains a foreign object, a pocket of air, or contrast media. The radiographer must consider these circumstances individually and determine how best to image the patient or part. Using the density control buttons may work in some cases, whereas in others it may be necessary to recenter the patient or part. Sometimes the best solution is a manual technique determined through use of a technique chart. AEC is not a replacement for a knowledgeable radiographer using critical thinking skills.

> **❗ Patient Protection Alert**
> *Patient Variability*
> Factors related to the patient affect the time of exposure reaching the IR and ultimately image quality. Increases or decreases in patient thickness result in changes in the time of exposure if the AEC system is functioning properly. Pathology, contrast media, foreign object, and pockets of gas are patient variables that may affect the proper exposure to the IR and ultimately image quality.

Collimation. The size of the x-ray field is a factor when AEC systems are used because the additional scatter radiation produced by failure to restrict the beam accurately may cause the detector to terminate the exposure prematurely. The detector is unable to distinguish transmitted radiation from scattered radiation and, as always, ends the exposure when a preset amount of exposure has been reached. Because the detector is measuring both types of radiation exiting the patient, the timer is turned off too soon when scatter is excessive, which results in underexposure of the area of interest.

Additionally, if the x-ray field size is collimated too closely, the detector does not receive sufficient exposure initially and may prolong the exposure time, which could result in overexposure. The radiographer should open the collimator to the extent that the part being radiographed is imaged appropriately but not so much as to cause the AEC device to terminate the exposure before the area being imaged is properly exposed.

> **Important Relationship**
> *Collimation and Automatic Exposure Control Response*
> Excessive or insufficient collimation may affect the amount of exposure reaching the IR. Insufficient collimation may result in excessive scatter reaching the detectors, resulting in the exposure time terminating too quickly. Excessive collimation may result in too long of an exposure time.

Image Receptor Variations. Different types of IRs cannot be interchanged easily once an AEC device is calibrated to terminate exposures at a preset level. When calibration is performed, it is done for a particular type of IR, including digital.

> **Important Relationship**
> *Type of Image Receptor and Automatic Exposure Control Response*
> The AEC system is calibrated to the type and speed class of the IR used. If an IR of a different type or speed is used, the detectors will not sense the difference, and the exposure time will terminate at the preset value, which may jeopardize image quality.

The AEC device cannot sense when the radiographer uses a different type or speed class of IR and instead produces an exposure based on the system for which it was calibrated, resulting in either too much or too little exposure for that IR. For example, if a 100 speed film-screen system is used with an AEC device instead of the appropriate 400 speed film-screen system, the resulting image will have too little density because the exposure stopped (as preset) for the more sensitive 400 speed system. Some radiographic units have AEC devices that can accommodate more than one speed of film-screen system. With these types of units, the control panel allows selection of a different film-screen system speed.

Calibration. As with any radiographic unit, it is imperative that systematic equipment testing be performed to ensure proper system performance. Calibration and quality control testing are essential procedures to maintain the proper functioning of the AEC system (Box 8-1).

For an AEC device to function properly, the radiographic unit, including the type of IR, and the AEC device must be calibrated to meet departmental standards. When a radiographic unit with AEC is first installed, the AEC device is calibrated (and at intervals thereafter). The purpose of calibration is to ensure that consistent and appropriate exposures to the IR are produced.

Failure to maintain regular calibration of the unit results in the lack of consistent and reproducible exposures to the detectors and could affect image quality. This situation ultimately leads to overexposure of the patient and poor efficiency of the imaging department as well as the possibility of improper interpretation of radiographs.

BOX 8-1 | Quality Control Check: Automatic Exposure Control

- The AEC device should provide consistent optical densities for variations in exposure factors, patient thicknesses, and detector selection. Several aspects of the AEC performance can be monitored with a densitometer by imaging a homogeneous patient equivalent phantom plus additional thickness plates.
- Consistency of exposures with varying mA, kVp, part thicknesses, and detector selection can be evaluated individually and in combination by imaging the phantom and measuring the resultant optical densities. Optical densities should be within ±0.2 for proper performance of the AEC device. In addition, reproducibility of exposures for a given set of exposure factors and selected detector should result in optical densities within ±0.10.

The radiographer must use AEC accurately regardless of the type of IR used. Failure to do so can result in overexposure of the patient to ionizing radiation or production of an image that is of poor quality. The visual cues of increased or decreased radiographic density present when using film-screen IRs are lacking in digital imaging. It cannot be overstated that when using digital IRs, the radiographer must be very conscientious about excessive radiation exposure to the patient. If a high amount of radiation reaches the digital IR, the image will probably appear diagnostic while the patient receives unnecessary exposure.

> **! Patient Protection Alert**
> *Anatomically Programmed Radiography and Patient Exposure*
> When using a preprogrammed set of exposure factors (APR), the radiographer must evaluate the appropriateness of the exposure technique factors selected. Adjustment of the preprogrammed exposure factors may be necessary for that patient or procedure.

During computer processing, image brightness can be adjusted following underexposure; however, there may be an increase in the visibility of quantum noise. The radiographer must monitor the exposure indicator as a means of detecting AEC malfunctions for digital IRs.

Tables 8-1 and 8-2 clarify the relationship between exposure technique factors and AEC for film-screen (see Table 8-1) and digital IRs (see Table 8-2).

ANATOMICALLY PROGRAMMED RADIOGRAPHY

Anatomic programming, or **anatomically programmed radiography (APR),** refers to a radiographic system that allows the radiographer to select a particular button on the control panel that represents an anatomic area; a preprogrammed set of exposure factors is displayed and selected for use. The appearance of these controls varies, depending on the unit (Figure 8-6), but the operation of all APR systems is based on the same principle. APR is controlled by an integrated circuit or computer chip that has been programmed with exposure factors for different projections and positions of different anatomic parts. Once an anatomic part and projection or position has been selected, the radiographer can adjust the exposure factors that are displayed.

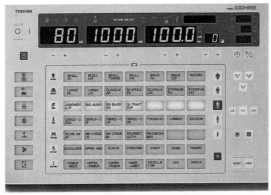

FIGURE 8-6 Anatomically programmed radiography selections are displayed on this console. The radiographer can choose from PA lungs, lateral skull, knee, and hand, among others. Each selection displays the preprogrammed technical factors that the radiographer can decide to use or adjust.

APR and AEC are not related in their functions, other than as systems for making exposures. However, these two different systems are commonly combined on radiographic units because of their similar dependence on integrated computer circuitry. APR and AEC often are used in conjunction with one another. A radiographer can use APR to select a projection or position for a specific anatomic part and view the kVp, mA, and exposure time for manual technique. When APR is used in conjunction with AEC on some radiographic units, the APR system not only selects and displays manual exposure factors, but also selects and displays the AEC detectors to be used for a specific radiographic examination. For example, pressing the Lungs PA button results in selection of 120 kVp, the upright Bucky, and the two outside AEC detectors. As with AEC, APR is a system that automates some of the work of radiography. However, the individual judgment and discretion of the radiographer is still required to use the APR system correctly for the production of optimal quality images.

TABLE 8-1	Film-Screen Radiography and AEC	
An upright PA chest exam done using the following factors produces an optimal image:		
400 speed film-screen system	AEC with 2 outside detectors	
120 kVp	upright Bucky	
400 mA	0 (normal) density	
Assuming all other factors remain the same, how would the following changes affect the density of the image?		

Change	Effect on Density in Area of Interest	Explanation
100 speed film-screen IR	↓	AEC is calibrated to the 400 speed film-screen system. The exposure ends when the exposure is sufficient for the 400 speed IR, which is not sufficient for the 100 speed IR.
Center detector selected	↑	The exposure time is increased. Because the thoracic spine lies over the center detector, the spine has appropriate density, but the lungs have too much density.
70 kVp	0	Changing the kVp does not affect the density, because AEC simply waits for the right number of photons to exit the patient. The exposure time will be increased and result in an increase in the actual mAs. However, the contrast is increased.
100 mA	0	Changing the mA does not affect the density because AEC simply waits for the right number of photons to exit the patient. However, the length of exposure is increased.
−2 density	↓	Changing the density selector changes the setting of the AEC so it turns off the exposure much sooner, resulting in reduced density.
Selecting the table Bucky setting but still using the upright Bucky	↑	The AEC device in the table Bucky is waiting for enough exit radiation to strike the detectors so that the exposure can be terminated. Because the x-ray beam is aimed at the upright Bucky, it is a very long exposure and results in increased density.
Patient has cardiac pacemaker positioned over detector	↑	The detector that is behind the pacemaker takes a long time to terminate the exposure because the radiation has to pass through the pacemaker. This results in increased density.

TABLE 8-2	Digital Imaging and AEC	

An upright PA chest exam is done as indicated in Table 8-1, except that now a computed radiography (CR) system is used instead of film-screen.

Assuming all other factors remain the same, unless indicated, how would the following changes affect the brightness of the image?

Change	Effect on Brightness in Area of Interest	Explanation
CR image receptor	0	The AEC is calibrated to the 400 speed film-screen system. The exposure ends when the exposure is sufficient for the 400 speed IR, which is suboptimal for the CR image receptor. The computer maintains the brightness, but quantum noise is apparent because of underexposure of the imaging plate.
Center detector selected*	0	Because the thoracic spine lies over the center detector, the imaging plate receives more exposure than is needed. The exposure indicator will reflect an increase in exposure to the imaging plate. The computer maintains the brightness but the image contrast is decreased because of excessive scatter, and the patient is overexposed.
70 kVp*	0	The length of exposure to the imaging plate will be increased and results in an increase in the actual mAs to maintain the exposure to the imaging plate. However, the contrast is increased due to the lower kVp.
100 mA*	0	The length of exposure is increased to maintain exposure to the imaging plate.
−2 density*	0	The exposure terminates much sooner, with one - half the exposure to the imaging plate. The exposure indicator will reflect a decrease in exposure to the imaging plate. The computer maintains the brightness, but quantum noise is apparent because of underexposure of the imaging plate.
Selecting the table Bucky setting but still using the upright Bucky*	0	Excessive radiation reaches the imaging plate because the detectors in the table Bucky are unable to terminate the exposure. The exposure indicator will reflect an increase in exposure to the imaging plate. The computer maintains the brightness but the image contrast is decreased because of excessive scatter, and the patient is overexposed.
Patient has cardiac pacemaker-positioned over detector*	0	The detector that is behind the pacemaker takes a long time to turn the exposure off because the radiation has to pass through the pacemaker. The exposure indicator will reflect an increase in exposure to the imaging plate. The computer maintains the brightness but the image contrast is decreased because of excessive scatter, and the patient is overexposed.

*AEC is now calibrated to the computed radiography system.

Important Relationship
Digital Image Receptors and the Automatic Exposure Control Response
Because the visual cues of increased or decreased radiographic density when using film-screen IRs are lacking in digital imaging, the radiographer must be very conscientious about excessive radiation exposure to the patient.

EXPOSURE TECHNIQUE CHARTS

Exposure technique charts are useful tools that assist the radiographer in selecting a manual exposure technique or when using AEC regardless of the type of IR. Exposure technique charts are equally valuable for film-screen or digital IRs. **Exposure technique charts** are preestablished guidelines used by the radiographer to select standardized manual or AEC exposure factors for each type of radiographic examination. Technique charts standardize the selection of exposure factors for the typical patient so that the quality of radiographic images is consistent. Additional information, such as collimation, AEC detector cell selection, and patient shielding, can be included in the technique chart.

> **!   Patient Protection Alert**
> *Exposure Technique Charts and Digital Imaging*
> Exposure technique charts are just as important, if not more so, when using digital IRs. Underexposure or overexposure of a film-screen IR can result in a radiograph with decreased or increased density. Because image brightness is controlled by computer processing, the visual cues for overexposure or underexposure are missing. Exposure technique charts are an effective tool in selecting appropriate exposure techniques for a quality digital image.

For each radiographic procedure, the radiographer consults the technique chart for the recommended exposure variables—kVp, mAs, type of IR, grid, and SID. Based on the thickness of the anatomic part to be radiographed, the radiographer selects the exposure factors presented in the technique chart. For example, if a patient is scheduled for a routine abdominal examination, the radiographer positions the patient and aligns the central ray to the patient and IR, measures the abdomen for a manual technique, and consults the chart for the predetermined standardized exposure variables.

Because many factors have an impact on the selection of appropriate exposure factors, technique charts are instrumental in the production of consistent quality radiographs, reduction in repeat radiographic studies, and reduction in patient exposure. The proper development and use of technique charts are keys to the selection of appropriate exposure factors.

> **Important Relationship**
> *Exposure Technique Charts and Radiographic Quality*
> Exposure technique charts are just as important for digital imaging because digital systems have a wide dynamic range and can compensate for exposure technique errors. Technique charts should be developed and used with all types of radiographic imaging systems to maintain patient radiation exposure *as low as reasonably achievable* (ALARA).

Conditions

A technique chart presents exposure factors that are to be used for a particular examination based on the type of radiographic equipment. Technique charts help ensure that consistent image quality is achieved throughout the entire radiology department; they also decrease the number of repeat radiographic studies needed and therefore decrease the patient's exposure.

Technique charts do not replace the critical thinking skills required of the radiographer. The radiographer must continue to use individual judgment and discretion in properly selecting exposure factors for each patient and type of examination. The primary task of the radiographer is to produce the highest-quality radiograph while delivering the least amount of radiation exposure. Technique charts are designed for the average or typical patient and do not account for unusual circumstances. Patient variability in terms of body build or physical condition or the presence of a pathologic condition requires the radiographer to problem solve when selecting exposure factors. These atypical conditions require accurate patient assessment and appropriate exposure technique adjustment by the radiographer.

A technique chart should be established for each x-ray tube, even if a single generator is used for more than one tube. For example, if a radiographic room has two x-ray tubes, one for a radiographic table and one for an upright Bucky unit, each tube should have its own technique chart because of possible inherent differences in the radiation output produced by each tube. Each portable radiographic unit must also have its own technique chart.

For technique charts to be effective tools in producing radiographs of consistent quality, departmental standards for radiographic quality should be established. In addition, standardization of exposure factors and the use of accessory devices are needed. For example, an adult knee can be radiographed adequately with or without the use of a grid. Although both radiographs might be acceptable, departmental standards may specify that the knee be radiographed with the use of a grid. These types of decisions should be made before technique chart development takes place so that the departmental standards can be clarified. Technique charts are then constructed using these standards, and radiographers should adhere to the departmental standards.

For technique charts to be effective, the radiographic system must be operating properly. A good quality control program for all radiographic equipment ensures monitoring of any variability in the performance of the equipment.

Accurate measurement of part thickness is a critical condition for the effective use of technique charts. The measured part thickness determines the selected kVp and mAs values for the radiographic examination. If the part is measured inaccurately, incorrect exposure factors may be selected. Measurement of part thickness must be standardized throughout the radiology department.

Calipers are devices that measure part thickness and should be readily accessible in every radiographic room (Figure 8-7). In addition, the technique chart should specify the exact location for measuring part thickness. Part measurement may be performed at the location of the central ray midpoint or the thickest portion of the area to be radiographed. Errors in part thickness measurement are common mistakes made when one is consulting technique charts.

Because the range of exposures to produce a quality digital image is wider (wide exposure latitude), precise measurement of the anatomic part is not as critical. Although the technique charts discussed in this chapter use patient measurement to determine the exposure factors to be selected, categorizing the typical patient according to size (small, medium, and large) should be sufficient when using digital IRs.

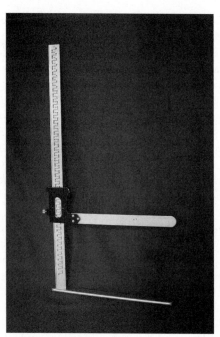

FIGURE 8-7 A caliper is used to measure part thickness.

Types of Technique Charts

Technique charts can vary widely in terms of their design, but they share some common characteristics. The primary exposure factors of kVp and mA and common accessory devices used, such as IR type and grid ratio, are included regardless of the type of technique chart used. Two primary types of exposure technique charts exist: fixed kVp/variable mAs and variable kVp/fixed mAs. Each type of chart has different characteristics, and both have advantages and disadvantages.

Variable kVp/Fixed mAs Technique Chart. The **variable kVp/fixed mAs technique chart** is based on the concept that kVp can be increased as the anatomic part size increases. Specifically, the baseline kVp is increased by 2 for every 1-cm (0.4-inch) increase in part thickness, whereas the mAs is maintained (Table 8-3). The baseline kVp is the original kVp value predetermined for the anatomic area to be radiographed. The baseline kVp is then adjusted for changes in part thickness.

Accurate measurement of part thickness is critical to the effective use of this type of technique chart. Part thickness must be measured accurately to ensure that the 2-kVp adjustment is applied appropriately. The radiographer consults the technique chart and prepares the exposure factors specified for the type of radiographic examination (i.e., mAs, SID, grid use, type of IR). The anatomic part is measured accurately, and the kVp is adjusted appropriately. For example, a standard exposure technique for a patient's knee measuring 10 cm (4 inches) is 63 kVp at 10 mAs, 400 speed film-screen IR, and use of a 12:1 table Bucky grid. A patient with a knee measuring 15 cm (6 inches) would require a change only in the kVp,

TABLE 8-3	Variable kVp/Fixed mAs Technique Chart

Anatomic part: *Knee*	IR: *400 speed*
Projection: *AP*	Tabletop/Bucky: *Bucky*
Measuring point: *Midpatella*	Grid ratio: *12:1*
SID: *40 inches*	Focal spot size: *Small*

cm	kVp	mAs
10	63	20
11	65	20
12	67	20
13	69	20
14	71	20
15	73	20
16	75	20
17	77	20
18	79	20

from 63 to 73 (2 kVp change for every 1-cm [approximately ½-inch] change in part thickness).

Important Relationship
Variable kVp/Fixed mAs Technique Chart
The variable kVp chart adjusts the kVp for changes in part thickness while maintaining a fixed mAs.

Determination of the baseline kilovoltage for each anatomic area has not been standardized. Historically, various methods have been used to determine the baseline kVp value. The goal is to determine a kVp value that adequately penetrates the anatomic part when using a 2-kVp adjustment for every 1-cm (approximately ½-inch) change in tissue thickness. The baseline kVp value can be determined experimentally with the use of radiographic phantoms (patient equivalent devices).

Developing a variable kVp technique chart that can be used effectively throughout the kilovoltage range has proved problematic. In addition, technology advances in imaging receptors may challenge the applicability of the variable kVp/fixed mAs type technique chart.

In general, changing the kVp values for variations in part thickness may be ineffective throughout the entire range of radiographic examinations. A variable kVp/fixed mAs chart may be most effective with pediatric patients or when small extremities, such as hands, toes, and feet, are being imaged. At low kVp levels, small changes in kVp may be more effective than changing the mAs.

This type of chart has the advantage of being easy to formulate because making kVp changes to compensate for different part sizes is simple. However, because kVp is variable, radiographic contrast may vary as well, and these types of charts tend to be less accurate for part size extremes. In addition, adequate penetration of the part is not assured.

Fixed kVp/Variable mAs Technique Chart. The fixed kVp/variable mAs technique chart (Table 8-4) uses the concept of selecting an optimal kVp value that is required for the radiographic examination and adjusting the mAs for variations in part thickness. **Optimal kVp** can be described as the kVp value that is high enough to ensure penetration of the part but not too high to diminish radiographic contrast. For this type of chart, the optimal kVp value for each part is indicated, and mAs is varied as a function of part thickness.

> **Important Relationship**
> *Fixed kVp/Variable mAs Technique Charts*
> Fixed kVp/variable mAs technique charts identify optimal kVp values and alter the mAs for variations in part thickness.

Optimal kVp values required for each anatomic area have not been standardized. Although charts identifying common kVp values for different anatomic areas can be found, experienced radiographers tend to develop their own optimal kVp values. The goal is to determine the kVp that penetrates the part without compromising radiographic contrast. Digital computer processing provides the opportunity to vary the image contrast displayed, and therefore the optimal kVp determined for digital IRs could be higher than the kVp for film-screen IRs. Specifying the optimal kVp value used in a fixed kVp/variable mAs technique chart encourages all radiographers to adhere to the departmental standards.

Once optimal kVp values are established, fixed kVp/variable mAs technique charts alter the mAs for variations in thickness of the anatomic part. Because x-rays are attenuated exponentially, a general guideline is for every 4- to 5-cm (1.6- to 2-inch) change in part thickness, the mAs should be adjusted by a factor of 2. Using the previous example for a patient's knee measuring 10 cm (4 inches) and an optimal kVp, the exposure technique would be 63 kVp at 10 mAs, 400 speed film-screen IR with a 12:1 table Bucky grid. A patient with a knee measuring 15 cm (6 inches)

TABLE 8-4	Fixed kVp/Variable mAs Technique Chart	
Anatomic part: *Knee*		IR: *400 speed*
Projection: *AP*		Tabletop/Bucky: *Bucky*
Measuring point: *Midpatella*		Grid ratio: *12:1*
SID: *40 inches*		Focal spot size: *Small*

cm	kVp	mAs
10-13	73	10
14-17	73	20
18-21	73	40

would require a change only in the mAs, from 10 to 20 (a 5-cm [2-inch] increase in part thickness requires a doubling of the mAs).

Accurate measurement of the anatomic part is important but is less critical compared with the precision needed with variable kVp charts. An advantage of fixed kVp/variable mAs technique charts is that patient groups can be formed around 4- to 5-cm (1.6- to 2-inch) changes. Patient thickness groups can be created instead of listing thickness changes in increments of 1 cm (approximately ½ inch).

The fixed kVp/variable mAs technique chart has the advantages of easier use, more consistency in the production of quality radiographs, greater assurance of adequate penetration of all anatomic parts, uniform radiographic contrast, and increased accuracy with extreme variation in size of the anatomic part.

Exposure Technique Chart Development

Radiographers can develop effective technique charts that assist in exposure technique selection. The steps involved in technique chart development are similar, regardless of the design of the technique chart. The primary tools needed are radiographic phantoms, calipers for accurate measurement, and a calculator. Once optimal radiographs are produced using these phantoms, exposure techniques can be **extrapolated** (mathematically estimated) for imaging other similar anatomic areas.

A critical component in technique chart development is to determine minimal kVp value that adequately penetrates the anatomic part to be radiographed. One available method is to use the concept of **comparative anatomy**, which can assist the radiographer in determining minimal kVp values. This concept states that different parts of the same size can be radiographed by use of the same exposure factors, provided that the minimal kVp value needed to penetrate the part is used in each case. For example, a radiographer knows what exposure factors to use with a particular radiographic unit for a knee that measures 10 cm (4 inches) in the AP aspect, but he or she now needs to radiograph a shoulder. The radiographer measures the shoulder in the AP aspect and determines that it measures 10 cm (4 inches). The radiographer does not have a technique for a shoulder for this radiographic unit. The concept of comparative anatomy states that the shoulder in this case can be radiographed successfully using the same technique that the radiographer has used for the 10-cm (4-inch) knee as long as the minimal kVp to penetrate the part has been used for the shoulder or knee.

The stages for development of exposure technique charts are similar regardless of the type of chart (Box 8-2). Patient-equivalent phantoms for sample anatomic areas provide a means for establishing standardized exposure factors. Using the concept of comparative anatomy assists the radiographer in extrapolating exposure techniques for similar anatomic areas. After the initial development of an exposure technique chart, the chart must be tested for accuracy and revised if necessary.

Poor radiographic quality may result when the exposure technique chart is not used properly. Radiographers need to problem solve by evaluating the numerous exposure variables that could have contributed to a poor-quality radiograph before assuming the chart is ineffective.

BOX 8-2	**How to Develop an Exposure Technique Chart**

1. Select a kVp value appropriate to the anatomic area to be radiographed. Determine the mAs value that produces the desired radiographic density.
2. Using a patient-equivalent phantom, produce several radiographs, varying the kVp and mAs values. Use the general rules for exposure technique adjustment (i.e., the 15% rule). Radiographic densities should be similar.
3. Evaluate the quality of the radiographs, and eliminate those deemed unacceptable.
4. Of the remaining acceptable radiographs, select those having the kVp value appropriate for the type of technique chart desired and according to departmental standards.
5. Extrapolate the exposure techniques (variable kVp or variable mAs) for changes in part thickness.
6. Use the concept of comparative anatomy to develop technique charts for similar anatomic areas.
7. Test the technique chart for accuracy, and revise if needed.

A commitment by management and staff to use exposure technique charts is critical to the consistent production of quality radiographs. Well-developed technique charts are of little use if radiographers choose not to consult them.

CHAPTER SUMMARY

- AEC systems are designed to produce optimal radiation exposure to the IR to produce a quality image.
- AEC uses detectors (typically ionization type) that measure the amount of radiation exiting the patient and terminate the exposure when it reaches a preset amount; this amount corresponds to the amount of radiation that is needed to produce optimal image quality.
- The kVp selected must penetrate the part and produce the desired scale of contrast. Increasing or decreasing the kVp causes the exposure time to be decreased or increased accordingly.
- Changing the mA, when available, causes the exposure time to be decreased or increased accordingly.
- In order for AEC to work accurately, the x-ray beam must be centered precisely to the anatomic area of interest, the correct detectors must be selected, and the anatomic part must cover the dimension of the detectors.
- The mAs readout displayed informs the radiographer of the total radiation exposure used for the procedure.
- Other AEC features can be manipulated or used: Density selectors allow for increased or decreased exposure to the IR; backup time (or mAs) provides a safety mechanism that prevents the exposure from exceeding a set amount; and the mAs readout displays exactly how much mAs was used to produce the image.
- Limitations of AEC systems include that they typically allow only one type of IR, and the minimum response time may be longer than the exposure needed.
- APR is another exposure system that allows selection of a specific body part and position, resulting in display of preprogrammed exposure factors. These may include AEC information.

- Exposure technique charts standardize the selection of exposure factors for the typical patient so that the quality of radiographic images is consistent.
- The variable kVp/fixed mAs technique chart is based on the concept that kVp can be increased as the anatomic part size increases. The baseline kVp is adjusted for changes in part thickness.
- The fixed kVp/variable mAs technique chart uses the concept of selecting an optimal kVp value that is required for the radiographic examination and adjusting the mAs for variations in part thickness.

REVIEW QUESTIONS

1. AEC devices work by measuring _____.
   A. radiation leaving the tube
   B. radiation that exits the patient
   C. radiation that is absorbed by the patient
   D. attenuation of primary radiation by the patient

2. How many detectors are typically found in an AEC system?
   A. One
   B. Two
   C. Three
   D. Four

3. Minimum response time refers to _____.
   A. the proper exposure time needed for an optimal exposure when an AEC device is used
   B. exposure time minus the amount of time the AEC detectors are measuring radiation
   C. the difference in exposure times between AEC systems and electronic timers
   D. the shortest exposure time possible when an AEC device is used

4. Which of the following statements about using AEC during digital imaging is true?
   A. Adjusting the mA value affects image brightness.
   B. Adjusting the kVp value affects image brightness.
   C. Adjusting the backup time affects image brightness.
   D. Adjusting the density controls affects the exposure to image receptor.

5. Which one of the following statements comparing ionization chamber AEC systems with phototimers is true?
   A. Ionization chamber systems are accurately called *phototimers*.
   B. Ionization chamber systems measure radiation before it interacts with the image receptor.
   C. Phototimers are more modern.
   D. Phototimers measure radiation before it interacts with the image receptor.

6. The purpose of the backup timer is to _____.
A. ensure a diagnostic exposure each time AEC is used
B. produce consistent levels of exposure on all radiographs
C. determine the exposure time that is used
D. limit unnecessary x-ray exposure

7. What happens if AEC is activated for a stretcher chest study?
A. An inappropriately short exposure occurs.
B. An inappropriately long exposure occurs.
C. An appropriate exposure probably occurs.
D. Underexposure of the radiograph occurs.

8. The purpose of anatomic programming is to _____.
A. present the radiographer with a preselected set of exposure factors
B. override AEC when the radiographer has made a mistake in its use
C. determine which AEC detectors should be used for a particular examination
D. prevent overexposure and underexposure of radiographs, which sometimes happen when AEC is used

9. Which statement concerning both AEC and APR is true?
A. The skilled use of both requires less knowledge of exposure factors on the part of the radiographer.
B. The use of both requires the radiographer to be less responsible for accurate centering of the anatomic part.
C. The individual judgment and discretion of the radiographer is still necessary when using these systems.
D. The tasks involved with practicing radiography generally are made more difficult with these systems.

10. When using AEC with digital imaging systems, assuming all other factors are correct, selecting the center chamber on a PA chest image results in _____.
A. decreased exposure in the lung area
B. increased exposure in the lung area
C. appropriate exposure in the lung area
D. increased quantum noise in the image

11. When using AEC with digital imaging systems, assuming all other factors are correct, selecting the minus 2 density on a PA chest image results in _____.
A. increased quantum noise
B. increased brightness in the lung area
C. appropriate brightness in the lung area
D. A and C

12. Using a film-screen system and AEC, a chest in the lateral position is imaged with 70 kVp instead of the typical 120 kVp. Compared with an optimal lateral chest image, this image would have _____.
    A. increased density
    B. decreased density
    C. increased contrast
    D. decreased contrast

13. What type of exposure technique system uses a fixed mAs regardless of part thickness?
    A. Fixed kVp
    B. Variable kVp
    C. Manual
    D. AEC

14. A primary goal of an exposure technique chart is to _____.
    A. extend the life of the x-ray tube
    B. improve the radiographer's accuracy
    C. produce quality images consistently
    D. increase the patient work flow

15. Which of the following is an important condition required for technique charts to be effective?
    A. Equipment must be calibrated to perform properly.
    B. One technique chart should be used for all radiographic units.
    C. All technologists should use the same mA setting.
    D. The chart should not be revised once it has been used.

Image Evaluation

OBJECTIVES

After completing this chapter, the reader will be able to perform the following:

1. Define all the key terms in this chapter.
2. State all the important relationships in this chapter.
3. Define the attributes of a good-quality radiographic image.
4. Identify exposure factors and their radiographic effect.
5. Identify factors that contribute to poor image quality.
6. Recognize common exposure indicator errors.
7. Identify factors that could contribute to quantum noise and artifacts.
8. Given a poor-quality image, identify the factors contributing to its effect.
9. Given exposure factors, explain their contribution to poor image quality.
10. Calculate exposure technique factors to improve image quality.

Previous chapters discussed how a radiographic image is formed; attributes describing the quality of the image; exposure technique factors; and methods of acquiring, processing, and displaying the image. The focus of this chapter is to apply the knowledge previously gained in evaluating image quality and develop problem-solving skills related to exposure technique factors. Criteria used for image evaluation or attributes of image quality are briefly reviewed. The remaining sections provide students the opportunity to evaluate image quality and problem solve to identify factors contributing to poor quality and strategies for improvement.

CRITERIA FOR IMAGE EVALUATION

A quality radiographic image accurately represents the anatomic area of interest, and its information is well visualized for diagnosis. The *visibility* of the anatomic structures and the *accuracy* of their structural lines recorded (sharpness) determine the overall quality of the radiographic image. Visibility of the recorded detail refers to the *brightness* or *density* of the image along with image contrast; the accuracy of the structural lines is achieved by maximizing the amount of *spatial resolution* or *recorded detail* and minimizing the amount of *distortion*. Visibility of the recorded detail is achieved by the proper balance of image brightness or density and contrast.

Brightness or Density

Brightness and *density* refer to the same image quality attribute but are defined differently. *Brightness* is defined as the amount of luminance (light emission) of a display monitor. *Density* is defined as the amount of overall blackness on the processed image. An area of increased brightness, if viewed on the computer monitor, shows decreased density on a film image. An area of decreased brightness visualized on a computer monitor has increased density on a film image.

A radiograph must have sufficient brightness or density to visualize the anatomic structures of interest (Figure 9-1). A radiograph that is too light has excessive brightness or insufficient density to visualize the structures of the anatomic part. Conversely, a radiograph that is too dark has insufficient brightness or excessive density, and the anatomic part cannot be well visualized (Figure 9-2). The radiographer must evaluate the overall brightness or density on the image to determine whether it is sufficient to visualize the anatomic area of interest. He or she then decides whether the radiograph is diagnostic or unacceptable.

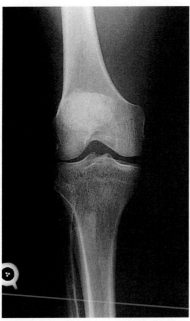

FIGURE 9-1 Radiograph demonstrating sufficient density.

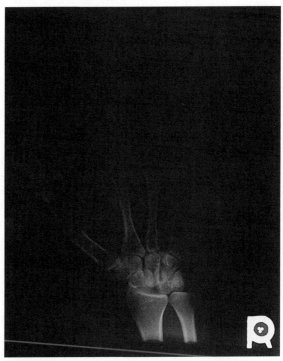

FIGURE 9-2 Radiograph demonstrating excessive density.

Contrast

In addition to sufficient brightness or density, the radiograph must exhibit differences in the adjacent brightness levels or densities in order to differentiate among the anatomic tissues. Because of these differences in brightness or density (i.e., contrast), the anatomic tissues are easily differentiated. Tissues that attenuate the x-ray beam similarly are more difficult to visualize because the brightness or densities are too alike to differentiate.

The level of radiographic contrast desired in an image is determined by the composition of the anatomic tissue to be radiographed and the amount of information needed to visualize the tissue for an accurate diagnosis. For example, the level of contrast desired in a chest image is different from the level of contrast required in an image of an extremity.

Radiographic contrast or *image contrast* is a term used in both digital and film-screen imaging to describe the variations in brightness and density. In digital imaging, the number of different shades of gray that can be stored and displayed by a computer system is termed *grayscale*. Because the digital image is processed and reconstructed in the computer as digital data, its contrast can be altered.

Radiographic film images are typically described by their scale of contrast or the range of densities visible. A film image with few densities but great differences among them is said to have high contrast. This is also described as *short-scale contrast*. A radiograph with a large number of densities but few differences among them is said to have low contrast. This is also described as *long-scale contrast*. Figure 9-3 shows an image with decreased contrast because of increased scatter radiation resulting in fog.

Spatial Resolution or Recorded Detail

The quality of a radiographic image depends on both the visibility and the accuracy of the anatomic structural lines recorded (sharpness). Adequate visualization of the anatomic area of interest (brightness/density and contrast) is just one component of radiographic quality. To produce a quality radiograph, the anatomic details must be recorded accurately and with the greatest amount of sharpness.

The ability of a radiographic image to demonstrate sharp lines determines the quality of the spatial resolution or recorded detail. The imaging process makes it impossible to produce a radiographic image without some degree of unsharpness. A radiographic image that has a greater amount of spatial resolution or recorded detail minimizes the amount of unsharpness of the anatomic structural lines. Figure 9-4 shows an image with decreased recorded detail because of motion unsharpness.

Distortion

Distortion results from the radiographic misrepresentation of either the size (magnification) or the shape of the anatomic part. When the part is distorted, spatial resolution or recorded detail is also reduced.

Radiographic images of objects are always magnified in relation to the true object size. The source-to-image receptor distance (SID) and object-to-image receptor distance (OID) play an important role in minimizing the amount of size distortion of the radiographic image.

When producing images of three-dimensional objects, some size distortion always occurs as a result of OID. The parts of the object that are farther away from the image receptor are represented radiographically with more size distortion than parts of the object that are closer to the image receptor. Even if the object is in close contact with the image receptor, some part of the object is still farther away from the image receptor than other parts of the object. SID also influences the total amount of magnification on the image. As SID increases, size distortion (magnification) decreases; as SID decreases, size distortion (magnification) increases.

In addition to size distortion, objects that are being imaged can be misrepresented radiographically by distortion of their shape. Shape distortion can appear in two different ways radiographically: elongation or foreshortening.

Shape distortion can occur from inaccurate central ray alignment of the tube, the part being radiographed, or the image receptor. Any misalignment of the central ray among these three factors—tube, part, or image receptor—alters the shape of the part recorded in the image (Figure 9-5).

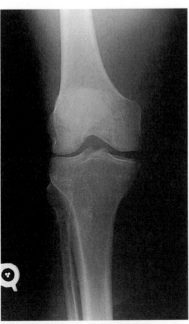

FIGURE 9-3 Radiograph demonstrating decreased contrast as a result of increased scatter radiation recorded as fog.

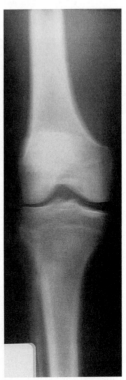

FIGURE 9-4 Radiograph demonstrating motion unsharpness.

The factors that determine the amount of image distortion are equally important for digital and film-screen imaging. Both SID and OID determine the amount of magnification of the anatomic structures on the image. In addition, improper alignment of the central ray, anatomic part, image receptor, or a combination of these components distorts the shape of the part, whether obtained with a digital or film-screen image receptor.

Quantum Noise

Image noise contributes no useful diagnostic information and serves only to detract from the quality of the image. Quantum noise is a concern in digital and film-screen imaging (quantum mottle) and is photon-dependent. Quantum noise is visible as brightness or density fluctuations on the image. The fewer the photons reaching the image receptor to form the image, the greater the quantum noise visible on the digital image.

Although quantum noise (mottle) can be a problem for both digital and film-screen imaging, it is more likely in digital imaging. As discussed previously, the digital computer system can adjust for low or high x-ray exposures during image acquisition. When the x-ray exposure to the image receptor is too low (decreased number of photons), computer processing alters the appearance of the digital image to make the brightness acceptable, but the image displays increased quantum noise (Figure 9-6).

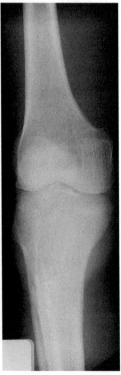

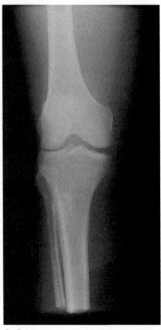

FIGURE 9-5 Radiograph demonstrating shape distortion.

FIGURE 9-6 Radiograph demonstrating increased quantum noise.

Exposure Indicator

An important feature of digital image processing is its ability to create an image with the appropriate amount of brightness (as described earlier) regardless of the exposure to the image receptor (within reason). As a result of the histogram analysis (described in Chapter 7), valuable information is provided to the radiographer regarding the exposure to the digital image receptor. The exposure indicator provides a numeric value indicating the level of radiation exposure to the digital image receptor. Box 9-1 lists common computed radiography (CR) exposure indicator values and their relationship to exposure intensity. Currently, exposure indicators are not standardized among vendors; however, the industry is working toward standardization of the exposure indicator.

In CR, the exposure indicator value represents the exposure level to the imaging plate, and the values are vendor-specific:

- Fuji and Konica use sensitivity (S) numbers, and the value is inversely related to the exposure to the plate. A 200 S number is the result of 1 mR of exposure to the plate. If the S number increases from 200 to 400, this would indicate a decrease in exposure to the IR by half. Conversely, a decrease in the S number from 200 to 100 would indicate an increase in exposure to the IR by a factor of 2, or doubling of the exposure.
- Carestream (Kodak) uses exposure index (EI) numbers; the value is directly related to the exposure to the plate, and the changes are logarithmic expressions. For example, a change in EI from 1500 to 1800, a difference of 300, is equal to a factor of 2 and represents twice as much exposure to the plate.
- Agfa uses log median (lgM) numbers; the value is directly related to exposure to the plate, and changes are also logarithmic expressions. For example, a change in lgM from 2.5 to 2.8, a change of 0.3, is equal to a factor of 2 and represents twice as much exposure to the IR.

Optimal ranges of the exposure indicator values are not standardized but are vendor-specific, and vary among the types of procedures, such as abdomen/chest versus extremity imaging.

Direct digital radiography imaging systems may also display an exposure indicator that varies according to the manufacturer's specifications. The radiographer should monitor the exposure indicator values as a guide for proper exposure techniques. If the exposure indicator value is within the acceptable range, adjustments can be made for contrast and brightness with postprocessing functions. However,

BOX 9-1	Computed Radiography Vendor-Specific Exposure Indicators			
		Value = 1 mR		
Vendor	**Exposure Indicator**	**exposure**	**2 × Exposure**	**½ Exposure**
Fuji and Konica	Sensitivity (S)	200	100	400
Carestream (Kodak)	Exposure index (EI)	2000	2300	1700
Agfa	Log median value (lgM)	2.5	2.8	2.2

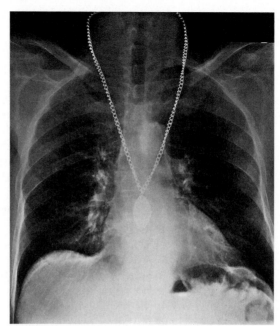

FIGURE 9-7 Radiograph demonstrating a patient artifact.

if the exposure is outside of the acceptable range, attempting to adjust the image data with postprocessing functions would not correct for improper receptor exposure and might result in noisy or suboptimal images that should not be submitted for interpretation. Overwriting the original image with a postprocessed replica at the radiographer's workstation may reduce the diagnostic and archival quality of the data and is not recommended.

For accurate computer processing of the latent image, the radiographer selects the appropriate anatomic part and projection. This step indicates to the computer which algorithm to use. If the radiographer selects a part other than the one imaged, a histogram analysis error may occur. In addition, any errors that occur, such as during data extraction from the IR or rescaling during computer processing, could affect the exposure indicator and provide a false value. It is important for radiographers not only to consider carefully the exposure indicator value but also to recognize its limitations.

Image Artifacts

An artifact is any unwanted image on a radiograph (Figure 9-7). Artifacts are detrimental to radiographs because they can make visibility of anatomy, a pathologic condition, or patient identification information difficult or impossible. They decrease the overall quality of the radiographic image. Various methods are used to classify artifacts. Generally, artifacts can be classified as *plus-density* and *minus-density*. Plus-density artifacts are greater in density than the area of the image immediately

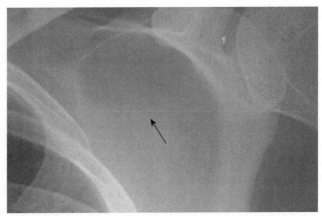

FIGURE 9-8 Radiograph demonstrating CR reader light guide artifact.

surrounding them. Minus-density artifacts are of less density than the area of the image immediately surrounding them.

Although the causes of some artifacts are the same regardless of the type of imaging system, others are specific to digital or film imaging. Artifacts from patient clothing and items imaged that are not a part of the area of interest are the same for both film and digital systems. The radiographer must be diligent in removing clothing or items that could obstruct visibility of the anatomic area of interest. Scatter radiation or fog and image noise have also been classified as radiographic artifacts because they add unwanted information to the image.

Artifacts specific to film-screen imaging are typically a result of film storage, handling, and chemical processing. Digital image artifacts can be a result of errors during extraction of the latent image (Figure 9-8) from the image receptor or performance of the electronic detectors.

EXPOSURE TECHNIQUE FACTORS

The following charts show the effect on image quality for changes in exposure technique factors. Because exposure technique factors affect the film image differently than the digital image, two charts are presented. Look for differences and similarities between exposure technique factors and their effect on digital and film image quality.

Image Quality

Film-Screen Image Receptors				
Factors	**Density**	**Contrast†**	**Recorded Detail**	**Distortion**
mAs				
• Increase	*Increase*	No effect	No effect	No effect
• Decrease	*Decrease*			
kVp				
• Increase	*Increase*	*Decrease*	No effect	No effect
• Decrease	*Decrease*	*Increase*		
OID				
• Increase	*Decrease*	*Increase**	*Decrease*	*Increase*
SID				
• Increase	*Decrease*	No effect	*Increase*	*Decrease*
• Decrease	*Increase*		*Decrease*	*Increase*
Focal Spot Size				
• Increase	No effect	No effect	*Decrease*	No effect
• Decrease			*Increase*	
Grid				
• Increase ratio	*Decrease*	*Increase*	No effect	No effect
• Decrease ratio	*Increase*	*Decrease*		
Beam Restriction				
• Increase	*Decrease*	*Increase*	No effect	No effect
• Decrease	*Increase*	*Decrease*		
Film-Screen Speed				
• Increase	*Increase*	No effect	*Decrease*	No effect
• Decrease	*Decrease*		*Increase*	
Patient Thickness				
• Increase	*Decrease*	*Decrease*	*Decrease*	*Increase*
• Decrease	*Increase*	*Increase*	*Increase*	*Decrease*
Patient Motion				
	No effect	No effect	*Decrease*	No effect
Central Ray				
• Increase angle	*Decrease*	No effect	*Decrease*	*Increase*

†Increase is higher contrast, and decrease is lower contrast.
*Increases (higher) contrast because of less scatter reaching image receptor; effect dependent on anatomic region, thickness, and amount of OID.

Digital Image Receptors				
Factors	**Brightness***	**Contrast*†**	**Spatial Resolution**	**Distortion**
mAs				
• Increase	No effect	No effect	No effect	No effect
• Decrease				
kVp				
• Increase	No effect	*Decrease*	No effect	No effect
• Decrease		*Increase*		
OID				
• Increase	No effect	*Increase‡*	*Decrease*	*Increase*
SID				
• Increase	No effect	No effect	*Increase*	*Decrease*
• Decrease			*Decrease*	*Increase*
Focal Spot Size				
• Increase	No effect	No effect	*Decrease*	No effect
• Decrease			*Increase*	
Grid				
• Increase ratio	No effect	*Increase*	No effect	No effect
• Decrease ratio		*Decrease*		
Beam Restriction				
• Increase	No effect	*Increase*	No effect	No effect
• Decrease		*Decrease*		
Patient Thickness				
• Increase	No effect	*Decrease*	*Decrease*	*Increase*
• Decrease		*Increase*	*Increase*	*Decrease*
Patient Motion				
	No effect	No effect	*Decrease*	No effect
Central Ray				
• Increase angle	No effect	No effect	*Decrease*	*Increase*

*Brightness and contrast can be adjusted by the computer.
†Increase is higher contrast, and decrease is lower contrast.
‡Increases (higher) contrast because of less scatter reaching image receptor; effect dependent on anatomic region, thickness, and amount of OID.

ACTIVITY 1

Image Quality
Digital

An optimal digital image of the hip was produced using the following exposure technique:

200 mA	12:1 grid ratio
50 ms	CR image receptor
70 kVp	8 × 12 collimation
40-inch SID	Patient thickness 10 cm
0.6 mm small focal spot	Minimal OID

Without compensation, the proposed changes are made one by one. On the following chart, indicate the effect, if any, each change has on the brightness, contrast, and spatial resolution of the radiographic image.

1. If the image brightness, contrast, or spatial resolution of the image is increased, mark a plus symbol (+) in the space provided.
2. If the image brightness, contrast, or spatial resolution of the image is decreased, mark a minus symbol (–) in the space provided.
3. If the image brightness, contrast, or spatial resolution of the image is unchanged, mark a 0 in the space provided.

Proposed individual change	Brightness	Contrast	Spatial Resolution
85 kVp			
1.25 mm focal spot size			
45" SID			
50 mA @ 0.20 s			
Patient thickness 6 cm			
Remove grid			
Increase OID 4"			
14 × 17 collimation			

ACTIVITY 2

Image Quality
Film

An optimal film radiograph of the pelvis was produced using the following exposure technique:

100 mA
0.5 s
70 kVp
40-inch SID
1.25 mm large focal spot
92° F development temperature
90-second processing time

12:1 grid ratio
400 speed F/S
14 × 17 collimation
Patient thickness 14 cm
Minimal OID

Without compensation, the proposed changes are made one by one. On the following chart, indicate the effect, if any, each change has on the density, contrast, and recorded detail of the radiographic image.
1. If the radiographic density, contrast, or recorded detail of the image is increased, mark a + in the space provided.
2. If the radiographic density, contrast, or recorded detail of the image is decreased, mark a – in the space provided.
3. If the radiographic density, contrast, or recorded detail of the image is unchanged, mark a 0 in the space provided.

Proposed Change	Density	Contrast	Recorded Detail
Increase SID to 48"			
Use 200 mAs			
Increase kVp to 80			
Film-screen relative speed 200			
Increase patient thickness to 18 cm			
10 × 12 collimation			
Change SID to 25"			
Use 200 mA @ ¼ s			
Development temperature decreased			
Patient moves during exposure			
17 × 17 collimation			
Angle tube 20 degrees			
Change to 8:1 grid ratio			
Use 50 mA station			
Use 0.6 mm focal spot size			
Increase OID 3"			

Activity 3

Image Quality Calculations
Mathematical Calculations

Exposure Technique Factor	Relationship Between Variables	Formula
mAs	↑ mA and ↓ second	mA × second = mAs
kVp 15% Rule	↑ kVp and ↓ mAs	kVp × 1.15 and mAs/2 kVp × .85 and mAs × 2
Inverse Square Law	↑ SID and ↓ Intensity	$\dfrac{\text{Intensity}_1 = (SID_2)^2}{\text{Intensity}_2 = (SID_1)^2}$
mAs/Distance Compensation Formula	↑ SID and ↑ mAs	$\dfrac{mAs_1 = (SID_1)^2}{mAs_2 = (SID_2)^2}$
Grid Conversion Factor No grid = 1 5:1 = 2 6:1 = 3 8:1 = 4 12:1 = 5 16:1 = 6	↑ Grid ratio and ↑ mAs	$\dfrac{mAs_1 = GCF_1}{mAs_2 = GCF_2}$
Patient Thickness	↑ Thickness and ↑ mAs	Every 4-5 cm change in thickness change mAs by a factor of 2
Film-screen Speed	↑ Speed (RS) and ↓ mAs	$\dfrac{mAs_1 = RS_2}{mAs_2 = RS_1}$
Magnification Factor	↑ OID and ↓ SID and ↑ mag Image size = Object size × MF	$MF = \dfrac{SID}{SOD}$ $\text{Object size} = \dfrac{\text{Image size}}{MF}$

Solve for the missing variable or calculate the new exposure factor to maintain exposure to the image receptor as in the initial exposure technique. Show all calculations.

mAs

mA = 100
time = 0.25 s
mAs =

mA =
time = 100 ms
mAs = 50

mA = 50
time =
mAs = 15

15% Rule

Initial kVp = 70
Initial mAs = 10
New kVp = 70 + 15% =
New mAs =

Initial kVp = 80
Initial mAs = 100
New kVp = 80 − 15% =
New mAs =

Initial kVp = 75
Initial mAs = 35
New kVp = 75 + 2(15%) =
New mAs =

mAs-Distance Conversions

Initial mA = 100
Initial SID = 40 inches
New SID = 72 inches
New mAs =

Initial time = 0.5 s
Initial SID = 60 inches
New SID = 25 inches
New mAs =

Initial mAs = 125
Initial SID = 56 inches
New SID = 40 inches
New mAs =

Grid Conversions

No grid, initial mAs = 10   12:1 grid, initial mAs = 50   5:1 grid, initial time = 0.05 s
Add 8:1 grid, new mAs =   6:1 grid, new mAs =   12:1 grid, new time =

Film-screen Speed (F/s Spd.)

Initial mAs = 25   Initial mAs = 10   Initial time = 0.25
Initial F/s Spd = 200   Initial F/s spd = 600   Initial F/s spd = 100
New F/s Spd = 400   New F/s Spd = 300   New F/s Spd = 50
New mAs =   New mAs =   New time =

Sample Activity

Image Quality Exposure Conversions

Calculate the new exposure factor to maintain a similar exposure to the image receptor as in the initial exposure technique. Show all calculations.

Initial Exposure Technique		New Exposure Technique
25 mAs		_____ mAs
65 kVp	TO	75 kVp
No grid		6:1 grid
40-inch SID		48-inch SID

Calculations:

a. *Increase from 65 to 75 kVp = 15% increase*

b. *Decrease mAs by ½ = 12.5 mAs*

c. *Add a 6:1 grid = increase mAs × 3 = 12.5 × 3 = 37.5 mAs*

d. *Increase SID from 40 inches to 48 inches =* $\dfrac{37.5}{X} = \dfrac{40^2}{48^2}$; *1600X = 86,400; X = 54 mAs*

e. *The new mAs to maintain a similar exposure to the image receptor as the initial technique is 54*

Activity 4

Image Quality Exposure Conversions

Initial Digital Exposure Technique		New Digital Exposure Technique
100 mAs		_____ mAs
80 kVp	TO	58 kVp
12:1 grid		No grid
56-inch SID		40-inch SID

Calculations:

Activity 5

Image Quality Exposure Conversions

Initial Film-Screen Exposure Technique
200 mA
0.05 s
65 kVp
6:1 grid
40-inch SID
400 F/S speed

TO

New Film-Screen Exposure Technique
____ mA
⅕ s
75 kVp
8:1 grid
56-inch SID
100 F/S speed

Calculations:

Image Evaluation

The ability to recognize exposure technique errors and their resultant effect on the radiographic image is an important problem-solving skill. The following exercises provide you an opportunity to apply the knowledge gained from previous chapters in identifying causes of poor-quality images for both digital and film-screen image receptors.

Activity 6

Image Evaluation
Matching:

One of the four computed radiography (CR) images is good quality, whereas the others are results of errors. Match each image with its corresponding statement:

1. Good-quality lateral skull image   _____

A.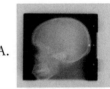

2. Imaging plate placed upside down   _____

B.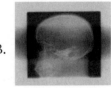

3. Grid placed upside down on imaging plate   _____

C.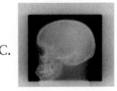

4. Grid removed with mAs adjustment   _____

D.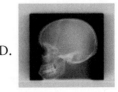

Activity 7

Image Evaluation
Multiple Choice:

Select the most likely exposure technique error responsible for the poor-quality image, and write your answer in the middle column:

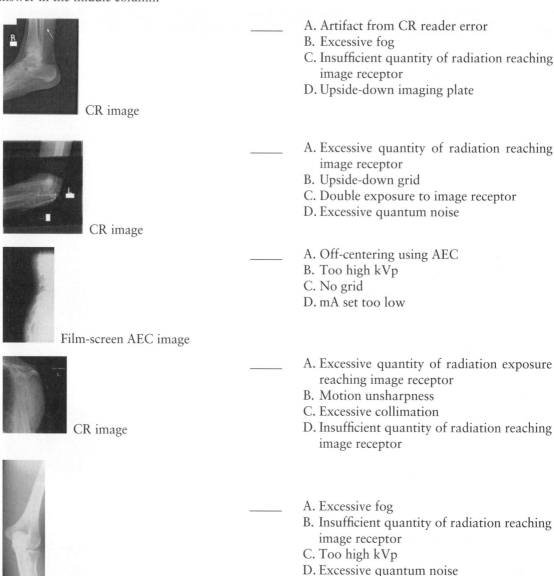

CR image

_____ A. Artifact from CR reader error
B. Excessive fog
C. Insufficient quantity of radiation reaching image receptor
D. Upside-down imaging plate

CR image

_____ A. Excessive quantity of radiation reaching image receptor
B. Upside-down grid
C. Double exposure to image receptor
D. Excessive quantum noise

Film-screen AEC image

_____ A. Off-centering using AEC
B. Too high kVp
C. No grid
D. mA set too low

CR image

_____ A. Excessive quantity of radiation exposure reaching image receptor
B. Motion unsharpness
C. Excessive collimation
D. Insufficient quantity of radiation reaching image receptor

Film-screen image

_____ A. Excessive fog
B. Insufficient quantity of radiation reaching image receptor
C. Too high kVp
D. Excessive quantum noise

Image Analysis

The ability to evaluate image quality and problem solve for improvement involves several skills. Knowledge of how exposure factors affect image quality individually and in combination is the first step to successful problem solving. In addition, the ability to calculate exposure factor changes accurately is necessary to improve image quality.

The following image quality exercises are opportunities to develop problem-solving skills by applying the knowledge learned from the previous chapters.

Sample Activity

Image Analysis
Film Image Evaluation: Image Quality Analysis

Radiograph 1
kVp = 75
F/S speed = 400
mAs = 10
Grid ratio = 12:1
SID = 40 inches
Focal spot = small
Optical density = 1.35

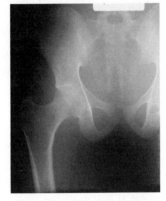

Radiograph 2
kVp = 86
F/S speed = 400
mAs = 2.5
Table top = no grid
SID = 45 inches
Focal spot = large
Optical density = 2.03

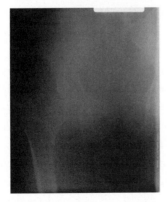

Evaluation:

➤ Visually compare Radiograph 1 and Radiograph 2, and comment on the quality of the density and contrast of Radiograph 2. State whether Radiograph 2 needs to be repeated and explain why.

➤ Evaluate each change in exposure factor, and discuss its appropriateness and how it affected the density or contrast, or both, of the image and patient exposure.

➤ Calculate the appropriate mAs value for each of the cumulative changes to determine why Radiograph 2 displays its level of density or contrast, or both.

➤ Identify the correct mAs value that should have been used for each of the exposure factor changes to maintain density as in Radiograph 1. Last, compare the actual mAs used in Radiograph 2 with the calculated mAs value that was needed to maintain density and contrast.

Calculate and Respond:

The kVp increased by 15% in Radiograph 2 and requires a decrease in mAs by a factor of 2:

$$\frac{10 \text{ mAs}}{2} = 5 \text{ mAs}$$

The grid was removed, and the mAs needs to decrease:

$$\frac{5 \text{ mAs}}{X} = \frac{5}{1}; \ 5X = 5; \ X = 1 \text{ mAs}$$

The SID was increased to 45 inches in Radiograph 2 and requires an increase in mAs:

$$\frac{1 \text{ mAs}}{X} = \frac{(40)^2}{(45)^2}; \ 1600X = 2,025; \ X = 1.27 \text{ mAs}$$

➤ In comparing Radiograph 2 with Radiograph 1, there is increased density on Radiograph 2. In the area of interest, Radiograph 2 had an OD of 2.03, which is at the high end of the diagnostic range. This image would be considered unacceptable and needs to be repeated because visibility of the area of interest is too low for diagnosis.

➤ Radiograph 2 has an increase in kVp of 15% (75 to 86), which would increase the density and decrease contrast; therefore, a decrease in mAs by a factor of 2 would be needed to compensate. The mAs would need to be 5 instead of 10. A higher kVp in the hip region is not typically used with film because it would decrease contrast and increase the proportion of scatter reaching the film. However, using a higher kVp requires the mAs to be decreased, and this would reduce patient exposure.

➤ The grid was removed, which would decrease contrast because more scatter radiation reached the film and density would be increased. Radiographic contrast would be decreased because of the excessive scatter reaching the film. The mAs would need to be decreased to compensate and should have been 1 instead of 5. A grid should be used with the hip because significant amounts of scatter will be produced and reach the film. However, removing the grid requires a decrease in mAs, and this would reduce patient exposure.

➤ The SID was increased to 45 inches in Radiograph 2 which would reduce the exposure to the image receptor and result in decreased density. The mAs would need to be increased from 1 to 1.27 mAs. In addition to reducing the exposure to the image receptor, increasing the SID will decrease magnification of the anatomic part and increase recorded detail.

➤ After all the changes in exposure factors, Radiograph 2 is too dark because 2.5 mAs was used instead of 1.27 mAs. In addition, the contrast was decreased by the increase in kVp and grid removal.

ACTIVITY 8

Image Analysis
Film Image Evaluation: Image Quality Analysis

Radiograph 1
kVp = 70
F/S speed = 400
mAs = 4
Grid ratio = 12:1
SID = 40 inches
Focal spot = small
Optical density = 1.04

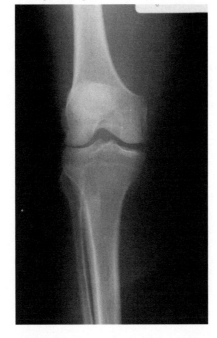

Radiograph 2
kVp = 60
F/S speed = 100
mAs = 6.3
Grid ratio = 6:1
SID = 34 inches
Focal spot = large
Optical density = 0.30

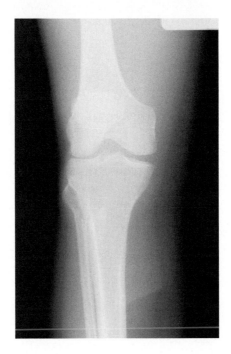

Evaluation:

➤ *Visually compare Radiograph 1 and Radiograph 2, and comment on the quality of the density, contrast, and sharpness of Radiograph 2. State whether Radiograph 2 needs to be repeated and explain why.*

➤ *Evaluate each change in exposure factor, and discuss its appropriateness and how it affected the density, contrast, or sharpness (even if not apparent) of the image and patient exposure.*

➤ *Calculate the appropriate mAs value for each of the cumulative changes to determine why Radiograph 2 displays its level of density, contrast, and sharpness.*

➤ *Identify the correct mAs value that should have been used for each of the exposure factor changes in order to maintain density as in Radiograph 1. Last, compare the actual mAs used in Radiograph 2 with the calculated mAs value that was needed to maintain density and contrast. In addition, make other exposure factor recommendations to improve the quality of the image.*

Calculate and Respond:

ACTIVITY 9

Image Analysis

Computed Radiography Image Evaluation (Recommended S number Between 100 and 300)

Radiograph 1

kVp = 81
mAs = 5
Focal spot = small
Grid ratio = 12:1
SID = 40 inches
Central ray perpendicular
S number = 156

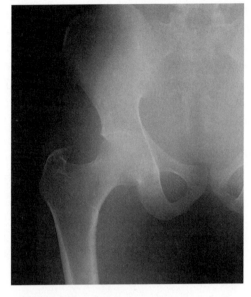

Radiograph 2

kVp = 59
mAs = 1.1
Focal spot = large
Table top = no grid
SID = 30 inches
Central ray angled 20 degrees caudad
S number = 620

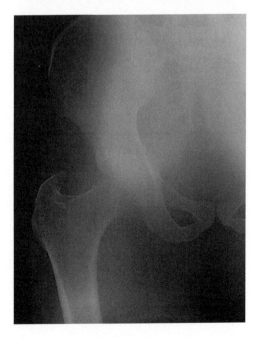

Evaluation:

➤ Visually compare Radiograph 1 and Radiograph 2, and comment on the quality of the contrast and spatial resolution of Radiograph 2. State whether Radiograph 2 should be repeated and explain why.

➤ Evaluate each change in exposure factor, and discuss its appropriateness and how it affected the exposure to the image receptor, contrast or spatial resolution or both (even if not apparent) of the image, and patient exposure.

➤ Calculate the appropriate mAs value for each of the cumulative changes to determine why Radiograph 2 displays its level of contrast, spatial resolution, and S number.

➤ Identify the correct mAs value that should have been used for each of the exposure factor changes in order to maintain the quality as in Radiograph 1. Last, compare the actual mAs used in Radiograph 2 with the calculated mAs value that was needed to maintain sufficient exposure to the image receptor. In addition, make other exposure factor recommendations to improve the quality of the image.

Calculate and Respond:

CHAPTER SUMMARY

- The visibility of the anatomic structures and the accuracy of their structural lines recorded (sharpness) determine the overall quality of the radiographic image.
- *Visibility* of the recorded detail refers to the *brightness* or *density* of the image along with image contrast; the accuracy of the structural lines is achieved by maximizing the amount of *spatial resolution* or *recorded detail* and minimizing the amount of *distortion*.
- *Brightness* and *density* refer to the same image quality attribute but are defined differently. *Brightness* is defined as the amount of luminance (light emission) of a display monitor. *Density* is defined as the amount of overall blackness on the processed image.
- An area of increased brightness, if viewed on the computer monitor, shows decreased density on a film image. An area of decreased brightness visualized on a computer monitor has increased density on a film image.
- In addition to sufficient brightness or density, the radiograph must exhibit differences in the adjacent brightness levels or densities in order to differentiate among the anatomic tissues.
- In digital imaging, the number of different shades of gray that can be stored and displayed by a computer system is termed *grayscale*. Because the digital image is processed and reconstructed in the computer as digital data, its contrast can be altered.
- A film image with few densities but many differences among them is said to have high contrast. A radiograph with numerous densities but few differences among them is said to have low contrast.
- A radiographic image that has a greater amount of spatial resolution or recorded detail minimizes the amount of unsharpness of the anatomic structural lines.
- Distortion results from the radiographic misrepresentation of either the size (magnification) or the shape of the anatomic part. When the part is distorted, spatial resolution or recorded detail is also reduced.
- Quantum noise (mottle) is visible as brightness or density fluctuations on the image. The fewer the photons reaching the image receptor to form the image, the greater the quantum noise visible on the digital image.
- The exposure indicator provides a numeric value indicating the level of radiation exposure to the digital image receptor.
- Artifacts are detrimental to radiographs because they can make visibility of anatomy, a pathologic condition, or patient identification information difficult or impossible.
- It is important for the radiographer to comprehend how exposure technique variables affect the radiation exposure to the image receptor and their individual and combined effect on the quality of the digital and film-screen image.

REVIEW QUESTIONS

1. *Visibility* of the recorded detail refers to what image quality attribute?
   A. Distortion
   B. Spatial resolution
   C. Brightness
   D. A and B

2. *Accuracy* of the structural lines refers to what image quality attribute?
   A. Distortion
   B. Spatial resolution
   C. Brightness
   D. A and B

3. How would a film radiograph with excessive density be described when viewed on a display monitor?
   A. Insufficient brightness
   B. Increased contrast
   C. Decreased spatial resolution
   D. Excessive brightness

4. Excessive radiation exposure to the image receptor would result in a digital image displayed with _____.
   A. excessive brightness
   B. acceptable brightness
   C. insufficient brightness
   D. increased quantum noise

5. Density fluctuations on a radiographic image could be a result of _____.
   A. artifacts
   B. distortion
   C. quantum mottle
   D. excessive exposure

6. Without exposure technique compensation, removing a grid would result in the film image displaying _____.
   (1) increased density
   (2) decreased recorded detail
   (3) decreased contrast
   A. 1 and 2 only
   B. 1 and 3 only
   C. 2 and 3 only
   D. 1, 2, and 3

7. Without exposure technique compensation, increasing the film-screen speed would result in the film image displaying _____.
   (1) increased density
   (2) decreased recorded detail
   (3) decreased contrast
   A. 1 and 2 only
   B. 1 and 3 only
   C. 2 and 3 only
   D. 1, 2, and 3

8. Without exposure technique compensation, increasing the SID would result in the digital image displaying:
   (1) decreased brightness
   (2) increased spatial resolution
   (3) decreased distortion
   A. 1 and 2 only
   B. 1 and 3 only
   C. 2 and 3 only
   D. 1, 2, and 3

9. The initial exposure technique for a good-quality radiograph is 15 mAs at 70 kVp, 40-inch (100-cm) SID, using 8:1 grid ratio. If the grid is removed and the SID reduced to 36 inches (90 cm), which of the following exposure techniques would best maintain the exposure to the image receptor?
   A. 3 mAs at 70 kVp
   B. 4.6 mAs at 70 kVp
   C. 7.5 mAs at 80 kVp
   D. 13.5 mAs at 70 kVp

10. Given an adequate exposure indicator value, a digital image of the hip is displayed with increased fog after the use of 20 mAs at 80 kVp without a grid. Which of the following exposure techniques would be best to improve the quality of the digital image?
    A. 40 mAs at 80 kVp, without a grid
    B. 10 mAs at 68 kVp, without a grid
    C. 20 mAs at 80 kVp and add a 12:1 ratio grid
    D. 50 mAs at 92 kVp and add a 12:1 ratio grid

Dynamic Imaging: Fluoroscopy

OBJECTIVES

After completing this chapter, the reader will be able to perform the following:

1. Define all the key terms in this chapter.
2. State all the important relationships in this chapter.
3. Differentiate between fluoroscopic and radiographic imaging.
4. Recognize the unique features of an image-intensified fluoroscopic unit and explain how the image is created and viewed.
5. Explain the process of brightness gain and conversion factor during image intensification.
6. Define automatic brightness control and state its function.
7. Explain how using the magnification mode affects image quality and patient exposure.
8. Identify common types of image degradation resulting from image-intensified fluoroscopy.
9. Differentiate among the types of television cameras used to convert the output phosphor image for viewing on a television monitor.
10. List the types of recording devices available for image-intensified fluoroscopy.
11. Compare and contrast features of image-intensified units from digital fluoroscopic units.
12. State radiation safety procedures used to reduce exposure to the patient and personnel.
13. Recognize the need for quality control on fluoroscopic units.

KEY TERMS

analog-to-digital converter (ADC)
automatic brightness control (ABC)
brightness gain
camera tube

charge-coupled device (CCD)
conversion factor
electrostatic focusing lenses
fluoroscopy
flux gain
image intensification

input phosphor
magnification mode
minification gain
output phosphor
photocathode
spatial resolution

The previous chapters discussed radiographic imaging to produce static radiographs of anatomic tissues. Imaging of the functioning or motion (dynamic) of anatomic structures is also needed for evaluation and is accomplished by fluoroscopy. For example, in order to visualize the stomach emptying its contents into the small bowel, images must be created in a continuous form for accurate evaluation of functioning. Most fluoroscopic procedures also require the use of contrast media to visualize internal structures and their functioning. This chapter discusses the components of fluoroscopic units, viewing and recording systems, and the digital fluoroscopy process in use today.

FLUOROSCOPY

Fluoroscopy allows imaging of the movement of internal structures. It differs from radiographic imaging by its use of a continuous beam of x-rays to create images of moving internal structures that can be viewed on a monitor. Internal structures, such as the vascular or gastrointestinal systems, can be visualized in their normal state of motion with the aid of special liquid or gas substances (contrast media) that are either injected or instilled.

In conventional fluoroscopy, the milliamperage (mA) used during imaging is considerably lower (0.5 to 5 mA) than radiographic mode, which is operated at a higher mA (100 to 1200 mA). A low mA provides for the increased time the fluoroscope is operated. Because the time of exposure is lengthened, the control panel includes a timer that buzzes audibly when 5 minutes of x-ray fluoroscopic time has been used. Another important feature of a fluoroscopic unit is the deadman switch. The continuous x-ray beam is activated by either a hand switch on the unit or a foot pedal that must be continuously depressed for the x-rays to be produced. Releasing the pressure applied to the pedal or switch terminates the radiation exposure.

Image Intensification

Image intensification (Figure 10-1) is the process in which the exit radiation from the anatomic area of interest interacts with the **input phosphor** (a light-emitting material, such as cesium iodide), for conversion to visible light. The light intensities are equal to the intensities of the exit radiation and are converted to electrons by a **photocathode** (photoemission). The electrons are focused by **electrostatic focusing lenses** and accelerated toward an anode to strike the **output phosphor** (coated with light-emitting crystals, such as zinc cadmium sulfide) and create a brighter image.

> **Important Relationship**
> *Image-Intensified Fluoroscopy*
> Dynamic imaging of internal anatomic structures can be accomplished with the use of an image intensifier. The exit radiation is absorbed by the input phosphor, converted to electrons, sent to the output phosphor, released as visible light, and converted to an electronic video signal for transmission to the television monitor.

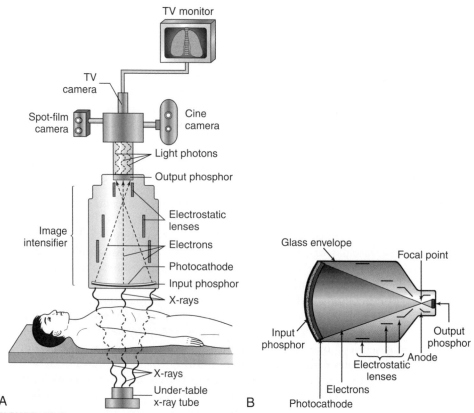

FIGURE 10-1 A, Fluoroscopic system used for dynamic imaging of internal structures. **B,** Major components of an image intensifier.

The image light intensities from the output phosphor are converted to an electronic video signal and sent to a television monitor for viewing. Figure 10-2 is an example of a typical radiographic and image-intensified fluoroscopic unit. Additional filming devices such as spot film or cine (movie film) can be attached to the fluoroscopic system to create permanent radiographic images of specific areas of interest.

Brightness Gain. A brighter image is a result of the high-energy electrons striking a small-output phosphor. Accelerating the electrons increases the light intensities at the output phosphor (**flux gain**). The reduction in size of the output phosphor image compared with the input phosphor image also increases the light intensities (**minification gain**). **Brightness gain** is the product of both flux gain and minification gain and results in a brighter image on the output phosphor.

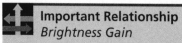

Important Relationship
Brightness Gain

A brighter image is created on the output phosphor when the accelerated electrons strike a smaller output phosphor.

Although the term *brightness gain* continues to be used, it is now common practice to express this increase in brightness with the term *conversion factor*. **Conversion factor** is an expression of the luminance at the output phosphor divided by the input exposure rate, and its unit of measure is the candela per square meter per milliroentgen per second ($cd/m^2/mR/s$). The numeric conversion factor value is roughly equal to 1% of the brightness gain value. For example, a brightness gain of 20,000 would have a conversion factor of 200. The higher the conversion factor or brightness gain value, the greater the efficiency of the image intensifier. See Box 10-1 for brightness gain and conversion factor formulas.

Automatic Brightness Control

The radiographer must also be familiar with **automatic brightness control (ABC)**, a function of the fluoroscopic unit that maintains the overall appearance of the fluoroscopic image (contrast and density) by automatically adjusting the kilovoltage peak (kVp), mA, or both. ABC generally operates by monitoring the current through the image intensifier or the output phosphor intensity and adjusting the exposure factor

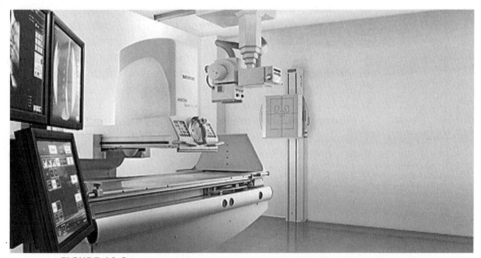

FIGURE 10-2 A typical radiographic and image-intensified fluoroscopic unit.

BOX 10-1 | **Brightness Gain and Conversion Factor Formulas**

$$\text{Brightness gain} = \text{Minification gain} \times \text{Flux gain}$$

$$\text{Flux gain} = \frac{\text{number of output light photons}}{\text{number of input x-ray photons}}$$

$$\text{Minification gain} = \left(\frac{d_i}{d_o}\right)^2$$

$$\text{Conversion factor} = \frac{\text{output phosphor illumination (cd/m}^2\text{)}}{\text{input exposure rate (mR/s)}}$$

if the monitored value falls below preset levels. The fluoroscopic unit allows the operator to select a desired brightness level, and this level is subsequently maintained by ABC. ABC is a little slow in its response to changes in patient tissue thickness and tissue density as the fluoroscopy tower is moved about over the patient; this is visible to the radiographer as a lag in the image brightness on the monitor as the tower is moved.

Magnification Mode

Another function of some image intensifiers is multifield mode or magnification mode. Most image intensifiers in use today have this capability. When operated in **magnification mode,** the voltage to the electrostatic focusing lenses is increased. This increase tightens the diameter of the electron stream, and the focal point is shifted farther from the output phosphor (Figure 10-3). The effect is that only the electrons from the center area of the input phosphor interact with the output phosphor and contribute to the image, giving the appearance of magnification. For example, a 30/23/15–cm trifocus image intensifier can be operated in any of those three modes. When operated in the 23-cm mode, only the electrons from the center 23 cm of the input phosphor interact with the output phosphor; the electrons about the periphery miss and do not contribute to the image. The same is true of the 15-cm mode. Selecting magnification mode automatically adjusts x-ray beam collimation to match the displayed tissue image and avoids irradiating tissue that does not appear in the image. The degree of magnification (magnification factor [MF]) may be found by dividing the full-size input diameter by the selected input diameter. For example: $MF = 30 \div 15 = 2\times$ magnification.

This magnification improves the operator's ability to see small structures (spatial resolution, discussed shortly) but at the expense of increasing patient dose. Remnant x-ray photons are converted to light and then to electrons and are focused on the

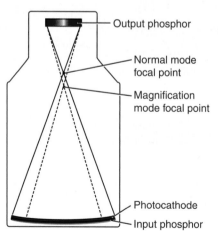

FIGURE 10-3 Magnification mode. When the image intensifier is operated in magnification mode, the voltage to the electrostatic focusing lenses is increased. This increase tightens the diameter of the electron stream, and the focal point is shifted farther from the output phosphor, resulting in a magnified image.

output phosphor. If fewer electrons are incident on the output phosphor, the output intensity decreases. To compensate, more x-ray photons are needed at the beginning of the process to produce more light, resulting in more electrons at the input end of the image intensifier. ABC automatically increases x-ray exposure to achieve this. Again, with an increase in x-rays used comes an increase in patient dose.

Important Relationship
Magnification Mode and Patient Dose
Operating the image intensifier in one of the magnification modes increases the operator's ability to see small structures but at the price of increasing radiation dose to the patient.

Magnification modes improve **spatial resolution,** which refers to the smallest structure that may be detected in an image. Spatial resolution is measured in line pairs per millimeter (Lp/mm), and typical fluoroscopic systems have spatial resolution capabilities of 4 to 6 Lp/mm but depend greatly on the rest of the imaging chain (i.e., the viewing and recording systems).

Distortion is also an issue with image-intensified fluoroscopy. In radiography, distortion is a misrepresentation of the true size or shape of an object. In the case of fluoroscopy, shape distortion can be a problem. In fluoroscopy, distortion is a result of inaccurate control or focusing of the electrons released at the periphery of the photocathode and the curved shape of the photocathode. The combined result is an unequal magnification (distortion) of the image, creating what is called a "pincushion appearance" (Figure 10-4). This problem also causes a loss of brightness around the periphery of the image, which is referred to as *vignetting.*

One last factor to consider with image intensifiers is noise. Image noise results when insufficient information is present to create the image. In the case of fluoroscopy, this lack of image-forming information ultimately goes back to an insufficient quantity of x-rays. If too few x-rays exit the patient and expose the input phosphor, not enough light is produced, which decreases the number of electrons released by the photocathode to interact with the output phosphor. A "grainy" or

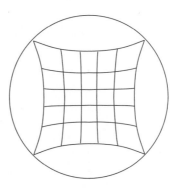

Image displaying
"pincushion" distortion

FIGURE 10-4 Pincushion distortion. Appearance of the pincushion effect. The circle represents the television monitor display, and the grid represents the effect on the image.

"noisy" image results (Figure 10-5). Although other factors in the fluoroscopic chain may contribute to noise, the solution generally comes back to increasing the mA (quantity of radiation). See Box 10-2 for common quality control tests specific to fluoroscopic equipment.

Viewing Systems

The original image intensifiers produced an image that was viewed using a mirror optics system—something akin to a sophisticated way of looking at the output phosphor with a "rearview mirror." Conventionally, the viewing system is now a closed-circuit television monitor system. To view the image from the output phosphor on a television monitor, it must first be converted to an electrical signal (often referred to as the *video signal*) by the television camera. Two devices are commonly used today to accomplish this: the camera tube and the charge-coupled device (CCD). The camera tube and CCD differ in their size and the readout process.

Television Cameras. Television cameras used in order to display the fluoroscopic image include the older camera tube (vidicon/Plumbicon) and the newer charge-coupled device (CCD). The **camera tube** has a vacuum tube approximately 15 cm (6 inches) in length that encloses an electron gun and a photoconductive target assembly (Figure 10-6). The diameter of the tube is the same size as the output phosphor. The light from the output phosphor arrives at the target assembly either by fiberoptics or by a lens system. A steady stream of electrons from the electron gun

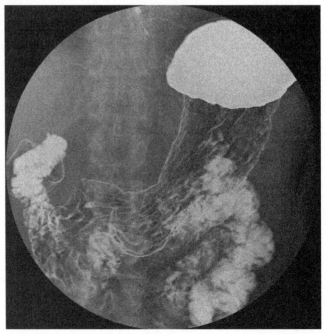

FIGURE 10-5 Quantum noise. If too few x-rays exit the patient and expose the input phosphor, not enough light is produced, which decreases the number of electrons released by the photocathode to interact with the output phosphor. A "grainy" or "noisy" image results.

BOX 10-2 | **Fluoroscopic Equipment Inspection Checklist**

Inspect:	Ensure that:
Bucky slot cover	When the Bucky is parked at the foot of the table, the metal cover should expand and cover the entire opening.
Protective curtain	The curtain should be in good condition and move freely into place when the tower is moved to the operating position.
Tower—locks, power assist, control panel	The electromagnetic locks are in good working order, the power assist moves the tower about easily in all directions, and all control panel indicator lights are operational.
Exposure switch (deadman switch)	The switch is not sticking and operates the x-ray tube only while in the depressed position. (Also test the switch with the tower in the park position; it should not activate the x-ray tube while parked.)
Collimator shutters	In the fully open position, the shutters should restrict the beam to the size of the input phosphor and be accurate to within ±3%.
Fluoroscopic timer	The timer should buzz audibly after 5 minutes of fluoroscopic "beam-on" time.
Monitor brightness	While exposing a penetrometer through a fluoroscopic phantom, the monitor image is adjusted to display as many of the penetrometer steps as possible.
Table tilt motion	The table tilts smoothly to its limit in both directions, and the angulation indicator is operational.

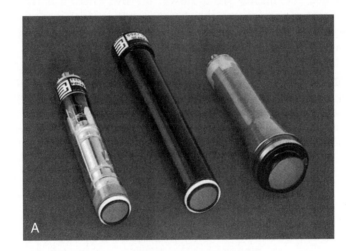

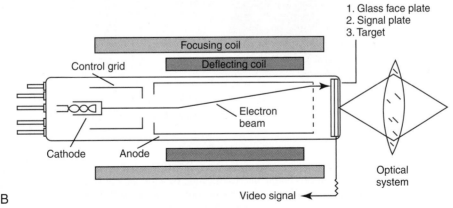

FIGURE 10-6 A, Vidicon-type camera tube. B, The vidicon tube has a vacuum tube that encloses an electron gun and a photoconductive target assembly. The electrical signal leaving the camera tube varies in strength proportionally based on the varying brightness of the image being scanned.

scans the target assembly very quickly, from left to right and top to bottom (raster pattern). As the stream of electrons bombard the target, anywhere there is light intensity from the output phosphor image there will be an electrical signal leaving the tube. A brighter or higher light intensity that is scanned results in the electrical signal leaving the camera tube with a higher strength. The darker or lower the light intensities scanned, the lower the strength of the electrical signal. The electrical signal leaving the camera tube varies in strength proportionally based on the varying brightness of the image being scanned. This electrical (video) signal goes to the television monitor to complete the display process.

The **charge-coupled device (CCD)** is a light-sensitive semiconducting device that generates an electrical charge when stimulated by light and stores this charge in a capacitor. The charge is proportional to the light intensity and is stored in rows of pixels. The CCD is a series of semiconductor capacitors, with each capacitor representing a pixel. Each pixel is composed of photosensitive material that dislodges electrons when stimulated by light photons. To digitize the charge from this device, the electrodes between each pixel, called *row gates,* are charged in sequence, moving the signal down the row where it is transferred into a capacitor. From the capacitors, the charge is sent as an electronic signal to the television monitor. In this way, each pixel is "read" individually and sent to the television monitor (Figure 10-7).

Compared with the vidicon-type camera tube, the CCD is read out by the charge in each pixel, whereas the vidicon is read out by an electronic beam. CCD TV cameras have some advantages over the camera tubes in that they are more sensitive to a wider range of light intensities and no geometric distortions of the display fluoroscopic image. The CCD is smaller in size than the vidicon camera tube and works well in digital imaging.

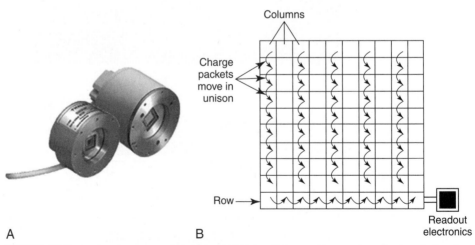

A   B

FIGURE 10-7 **A,** The charge-coupled device (CCD) is a light-sensitive semiconducting device that generates an electrical charge when stimulated by light and stores this charge in a capacitor. **B,** To digitize the charge from the CCD, the electrodes between each pixel, called *row gates,* are charged in sequence, moving the signal down the row where it is transferred into a capacitor. From the capacitors, the charge is sent as an electronic signal to the television monitor.

Coupling of Devices. As mentioned earlier, the camera tube or CCD may be coupled to the output phosphor of the image intensifier by either a fiberoptic bundle or an optical lens system. The fiberoptic bundle is simply a bundle of very thin optical glass filaments. This system is very durable and simple in design but does not allow for spot filming.

The optical lens system is a series of optical lenses that focus the image from the output phosphor on the television camera (camera tube or CCD). When spot filming is desired, a beam-splitting mirror (a partially silvered mirror that allows some light to pass through and reflects some in a new direction) is moved into the path of the output image and diverts some of the light to the desired spot-filming device (e.g., photospot or cine camera) (Figure 10-1). This system, although allowing for spot filming of this type, is more susceptible to rough handling, which may cause maladjustment of the mirror and lenses and result in a blurred image.

Television Monitor. The varying electrical (video) signals reach the television display monitor (cathode ray tube [CRT]) almost instantaneously. The CRT (Figure 10-8) includes an electron gun that scans the phosphor layer found on the inside of the glass front of the monitor, again in the raster pattern. As the video signal increases and decreases, so does the amount of electrons emitted from the electron gun. The greater the number of electrons leaving the gun, the brighter the fluorescence of the phosphor, resulting in a bright spot on the display monitor. The lower the video signal, the fewer electrons emitted from the gun, and the lower the brightness of the displayed image.

In essence, the television monitor is reconstructing the image from the output phosphor as a visible image. The image is created on the fluorescent screen one line at a time starting in the upper left-hand corner and moving to the right (active trace).

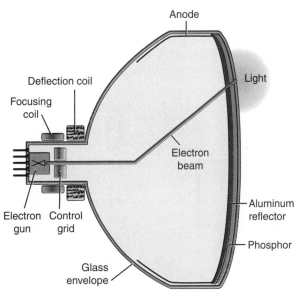

FIGURE 10-8 CRT television monitor. The television monitor reconstructs the image from the output phosphor as a visible image. The CRT includes an electron gun that scans the phosphor layer found on the inside of the glass front of the monitor in a raster pattern.

It then blanks (turns off) and returns to the left side (horizontal retrace). This process continues to the bottom of the screen. It then returns to the top (vertical retrace) and begins again by placing a line between each of the previous ones. This action creates a television frame. Typical television monitors are called *525-line systems* because the traces create a 525-line frame. High-resolution monitors have 1024 lines per frame. However, the monitor continues to be the weak link in terms of resolution of the fluoroscopic chain. The image intensifier is capable of resolving approximately 5 Lp/mm, whereas the monitor can display only 1 to 2 Lp/mm.

> **Important Relationship**
> *Coupling Systems and the Television Monitor*
> The camera tube and CCD are devices that couple the image intensifier to the television monitor to convert the image from the output phosphor to an electronic (video) signal that can be reconstructed on the television monitor.

Recording Systems

Cassette spot filming has been a standard of conventional fluoroscopic imaging for many years (Figure 10-9). This is a static imaging process in which a standard radiographic cassette is used to obtain an image. With this system, the cassette is loaded into the lower part of the fluoroscopic tower and "parked" in a protective envelope in the back. When the spot-film exposure button is pressed, the cassette is moved into position between the patient and image intensifier, and the machine shifts from fluoroscopic to radiographic mode and exposes the film. In the shift to radiographic mode, the mA increases from one of the 0.5 to 5 mA fluoroscopic modes to one of the 100 to 1200 mA radiographic modes. Because this method of imaging uses radiographic mode, it uses a much higher radiation dose to the patient than the other methods. As an alternative to exposing the entire film, the tower is generally equipped with a series of masking shutters that can "divide" the cassette and allow for numerous exposures on one cassette, such as two exposures on one cassette, four

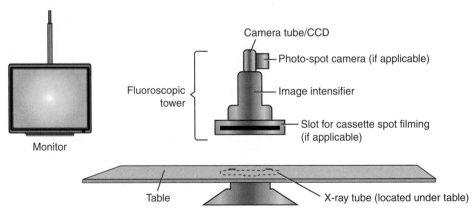

FIGURE 10-9 A typical image intensified fluoroscopic unit showing two types of recording systems, cassette spot filming and photo-spot camera.

on one, and six on one. In each setting, the image is smaller and organized as one of multiple images on one film.

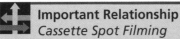
Important Relationship
Cassette Spot Filming
Cassette spot-film devices are one means of recording static images during a fluoroscopic examination. The unit shifts to radiographic mode (using a higher mA), and the radiation dose to the patient is much higher than in fluoroscopic mode.

Film cameras (sometimes called *photo-spot cameras*) have also been a mainstay of conventional fluoroscopy. Refer back to Figure 10-9. They most commonly use 105-mm "chip" film or 70-mm roll film. The photo-spot camera is also a static imaging system that is used with an optical lens system incorporating a beam-splitting mirror. When the spot-film exposure switch is pressed, the beam-splitting mirror is moved into place, diverting some of the beam toward the photo camera and exposing the film. This device is using the visible light image from the output phosphor of the image intensifier and is exposing the 105-mm (or 70-mm) film photographically, similar to a 35-mm film camera used in photography. This system allows for very fast imaging of up to 12 frames per second, and because it is "photographing" the image off of the output phosphor of the image intensifier, it requires approximately half the radiation dose of the cassette spot-filming system.

With conventional fluoroscopy, videotape recording is an option when dynamic imaging is desired. This process uses a VHS videotape recorder (or a high-resolution VHS-S videotape recorder) connected to the television monitor. From this point, it operates much the same as a VHS home system (VCR). During fluoroscopic examinations, the "record" button is pressed on the system, and it records the image from the monitor. Although not typically used in today's fluoroscopic systems, such imaging is useful in functional studies of the esophagus or for placement of catheters or medical devices.

As more departments transition to fully digital environments and eliminate film and chemical processing, a greater dependence is placed on digital imaging and storage means. Without chemical processing and film, the cassette spot filming and the photo-spot imaging go away. If the fluoroscopic signal is in digital form, the size of the data files makes it impossible to record any length of dynamic images on VHS tape.

DIGITAL FLUOROSCOPY

Similar to conventional fluoroscopy, digital fluoroscopy has evolved over time. The early versions of digital fluoroscopy used the conventional fluoroscopic chain but added an analog-to-digital converter (ADC) and computer between the TV camera and the monitor (Figure 10-10). An **analog-to-digital converter (ADC)** is a device that takes the video (analog) signal and divides it into a number of bits (1's and 0's) that the computer "understands." The number of bits into which the signal is divided determines the contrast resolution (number of gray shades) of the system. The ADC is necessary for the computer to process and display the image. Once in

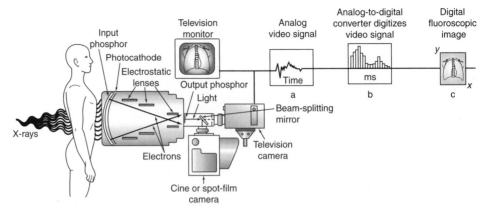

FIGURE 10-10 Analog and digital signals in fluoroscopy. The video signal from the television camera is analog, where the voltage signal varies continuously. This analog signal is sampled *(a)*, producing a stepped representation of the analog video signal *(b)*. The numeric values of each step are stored *(c)*, producing a matrix of digital image data. The binary representation of each pixel value in the matrix is stored and can be manipulated by a computer. The value of each pixel can be mapped to a brightness level for viewing on a display monitor or to an optical density for hard copy on film.

digital form, the image can be postprocessed and stored in that format or printed onto film using a dry laser printer.

The incorporation of a CCD into this setup improved digital fluoroscopy further. The CCD eliminated some of the problems associated with the camera tube. The CCD is more light-sensitive and exhibits less noise and no spatial distortion. It also has a higher spatial resolution and requires less radiation in the system, reducing patient dose.

A more recent advance in digital fluoroscopy is the introduction of a flat-panel detector in place of an image intensifier. Two forms of flat-panel detectors may be used for fluoroscopic applications: the cesium iodide amorphous silicon indirect-capture detector and the amorphous selenium direct-capture detector. Both are described in Chapter 6; refer back to that chapter to review their design and function. For use as a dynamic digital detector (i.e., in digital fluoroscopy applications), there are a few differences. Generally, the digital detectors must respond in rapid sequences to create a dynamic image. Current dynamic digital detectors are capable of up to 60 frames per second. To accomplish this, rapid readout speeds (how the active matrix processes the image data) are necessary.

The flat panel is designed as a two-dimensional rectilinear array of pixels that can be electronically processed line by line in a fraction of a second. For fluoroscopic applications, very-low-noise flat-panel detector systems are needed. Fluoroscopy generally operates at a low-dose output such that any operational noise degrades the fluoroscopic image, making noise a greater factor in detectors used for this application. Application-specific integrated circuits are used to minimize noise and amplify signal from the active matrix. These circuits are particularly important in fluoroscopic applications because they minimize noise, maximize readout speed, and allow for switching from low-dose to high-dose inputs (for spot imaging). Another consideration with low-dose fluoroscopic applications is the maintenance of a large fill factor (the area of each pixel that is sensitive to x-ray detection materials). With general radiography that uses a larger dose output, this is generally not a problem, but it becomes a problem with fluoroscopic applications, in particular with indirect-capture detectors. Other features, such as a light-emitting diode array "backlighting system," have also been incorporated to erase the detector between frames to prevent "ghosting" caused by any residual exposure charge from the previous frame.

The use of flat-panel detectors in place of an image intensifier offers several advantages. The first is a reduction in size, bulk, and weight of the fluoroscopic tower. A flat-panel detector has a compact construction, allowing easier manipulation of the tower, greater flexibility of movement, and greater access to the patient during the examination. Flat-panel detectors also replace the spot filming and other recording devices. They are capable of operating in radiographic mode so that in many cases additional radiographic images are not needed. The images, both dynamic and static, are recorded by the system and can be readily archived with the patient record in a picture archiving and communication system (PACS). Flat-panel detectors do not degrade with age; are more durable; present a rectangular field providing more information; and have better contrast resolution, wider dynamic range, and all of the postprocessing options common to digital images. Finally, flat-panel detectors do not exhibit most image artifacts such as veiling glare (reduces image contrast) and peripheral distortion (pincushion distortion) seen with image intensifiers. They can do all of this with a 50% lower radiation dose to the patient.

Important Relationship
Digital Fluoroscopic Systems

The use of a flat-panel detector in place of an image intensifier offers several advantages, such as a reduction in the size, bulk, and weight of the fluoroscopic tower, allowing for easier manipulation of the tower and greater access to the patient during the examination. Flat-panel detectors also replace the spot filming and other recording devices, and, because they are capable of operating in radiographic mode, in many cases additional radiographic images are not needed. The images, both dynamic and static, can also be readily archived with the patient record in a PACS.

The mA used to operate a digital fluoroscopic unit is similar to the mA used in the radiographic mode, in the hundreds, as opposed to conventional fluoroscopy in the low mA range. In addition, the x-ray beam is not operated continuously, but rather it is automatically pulsed to reduce the heat loading on the tube.

RADIATION SAFETY

Radiation safety is just as important during fluoroscopic imaging as it is with radiographic imaging. Because conventional fluoroscopy uses a continuous stream of x-rays, the exposure should be pulsed intermittently; this is more important during image-intensified fluoroscopy because the operator controls the exposure by a hand switch or foot pedal. Applying pressure to the exposure switch or pedal intermittently significantly reduces patient and personnel exposure and reduces the heat load on the x-ray tube. Digital fluoroscopy uses a controlled pulsed x-ray exposure, and the operator is not required to release pressure intermittently.

TABLE 10-1	**Methods of Reducing Patient and Personnel Exposure During Fluoroscopy**

- During image-intensified fluoroscopy, the operator should intermittently pulse the continuous x-ray exposure.
- Reducing the amount of x-ray fluoroscopic time reduces patient and personnel exposure.
- Monitor and document the amount of total x-ray fluoroscopic time displayed in 5-minute increments on the control panel.
- The intensity of x-ray exposure at the tabletop should not exceed 10 R per minute for units equipped with ABS and 5 R per minute for units without ABS.
- The SSD should be not less than 38 cm (15 inches) for stationary fluoroscopic units and not less than 30 cm (12 inches) on mobile fluoroscopic units.
- Personnel in the fluoroscopic room during procedures should increase their distance from the patient to reduce exposure to scatter radiation.
- Personnel should wear appropriate lead shielding during fluoroscopic procedures.
- The Bucky slot cover must contain at least 0.25 mm of lead equivalent and cover the opened space on the side of the table.
- A protective curtain placed between the patient and operator must have at least 0.25 mm of lead equivalent.

Time, distance, and shielding are the standard radiation safety practices used during fluoroscopic imaging. Reducing the x-ray exposure time reduces the exposure to the patient and any personnel remaining in the room. The control panel timer produces an audible noise when 5 minutes of x-ray fluoroscopic time has been used. It is the operator's responsibility to minimize the x-ray fluoroscopy, and the radiographer should document the total amount of x-ray fluoroscopic time used during the procedure. In addition, the intensity of the x-ray exposure at the tabletop should not exceed 10 R per minute for units equipped with ABC and 5 R per minute for units without ABC. Whenever the patient's exposure is reduced, personnel exposure also is reduced.

The source-to-skin distance (SSD) should be not less than 38 cm (15 inches) for stationary fluoroscopic units and not less than 30 cm (12 inches) on a mobile fluoroscopic unit. In addition, outside of the operator, personnel should increase their distance from the patient to reduce exposure to scatter radiation from the patient.

In addition to all personnel in the room wearing lead aprons, two additional types of shielding are required during fluoroscopy. Because the Bucky tray is positioned at the end of the table for operation of the under-table x-ray tube, a Bucky slot cover with at least 0.25 mm of lead equivalent should automatically cover the opened space at the side of the table. In addition, a protective curtain with at least 0.25 mm of lead equivalent must be placed between the patient and the operator to reduce exposure to the operator. Table 10-1 lists methods of reducing patient and personnel exposure during fluoroscopy.

QUALITY CONTROL

Quality control programs are vitally important for all ionizing radiation–producing equipment to monitor equipment performance and minimize patient dose. Fluoroscopic equipment is used extensively in health care and contributes significantly

BOX 10-3	**Quality Control Check: Fluoroscopic Equipment**

- **Fluoroscopic exposure rates:** Fluoroscopic exposure rate should not exceed 10R/min for units with automatic brightness stabilization (ABS) systems and 5 R/min for those without ABS systems.
- **High-Contrast Resolution:** The system's ability to resolve small, thin, black and white area and is a measure of spatial resolution. Imaging a High-Contrast Resolution Test tool, an image intensifier with a 9-inch input phosphor should resolve at least 20 to 24 holes per inch in the center of the image and 20 holes per inch at the edge.
- **Low-Contrast Resolution:** The system's ability to resolve relatively large objects that are similar in beam attenuation to their surrounding tissue. Imaging a Low-Contrast Resolution Test Tool, the fluoroscopic system should visualize at least the largest holes and some visualization of the smaller holes.
- **Distortion:** Observe the fluoroscopic image of a wire mesh pattern for any distortion such as pincushion.
- **Image Lag:** Observe a phantom image for any blurring as a result of lag while moving the image intensifier.

to the radiation dose received by the general population. Quality control is a team effort among the radiographer, radiologist, and medical physicist. Although some equipment monitoring and data may be collected by a radiographer, performance tests and their interpretation are typically performed by a medical physicist. However, the radiographer should be familiar with the monitoring and testing necessary to ensure that the fluoroscopic unit is operating correctly.

The radiographer, in particular, a quality control radiographer, may be responsible for the operational inspection of the equipment. This inspection should be conducted using a checklist of the items found in Box 10-2 and conducted at least every 6 months. This radiographer may also be responsible for an inspection of the imaging suite itself to examine the general physical condition of the room, unit, supporting electrical cables, and control booth, noting any wear or deteriorating condition. This inspection of the physical condition should be placed on the same schedule and conducted along with the operational inspection.

The other important part of the quality program is the performance inspection and testing of the equipment (Box 10-3 lists a few common fluoroscopic quality control tests). Although a quality control radiographer may perform some of these tests, an appropriately trained and licensed medical physicist should conduct and interpret this portion of the program and oversee the entire quality control monitoring program.

CHAPTER SUMMARY

- Fluoroscopy allows imaging of the movement of internal structures by its use of a continuous beam of x-rays.
- Image intensification provides a brighter image for viewing. The exit radiation is absorbed by the input phosphor, converted to electrons, sent to the output phosphor, released as visible light, and converted to an electronic video signal for transmission to the television monitor.

- Brightness gain is the product of flux gain and minification gain and results in a brighter image on the output phosphor.
- Automatic brightness control (ABC) maintains the overall appearance of the image by monitoring the current through the image intensifier or the output phosphor intensity and adjusting exposure factors if the monitored values fall below preset levels.
- Image intensifiers provide a multifield mode that magnifies the image. When operating the unit in the magnification mode, spatial resolution improves, but patient exposure increases.
- To view the fluoroscopic image on a television monitor, it must be converted to an electrical signal by a camera tube or charge-coupled device (CCD).
- Cassette spot film, photo-spot cameras, cine film, and videotape recording all are methods producing static images during image-intensified fluoroscopy.
- Cassette spot filming shifts to the radiographic mode using a higher mA and increases patient exposure.
- Digital fluoroscopy can be accomplished by attaching an analog-to-digital converter (ADC) between the camera tube or CCD and the television monitor.
- Digital fluoroscopy may also use a flat-panel detector in place of an image intensifier. The use of flat-panel detectors in place of an image intensifier offers several advantages, such as a reduction in the size, bulk, and weight of the fluoroscopic tower, allowing for easier manipulation of the tower and greater access to the patient during the examination.
- Flat-panel detectors also replace the spot filming and other recording devices, and because they are capable of operating in radiographic mode, in many cases additional radiographic images are not needed.
- Image-intensified fluoroscopy uses a lower mA (0.5 to 5 mA), whereas digital fluoroscopy uses a higher mA (100 to 1200 mA). Digital fluoroscopy uses a pulsed x-ray beam, whereas image intensifiers operate as a continuous x-ray beam exposure unless the operator produces intermittent x-ray exposures.
- Radiation safety practices include reducing the amount of fluoroscopic time and shielding the operator by the Bucky slot cover and a protective curtain placed between the patient and the operator. The source-to skin-distance (SSD) should be not less than 38 cm (15 inches) for stationary fluoroscopic units and not less than 30 cm (12 inches) on a mobile fluoroscopic unit, and the intensity of the x-ray exposure at the tabletop should not exceed 10 R/minute.
- Quality control procedures are important to monitoring the performance of the fluoroscopic unit.

REVIEW QUESTIONS

1. In conventional fluoroscopy, the milliamperage range is typically:
   A. 0.5 to 5 mA
   B. 20 to 50 mA
   C. 100 to 300 mA
   D. 400 to 600 mA

2. During fluoroscopy, releasing the pressure applied to the pedal or switch terminates the radiation exposure and is known as the _____.
   A. fluoroscopic timer
   B. intensification switch
   C. activation switch
   D. deadman switch

3. What component of the image intensifier converts the exit or remnant radiation into visible light?
   A. Output phosphor
   B. Photocathode
   C. Input phosphor
   D. Electrostatic focusing lenses

4. What component of the image intensifier converts the visible light to electrons?
   A. Output phosphor
   B. Photocathode
   C. Input phosphor
   D. Electrostatic focusing lenses

5. In conventional fluoroscopy, in order to view the images on a television monitor, the light intensities are converted by a _____.
   A. camera tube
   B. electrostatic lens
   C. charge-coupled device
   D. A or C

6. Brightness gain is a product of _____.
   A. minification gain and automatic brightness control
   B. flux gain and automatic brightness control
   C. minification gain and flux gain
   D. automatic brightness control and milliamperage

7. The numeric conversion factor value is equal to _____ of the brightness gain value.
   A. 0.001
   B. 0.01
   C. 0.1
   D. 1.0

8. A brightness gain of 40,000 would have a conversion factor of _____.
   A. 40
   B. 400
   C. 4000
   D. 40,000

9. A disadvantage of using the magnification mode during fluoroscopy is _____.
   A. decreased spatial resolution
   B. increased patient exposure
   C. decreased density
   D. decreased contrast

10. When spot filming during conventional fluoroscopic image intensification, the radiation dose to the patient is decreased.
    A. True
    B. False

11. In digital fluoroscopy, the x-ray beam is operated in a continuous mode similar to conventional fluoroscopy.
    A. True
    B. False

12. When operating a stationary fluoroscopic unit, the source-to-skin distance (SSD) should not be less than _____.
    A. 25 cm (10 inches)
    B. 30 cm (12 inches)
    C. 38 cm (15 inches)
    D. 45 cm (18 inches)

13. For fluoroscopic units with automatic brightness control (ABC), the x-ray exposure at the tabletop should not exceed _____.
    A. 0.01 R/minute
    B. 0.1 R/minute
    C. 1.0 R/minute
    D. 10 R/minute

14. The Bucky slot cover must have lead equivalent of _____.
    A. 0.10 mm
    B. 0.25 mm
    C. 0.50 mm
    D. 2.5 mm

15. Which of the following standard safety practices is NOT used to reduce radiation exposure to the operator during fluoroscopy?
    A. Distance
    B. Time
    C. Shielding
    D. All of the above are used

Summary of Important Relationships

Chapter 1: Radiation and Its Discovery

The Dual Nature of X-ray Energy
X-rays act like both waves and particles. (See p. 6)

Wavelength and Frequency
Wavelength and frequency are inversely related. Higher-energy x-rays have decreased wavelength and increased frequency. Lower-energy x-rays have increased wavelength and decreased frequency. (See p. 7)

Chapter 2: The X-Ray Beam

Filament
The filament is the source of electrons during x-ray production. (See p. 13)

Target
The target is the part of the anode that is struck by the focused stream of electrons coming from the cathode. The target stops the electrons and creates the opportunity for the production of x-rays. (See p. 14)

Tungsten
Because tungsten has a high atomic number (74) and a high melting point (3400° C [6152° F]), it efficiently produces x-rays. (See p. 15)

Dissipating Heat
As heat is produced when the x-ray exposure is made, it is transferred to the insulating oil that surrounds the x-ray tube. (See p. 15)

Rotating Anodes
Rotating anodes can withstand higher heat loads than stationary anodes because the rotation causes a greater physical area, or focal track, to be exposed to electrons. (See p. 16)

Production of X-rays
As electrons strike the target, their kinetic energy is transferred to the tungsten atoms in the anode to produce x-rays. (See p. 17)

Interactions That Produce X-ray Photons
Bremsstrahlung interactions and characteristic interactions both produce x-ray photons. (See p. 18)

Bremsstrahlung Interactions
Most x-ray interactions in the diagnostic energy range are bremsstrahlung. (See p. 19)

Characteristic Interactions
Characteristic x-rays can be produced in a tungsten target only when the kVp is set at 70 or greater because the binding energy of the K-shell electron is 69.5 keV. (See p. 20)

Thermionic Emission
When the tungsten filament gains enough heat *(therm)*, the outer-shell electrons *(ions)* of the filament atoms are boiled off, or emitted, from the filament. (See p. 21)

Tube Current
Electrons flow in only one direction in the x-ray tube—from cathode to anode. This flow of electrons is called the *tube current* and is measured in milliamperes (mA). (See p. 23)

Energy Conversion in the X-ray Tube
As electrons strike the anode target, approximately 99% of their kinetic energy is converted to heat, whereas only 1% (approximately) of their energy is converted to x-rays. (See p. 23)

Kilovoltage and the Speed of Electrons
The speed of the electrons traveling from the cathode to the anode increases as the kilovoltage applied across the x-ray tube increases. (See p. 24)

Speed of Electrons and Quality of X-rays
The speed of the electrons in the tube current determines the quality or energy of the x-rays that are produced. The quality or energy of the x-rays that are produced determines the penetrability of the primary beam. (See p. 25)

kVp and Beam Penetrability
As kVp increases, beam penetrability increases; as kVp decreases, beam penetrability decreases. (See p. 25)

Milliamperage, Tube Current, and X-ray Quantity
The quantity of electrons in the tube current and quantity of x-rays produced are directly proportional to the milliamperage. (See p. 27)

Exposure Time, Tube Current, and X-ray Quantity
The quantity of electrons that flows from cathode to anode and the quantity of x-rays produced are directly proportional to the exposure time. (See p. 29)

Quantity of Electrons, X-rays, and mAs
The quantity of electrons flowing from the cathode to the anode and the quantity of x-rays produced are directly proportional to mAs. (See p. 29)

Line Focus Principle
The line focus principle describes the relationship between the actual focal spot, where the electrons in the tube current bombard the target, and the effective focal spot, that same area as seen from directly below the tube. (See p. 30)

Anode Angle and Effective Focal Spot Size
Based on the line focus principle, the smaller the anode angle, the smaller the effective focal spot size. (See p. 30)

Anode Heel Effect
X-rays are more intense on the cathode side of the tube. The intensity of the x-rays decreases toward the anode side. (See p. 32)

Low-Energy Photons, Patient Dose, and Image Formation
Low-energy photons serve only to increase patient dose and do not contribute to image formation. (See p. 33)

Chapter 3: Image Formation and Radiographic Quality

Differential Absorption and Image Formation
A radiographic image is created by passing an x-ray beam through the patient and interacting with an image receptor, such as an imaging plate in computed radiography (CR). The variations in absorption and transmission of the exiting x-ray beam structurally represent the anatomic area of interest. (See p. 44)

X-ray Photon Absorption
During attenuation of the x-ray beam, the photoelectric effect is responsible for total absorption of the incoming x-ray photon. (See p. 45)

X-ray Beam Scattering
During attenuation of the x-ray beam, the incoming x-ray photon may lose energy and change direction as a result of the Compton effect. (See p. 46)

Factors Affecting Beam Attenuation
Increasing tissue thickness, atomic number, and tissue density increase x-ray beam attenuation because more x-rays are absorbed by the tissue. Increasing the quality of the x-ray beam decreases beam attenuation because the higher-energy x-rays penetrate the tissue. (See p. 48)

X-ray Interaction with Matter

When the diagnostic primary x-ray beam interacts with anatomic tissues, three processes occur: absorption, scattering, and transmission. (See p. 49)

Image Brightness or Densities

The range of image brightness or densities visible after processing is a result of the variation in x-ray absorption and transmission as the x-ray beam passes through anatomic tissues. (See p. 50)

Creating the Latent Image

The process of differential absorption for image formation is the same for digital and film-screen imaging. The varying x-ray intensities exiting the anatomic area of interest form the latent image. (See p. 51)

Brightness or Density and Radiographic Quality

A radiographic image must have sufficient brightness or density to visualize the anatomic structures of interest. (See p. 52)

Differentiating Among Anatomic Tissues

The ability to distinguish among types of tissues is determined by the differences in brightness levels or densities in the image or contrast. Anatomic tissues that attenuate the beam similarly have low subject contrast. Anatomic tissues that attenuate the beam very differently have high subject contrast. (See p. 55)

Sharpness of Anatomic Detail

The accuracy of the anatomic structural lines recorded in the radiographic image is determined by its spatial resolution and recorded detail. (See p. 58)

Size Distortion

Radiographic images of objects are always magnified in terms of the true object size. The SID and OID play an important role in minimizing the amount of size distortion or magnification created. (See p. 60)

Shape Distortion

Shape distortion can occur from inaccurate central ray (CR) alignment of the tube, the part being radiographed, or the image receptor. *Elongation* refers to images of objects that appear longer than the true objects. *Foreshortening* refers to images that appear shorter than the true objects. (See p. 61)

Number of Photons and Quantum Noise

Decreasing the number of photons reaching the image receptor may increase the amount of quantum noise within the radiographic image; increasing the number of photons reaching the image receptor may decrease the amount of quantum noise within the radiographic image. (See p. 62)

Dynamic Range and Digital Image Receptors
Digital image receptors can accurately detect a wide range of exit radiation intensities (wide dynamic range), and therefore anatomic tissues can be better visualized. (See p. 65)

Pixel Bit Depth and Contrast Resolution
The greater the pixel bit depth (i.e., 14-bit), the more precise the digitization of the analog signal, and the greater the number of shades of gray available for image display. Increasing the number of shades of gray available to display on a digital image improves its contrast resolution. (See p. 68)

Pixel Density and Pitch and Spatial Resolution
Increasing the pixel density and decreasing the pixel pitch increases spatial resolution. Decreasing pixel density and increasing pixel pitch decreases spatial resolution. (See p. 68)

Light Transmittance and Optical Density
As the percentage of light transmitted decreases, the optical density increases; as the percentage of light transmitted increases, the optical density decreases. (See p. 70)

Optical Density and Light Transmittance
For every 0.3 change in optical density, the percentage of light transmitted has changed by a factor of 2. A 0.3 increase in optical density results from a decrease in the percentage of light transmitted by half, whereas a 0.3 decrease in optical density results from an increase in the percentage of light transmitted by a factor of 2. (See p. 70)

Exposure Intensity and Optical Density
Increasing the exposure intensity to the film-screen image receptor will increase the optical density, while decreasing the exposure intensity to the film-screen image receptor will decrease the exposure intensity. (See p. 71)

Dynamic Range and Film-Screen Imaging
The range of exposure intensities that film can accurately detect is limited (limited dynamic range). This renders film more susceptible to overexposure and underexposure and restricts its ability to display tissues that vary greatly in x-ray attenuation. (See p. 72)

Chapter 4: Exposure Technique Factors

mAs and Quantity of Radiation
As the mAs is increased, the quantity of radiation reaching the IR is increased. As the mAs is decreased, the amount of radiation reaching the IR is decreased. (See p. 79)

Milliamperage and Exposure Time
Milliamperage and exposure time have an inverse proportional relationship when maintaining the same mAs. (See p. 80)

mAs and Digital Image Brightness

The amount of mAs does not have a direct effect on image brightness when using digital IRs. During computer processing, image brightness is maintained when the mAs is too low or too high. A lower-than-needed mAs produces an image with increased quantum noise, and a higher-than-needed mAs exposes the patient to unnecessary radiation. (See p. 80)

Exposure Indicator Value

A numeric value or exposure indicator is displayed on the processed digital image that indicates the level of x-ray exposure received (incident exposure) to the IR. If the exposure indicator value falls outside of the manufacturer's suggested range, image quality or patient exposure or both could be compromised. (See p. 81)

mAs and Film-Screen Density

The amount of mAs has a direct effect on the amount of radiographic density produced when using a film-screen IR. The minimum change needed to correct for a density error is determined by multiplying or dividing the mAs by 2. (See p. 82)

kVp and the Radiographic Image

Increasing or decreasing the kVp changes the amount of radiation exposure to the IR and the contrast produced within the image. (See p. 83)

Exposure Errors in Digital Imaging

kVp and mAs exposure errors should be reflected in the exposure indicator value; however, image brightness can be maintained during computer processing. (See p. 83)

Exposure Errors and Film-Screen Imaging

kVp directly affects the density produced on a film-screen image; however, its effect is not equal throughout the range of kVp (low, middle, and high). (See p. 83)

kVp and the 15% Rule

A 15% increase in kVp has the same effect on exposure to the IR as doubling the mAs. A 15% decrease in kVp has the same effect on exposure to the IR as decreasing the mAs by half. (See p. 85)

kVp and Radiographic Contrast

A high kVp results in less absorption and more transmission in the anatomic tissues, which results in less variation in the x-ray intensities exiting the patient (lower subject contrast), producing a low-contrast image. A low kVp results in more absorption and less x-ray transmission but with more variation in the x-ray intensities exiting the patient (higher subject contrast), resulting in a high-contrast image. (See p. 86)

Kilovoltage and Digital Image Quality

Assuming that the anatomic part is adequately penetrated, changing the kVp affects the radiation exposure to the digital IR similarly to changing the mAs, but dissimilar to mAs, kVp also affects image contrast. However, image brightness and contrast are primarily controlled during computer processing. (See p. 87)

Kilovoltage, Scatter Radiation, and Radiographic Contrast
At higher kVp, a greater proportion of Compton scattering occurs compared with x-ray absorption (photoelectric effect), which decreases radiographic contrast. Decreasing the kVp decreases the proportion of Compton scattering and increases radiographic contrast. (See p. 87)

Focal Spot Size and Recorded Detail
As focal spot size increases, unsharpness increases, and recorded detail decreases; as focal spot size decreases, unsharpness decreases, and recorded detail increases. (See p. 89)

SID and X-ray Beam Intensity
As SID increases, the x-ray beam intensity is spread over a larger area. This decreases the overall intensity of the x-ray beam reaching the IR. (See p. 90)

SID and mAs
Increasing the SID requires that the mAs be increased to maintain exposure to the IR, and decreasing the SID requires a decrease in the mAs to maintain exposure to the IR. (See p. 91)

SID, Size Distortion, and Recorded Detail
As SID increases, size distortion (magnification) decreases, and recorded detail or spatial resolution increases; as SID decreases, size distortion (magnification) increases, and recorded detail or spatial resolution decreases. (See p. 91)

OID, Size Distortion, and Recorded Detail or Spatial Resolution
Increasing the OID increases magnification and decreases the recorded detail or spatial resolution, whereas decreasing the OID decreases magnification and increases the recorded detail or spatial resolution. (See p. 93)

Grids, Scatter, and Contrast
Placing a grid between the anatomic area of interest and the IR absorbs scatter radiation exiting the patient and increases radiographic contrast. (See p. 98)

Grids and Image Receptor Exposure
Adding, removing, or changing a grid requires an adjustment in mAs to maintain radiation exposure to the IR. (See p. 98)

Beam Restriction and Image Receptor Exposure
Changes in beam restriction alter the amount of tissue irradiated and therefore affect the amount of exposure to the IR. The effect of collimation is greater when imaging large anatomic areas, performing examinations without a grid, and using a high kVp. (See p. 99)

Chapter 5: Scatter Control

kVp and Scatter
The amount and energy of scatter radiation exiting the patient depends, in part, on the kVp selected. Examinations using higher kVp produce a greater proportion of higher-energy scattered x-rays compared with examinations using low kVp. (See p. 114)

X-ray Beam Field Size, Thickness of the Part, and Scatter
The larger the x-ray beam field size, the greater the amount of scatter radiation produced. The thicker the part being imaged, the greater the amount of scatter radiation produced. (See p. 115)

Volume of Tissue Irradiated and Scatter
The volume of tissue irradiated is affected by both the part thickness and the x-ray beam field size. Therefore, the greater the volume of tissue irradiated, because of either or both factors, the greater the amount of scatter radiation produced. (See p. 115)

Beam Restriction and Patient Dose
As beam restriction or collimation increases, field size decreases, and patient dose decreases. As beam restriction or collimation decreases, field size increases, and patient dose increases. (See p. 116)

Collimation and Scatter Radiation
As collimation increases, the field size decreases, and the quantity of scatter radiation decreases; as collimation decreases, the field size increases, and the quantity of scatter radiation increases. (See p. 116)

Collimation and Radiographic Contrast
As collimation increases, the quantity of scatter radiation decreases, and radiographic contrast increases; as collimation decreases, the quantity of scatter radiation increases, and radiographic contrast decreases. (See p. 117)

Collimation and Exposure to the Image Receptor
As collimation increases, exposure to the IR decreases; as collimation decreases, exposure to the IR increases. (See p. 117)

Scatter Radiation and Image Quality
Scatter radiation adds unwanted exposure to the IR and decreases image quality. (See p. 123)

Grid Ratio and Radiographic Contrast
As grid ratio increases for the same grid frequency, scatter cleanup improves, and radiographic contrast increases; as grid ratio decreases for the same grid frequency, scatter cleanup is less effective, and radiographic contrast decreases. (See p. 125)

Focused versus Parallel Grids
Focused grids have lead lines that are angled to match approximately the divergence of the primary beam. Thus, focused grids allow more transmitted photons to reach the IR than parallel grids. (See p. 126)

Grid Ratio and Exposure to Image Receptor
As grid ratio increases, exposure to IR decreases; as grid ratio decreases, exposure to IR increases. (See p. 129)

Grid Ratio and Patient Dose
As grid ratio increases, patient dose increases; as grid ratio decreases, patient dose decreases. (See p. 131)

Upside-Down Focused Grids and Grid Cutoff
Placing a focused grid upside-down on the IR causes the lateral edges of the radiograph to be very underexposed. (See p. 133)

Off-Level Error and Grid Cutoff
Angling the x-ray tube across the grid lines or angling the grid itself during exposure produces an overall decrease in exposure on the radiograph. (See p. 134)

Off-Center Error and Grid Cutoff
If the center of the x-ray beam is not aligned from side to side with the center of a focused grid, grid cutoff occurs. (See p. 134)

Off-Focus Error and Grid Cutoff
Using an SID outside of the focal range creates a loss of exposure at the periphery of the radiograph. (See p. 134)

Air Gap Technique and Scatter Control
The air gap technique is an alternative to using a grid to control scatter reaching the IR. By moving the IR away from the patient, more of the scatter radiation will miss the IR. The greater the gap, the less scatter reaches the IR. (See p. 138)

Chapter 6: Image Receptors and Image Acquisition

Computed Radiography Digital Image Receptors
The CR latent image is acquired in the PSP layer of the IP. Most of the energy from the exit radiation intensities is stored in the PSP for extraction in the reader unit. (See p. 145)

Sampling Frequency and Spatial Resolution
Increasing the sampling frequency results in a smaller sampling and pixel pitch, which improves the spatial resolution of the digital image. Decreasing the sampling frequency results in a larger sampling and pixel pitch and decreased spatial resolution. (See p. 147)

Imaging Plate Size and Matrix Size

For a fixed matrix size CR system, using a smaller IP for a given field of view (FOV) results in improved spatial resolution of the digital image. Increasing the size of the IP for a given FOV results in decreased spatial resolution. (See p. 148)

Digital Detectors and Dynamic Range

Digital IRs have a large dynamic range; that is, they can capture accurately a wide range of x-ray intensities exiting the patient. The computer then processes the raw pixel data to compensate for exposure errors and create a radiographic image. However, lower or higher than necessary exposure techniques do not guarantee a quality digital image with reasonable radiation exposure to the patient. (See p. 154)

Signal-to-Noise Ratio and Image Quality

Increasing the SNR increases the visibility of anatomic details, whereas decreasing the SNR decreases the visibility of anatomic details. (See p. 155)

Sensitivity Specks and Latent Image Centers

Sensitivity specks serve as the focal point for the development of latent image centers. After exposure, these specks trap the free electrons and then attract and neutralize the positive silver ions. After enough silver is neutralized, the specks become a latent image center and are converted to metallic silver after chemical processing. (See p. 156)

Silver Halide and Film Sensitivity

As the number of silver halide crystals increases, film sensitivity or speed increases; as the size of the silver halide crystals increases, film sensitivity or speed increases. A faster film speed requires less radiation exposure to produce a specific density. (See p. 157)

Screen Speed and Recorded Detail

As screen speed is increased, recorded detail is decreased; as screen speed decreases, recorded detail increases. (See p. 160)

Screen Speed, Light Emission, and Patient Dose

The faster an intensifying screen, the more light is emitted for the same intensity of x-ray exposure. As screen speed increases, less radiation is necessary, and radiation dose to the patient is decreased; as screen speed decreases, more radiation is necessary, and radiation dose to the patient is increased. (See p. 161)

Film-Screen System Speed and mAs

Increasing the film-screen speed requires a decrease in the mAs to maintain density. Decreasing the film-screen speed requires an increase in the mAs to maintain density. (See p. 162)

Chapter 7: Image Processing and Display

Histogram Analysis
With digital systems, the computer creates a histogram of the data set. The histogram is a graph of the exposure received to the pixel elements and the prevalence of the exposures within the image. This created histogram is compared with a stored histogram model for that anatomic part; VOIs are identified, and the image is displayed. (See p. 169)

Exposure Indicators
The radiographer should strive to select techniques that result in exposure indicator values within the indicated optimum range for that digital imaging system. However, the radiographer also needs to recognize the limitations of exposure indicators in providing accurate information. (See p. 171)

Lookup Tables
Lookup tables provide the means to alter the original pixel values to improve the brightness and contrast of the image. (See p. 171)

Window Level and Image Brightness
A direct relationship exists between window level and image brightness on the display monitor. Increasing the window level increases the image brightness; decreasing the window level decreases the image brightness. (See p. 178)

Window Width and Image Contrast
A narrow (decreased) window width displays higher radiographic contrast, whereas a wider (increased) window width displays lower radiographic contrast. (See p. 180)

Developing or Reducing Agents
The developing agents are responsible for reducing the exposed silver halide crystals to metallic silver, visualized as radiographic densities. Phenidone is responsible for creating the lower densities, and hydroquinone is responsible for creating the higher densities. Their combined effect results in the range of visible densities on the radiograph. (See p. 184)

Clearing the Unexposed Crystals
The fixing agent, ammonium thiosulfate, is responsible for removing the unexposed crystals from the emulsion. (See p. 185)

Archival Quality of Radiographs
Maintaining the archival (long-term) quality of radiographs requires that most of the fixing agent be removed (washed) from the film. Staining or fading of the permanent image results when too much thiosulfate remains on the film. (See p. 186)

Archival Quality of Radiographs
Permanent radiographs must retain moisture of 10% to 15% to maintain archival quality. Excessive drying can cause the emulsion layers to crack. (See p. 186)

Replenishment and Solution Performance

The replenishment system provides fresh chemicals to the developing and fixing solutions to maintain their chemical activity and volume when they become depleted during processing. (See p. 187)

Developer Temperature and Radiographic Quality

Variations in developer temperature adversely affect the quality of the radiographic image. Increasing developer temperature increases the density, and decreasing developer temperature decreases the density. Radiographic contrast also may be adversely affected by changes in the developer temperature. (See p. 188)

Silver Recovery

Silver is a natural resource, is a heavy metal that can be toxic to the environment, and needs to be removed from the used fixer. (See p. 193)

Chapter 8: Exposure Technique Selection

Principle of Automatic Exposure Control Operation

Once a predetermined amount of radiation is transmitted through a patient, the x-ray exposure is terminated. This determines the exposure time and therefore the total amount of radiation exposure to the IR. (See p. 199)

Radiation-Measuring Devices

Detectors are the AEC devices that measure the amount of radiation transmitted. The radiographer selects the combination of the three detectors to use. (See p. 200)

Function of the Ionization Chamber

The ionization chamber interacts with exit radiation before it reaches the IR. Air in the chamber is ionized, and an electrical charge that is proportional to the amount of radiation is created. (See p. 201)

Automatic Exposure Control and mAs Readout

If the radiographic unit has an mAs readout display, the radiographer should take note of the reading after the exposure is made. This information can be invaluable. (See p. 202)

kVp Levels and Automatic Exposure Control Response

The radiographer must set the kVp value as needed to ensure adequate penetration and to produce the appropriate level of contrast. The kVp selected determines the length of exposure time when using AEC. A low kVp requires more exposure time to reach the predetermined amount of exposure. A high kVp decreases the exposure time to reach the predetermined amount of exposure and reduces the overall radiation exposure to the patient. (See p. 203)

mA Level and Automatic Exposure Control Response

If the radiographer can set the mA level when using AEC, it will affect the time of exposure for a given procedure. Increasing the mA decreases the exposure time to reach the predetermined amount of exposure. Decreasing the mA increases the exposure time to reach the predetermined amount of exposure. (See p. 203)

Function of Backup Time

Backup time, the maximum exposure time allowed during an AEC examination, serves as a safety mechanism when AEC is not used properly or is not functioning properly. (See p. 204)

Setting Backup Time

Backup time should be set at 150% to 200% of the expected exposure time. This allows the properly used AEC system to terminate the exposure appropriately but protects the patient and tube from excessive exposure if a problem occurs. (See p. 204)

Detector Selection

The combination of detectors affects the amount of exposure reaching the IR. If the area of radiographic interest is not directly over the selected detectors, that area likely will be overexposed or underexposed. When performing any radiographic study where the IR is located outside of the Bucky, the AEC system should be deactivated, and a manual technique should be used. (See p. 207)

Patient Centering

Accurate centering of the area of interest over the detectors is critical to ensure proper exposure to the IR. If the area of interest is not properly centered to the detectors, overexposure or underexposure may occur. (See p. 207)

Collimation and Automatic Exposure Control Response

Excessive or insufficient collimation may affect the amount of exposure reaching the IR. Insufficient collimation may result in excessive scatter reaching the detectors, resulting in the exposure time terminating too quickly. Excessive collimation may result in too long of an exposure time. (See p. 209)

Type of Image Receptor and Automatic Exposure Control Response

The AEC system is calibrated to the type and speed class of the IR used. If an IR of a different type or speed is used, the detectors will not sense the difference, and the exposure time will terminate at the preset value, which may jeopardize image quality. (See p. 210)

Digital Image Receptors and the Automatic Exposure Control Response

Because the visual cues of increased or decreased radiographic density when using film-screen IRs are lacking in digital imaging, the radiographer must be very conscientious about excessive radiation exposure to the patient. (See p. 211)

Exposure Technique Charts and Radiographic Quality

Exposure technique charts are just as important for digital imaging because digital systems have a wide dynamic range and can compensate for exposure technique errors. Technique charts should be developed and used with all types of radiographic imaging systems to maintain patient radiation exposure *as low as* reasonably *achievable* (ALARA). (See p. 214)

Variable kVp/Fixed mAs Technique Chart

The variable kVp chart adjusts the kVp for changes in part thickness while maintaining a fixed mAs. (See p. 217)

Fixed kVp/Variable mAs Technique Charts

Fixed kVp/variable mAs technique charts identify optimal kVp values and alter the mAs for variations in part thickness. (See p. 218)

Chapter 10: Dynamic Imaging: Fluoroscopy

Image-Intensified Fluoroscopy

Dynamic imaging of internal anatomic structures can be accomplished with the use of an image intensifier. The exit radiation is absorbed by the input phosphor, converted to electrons, sent to the output phosphor, released as visible light, and converted to an electronic video signal for transmission to the television monitor. (See p. 253)

Brightness Gain

A brighter image is created on the output phosphor when the accelerated electrons strike a smaller output phosphor. (See p. 254)

Magnification Mode and Patient Dose

Operating the image intensifier in one of the magnification modes increases the operator's ability to see small structures but at the price of increasing radiation dose to the patient. (See p. 257)

Coupling Systems and the Television Monitor

The camera tube and CCD are devices that couple the image intensifier to the television monitor to convert the image from the output phosphor to an electronic (video) signal that can be reconstructed on the television monitor. (See p. 262)

Cassette Spot Filming

Cassette spot-film devices are one means of recording static images during a fluoroscopic examination. The unit shifts to radiographic mode (using a higher mA), and the radiation dose to the patient is much higher than in fluoroscopic mode. (See p. 263)

Digital Fluoroscopic Systems

The use of a flat-panel detector in place of an image intensifier offers several advantages, such as a reduction in the size, bulk, and weight of the fluoroscopic tower, allowing for easier manipulation of the tower and greater access to the patient during the examination. Flat-panel detectors also replace the spot filming and other recording devices, and, because they are capable of operating in radiographic mode, in many cases additional radiographic images are not needed. The images, both dynamic and static, can also be readily archived with the patient record in a PACS. (See p. 265)

Summary of Mathematical Applications

Chapter 2: The X-Ray Beam

Calculating mAs

$$mAs = mA \times seconds$$

Examples:

$$200 \text{ mA} \times 0.25 \text{ s} = 50 \text{ mAs}$$

$$500 \text{ mA} \times 2 / 5 \text{ s} = 200 \text{ mAs}$$

$$800 \text{ mA} \times 100 \text{ ms (milliseconds or 0.1 second)} = 80 \text{ mAs}$$

(See p. 29)

Calculating Heat Units

An exposure is made with a three-phase x-ray unit using 600 mA, and 0.05 second, 75 kVp. How many heat units are produced from this exposure?

$$HU = mA \times time \times kVp \times generator \text{ factor}$$

$$HU = 600 \times 0.05 \times 75 \times 1.35$$

$$= 3037.5 \text{ HU}$$

(See p. 36)

Chapter 4: Exposure Technique Factors

Adjusting Milliamperage or Exposure Time

$$200 \text{ mA} \times 0.1 \text{ s} = 20 \text{ mAs}$$

To increase the mAs to 40, you could use:

$$400 \text{ mA} \times 0.1 \text{ s} = 40 \text{ mAs}$$

$$200 \text{ mA} \times 0.2 \text{ s} = 40 \text{ mAs}$$

(See p. 79)

Adjusting Milliamperage and Exposure Time to Maintain mAs

$$200 \text{ mA} \times 100 \text{ ms } (0.1 \text{ s}) = 20 \text{ mAs}$$

To maintain the mAs, use:

$$400 \text{ mA} \times 50 \text{ ms } (0.05 \text{ s}) = 20 \text{ mAs}$$

$$100 \text{ mA} \times 200 \text{ ms } (0.2 \text{ s}) = 20 \text{ mAs}$$

(See p. 80)

Using the 15% Rule

To increase exposure to the IR, multiply the kVp by 1.15 (original kVp + 15%):

$$75 \text{ kVp} \times 1.15 = 86 \text{ kVp}$$

To decrease exposure to the IR, multiply the kVp by 0.85 (original kVp – 15%):

$$75 \text{ kVp} \times 0.85 = 64 \text{ kVp}$$

To maintain exposure to the IR, when increasing the kVp by 15% (kVp × 1.15), divide the original mAs by 2:

$$75 \text{ kVp} \times 1.15 = 86 \text{ kVp and mAs/2}$$

When decreasing the kVp by 15% (kVp × 0.85), multiply the mAs by 2:

$$75 \text{ kVp} \times 0.85 = 64 \text{ and mAs} \times 2$$

(See p. 85)

Inverse Square Law Formula

$$\frac{I_1}{I_2} = \frac{(D_2)^2}{(D_1)^2}$$

The intensity of radiation at an SID of 40 inches is equal to 400 mR. What is the intensity of radiation when the distance is increased to 72 inches?

$$\frac{400 \text{ mR}}{X} = \frac{(72)^2}{(40)^2} \quad 400 \text{ mR} \times 1600 = 640,000 = 5184X;$$

$$\frac{640,000}{5184} = X; \quad 123.5 \text{ mRX} = X$$

(See p. 90)

mAs/Distance Compensation Formula

$$\frac{mAs_1}{mAs_2} \quad \frac{(SID_1)^2}{(SID_2)^2}$$

Optimal exposure to the IR is achieved at an SID of 40 inches using 25 mAs. The SID must be increased to 72 inches. What adjustment in mAs is needed to maintain exposure to the IR?

$$\frac{25}{X} = \frac{(40)^2}{(72)^2}; \quad 1600X = 129,600; \quad \frac{129,600}{1600}; \quad X = 81 \text{ mAs}_2$$

(See p. 91)

Magnification Factor

An anteroposterior projection (AP) of the knee is produced with an SID of 40 inches and an OID of 3 inches (SOD is equal to 37 inches). What is the MF?

$$SOD = SID - OID \quad MF = \frac{40}{37}; \quad MF = 1.081$$

$$37 = 40 - 3$$

(See p. 95)

Determining Object Size

On an AP image of a knee taken with an SID of 40 inches and an OID of 3 inches (SOD = 37 inches), the size of a lesion measures 0.5 inch in diameter on the radiograph. The MF has been determined to be 1.081. What is the object size of this lesion?

$$\frac{40}{37} = 1.081 \text{ MF} \quad \text{Object size} = \frac{0.5 \text{ inch}}{1.081}$$

The object size is 0.463 inch.
(See p. 96)

Adjusting mAs for Changes in Grid

A quality radiograph is obtained using 5 mAs at 70 kVp without using a grid. What new mAs is needed when adding a 12:1 grid to maintain the same exposure to the IR?

$$\frac{5 \text{ mAs}}{X} = \frac{1}{5}; \quad 1X = 25; X = 25 \text{ mAs}$$

The new mAs produces an exposure comparable with the IR.
(See p. 99)

Chapter 5: Scatter Control

Calculating Grid Ratio

What is the grid ratio when the lead strips are 2.4 mm high and separated by 0.2 mm?

$$\text{Grid ratio} = \frac{h}{D}$$

$$\text{Grid ratio} = \frac{2.4}{0.2} = 12 \ \text{ or } 12\!:\!1$$

(See p. 124)

Adding a Grid

If a radiographer produced a shoulder radiograph with a nongrid exposure using 3 mAs and next wanted to use a 12:1 ratio grid, what mAs should be used to produce the same exposure to the IR?

Nongrid exposure = 3 mAs

$$\text{GCF (for 12:1 grid)} = 5 \ (\text{from Table 5-2})$$

$$\text{GCF} = \frac{\text{mAs with the grid}}{\text{mAs without the grid}}$$

$$3 = \frac{\text{mAs with the grid}}{5}$$

$$15 = \text{mAs with the grid}$$

When adding a 12:1 ratio grid, the mAs must be increased by a factor of 5, in this case to 15 mAs.

(See p. 130)

Removing a Grid

If a radiographer produced a knee radiograph using a 8:1 ratio grid and 10 mAs and on the next exposure wanted to use a nongrid exposure, what mAs should be used to produce the same exposure to the IR?

Grid exposure = 10 mAs

GCF (for 8:1 grid) = 4 (from Table 5-2)

$$\text{GCF} = \frac{\text{mAs with the grid}}{\text{mAs without the grid}}$$

$$4 = \frac{10 \text{ mAs}}{\text{mAs without the grid}}$$

$$2.5 = \text{mAs without the grid}$$

When removing an 8:1 ratio grid, the mAs must be decreased by a factor of 4, in this case to 2.5 mAs.

(See p. 130)

Decreasing the Grid Ratio

If a radiographer used 40 mAs with a 12:1 ratio grid, what mAs should be used with a 6:1 ratio grid to produce the same exposure to the IR?

Exposure 1: 40 mAs, 12:1 grid, GCF = 5

Exposure 2: _____ mAs, 6:1 grid, GCF = 3

$$\frac{mAs_1}{mAs_2} = \frac{GCF_1}{GCF_2}$$

$$\frac{40}{mAs_2} = \frac{5}{3}$$

$$mAs_2 = 24$$

Decreasing the grid ratio requires less mAs.

(See p. 131)

Increasing the Grid Ratio

If a radiographer performed a routine portable pelvic examination using 40 mAs with an 8:1 ratio grid, what mAs should be used if a 12:1 ratio grid is substituted?

Exposure 1: 40 mAs, 8:1 grid, GCF = 4

Exposure 2: _____ mAs, 12:1 grid, GCF = 5

$$\frac{mAs_1}{mAs_2} = \frac{GCF_1}{GCF_2}$$

$$\frac{40}{mAs_2} = \frac{4}{5} = 50 \; mAs_2$$

Increasing the grid ratio requires additional mAs.

(See p. 131)

Chapter 6: Image Receptors and Image Acquisition

Adjusting mAs for Changes in Film-Screen System Speed

A quality radiograph is obtained using 10 mAs at 65 kVp and 100-speed film-screen system. What new mAs is used to maintain radiographic density when changing to a 400-speed film-screen system?

$$\frac{10 \; mAs}{X} = \frac{400 \; Speed}{100 \; Speed}$$

$$10 \; mAs \times 100; 1000 = 400X; \; \frac{1000}{400} = 2.5 \; mAs = X$$

(See p. 163)

Summary of Patient Protection Alerts

Chapter 2: The X-ray Beam

Beam Filtration
Low-energy photons, created during x-ray production, are unable to penetrate the patient. Patients are protected from unnecessary exposure to this low-energy radiation by having inherent and added filtration in the path of the x-ray beam. (See p. 33)

Chapter 4: Exposure Technique Factors

Excessive Radiation Exposure and Digital Imaging
Although the computer can adjust image brightness for technique exposure errors, routinely using more radiation than required for the procedure in digital radiography unnecessarily increases patient exposure. Even though the digital system can adjust for overexposures, it is an unethical practice to overexpose a patient knowingly. (See p. 83)

kVp/mAs
Whenever possible, a higher kilovoltage and lower mAs should be used to reduce patient exposure. Increasing kilovoltage requires less mAs to maintain the desired exposure to the IR and decreases the radiation dose to the patient. For example, changing from 75 to 86 when imaging a pelvis is a 15% increase in kVp and would require half the mAs needed for the original 75 kVp. Higher kVp increases the beam penetration, and therefore less radiation is needed to achieve a desired exposure to the IR. (See p. 85)

Grid Selection
Decisions regarding the use of a grid and grid ratio should be made by balancing image quality and patient protection. To keep patient exposure as low as possible, grids should be used only when appropriate, and the grid ratio should be the lowest that would provide sufficient contrast improvement. (See p. 99)

Beam Restriction

In performing a radiographic examination, the radiographer should be aware of the anatomic area of interest and limit the x-ray field size to just beyond this area. Collimating to the appropriate field size is a basic method for protecting the patient from unnecessary exposure. (See p. 99)

Chapter 5: Scatter Control

Appropriate Beam Restriction

In performing a radiographic examination, the radiographer should be aware of the anatomic area of interest and limit the x-ray field size to just beyond this area. Collimating to the appropriate field size is a basic method for protecting the patient from unnecessary exposure. (See p. 116)

Limit Field Size to Image Receptor Size

Whether or not automatic collimation is being used, the radiographer should always be sure that the size of the x-ray field is the same as or less than the size of the IR except for digital flat panel detectors. When using a digital flat panel detector, the x-ray field size should be restricted to the anatomic area of interest. These digital IRs are typically one size and, in many instances, larger than the anatomic area of interest. Therefore, it is even more crucial for the radiographer to collimate appropriately for the imaging procedure so that the patient is not unnecessarily exposed to radiation. (See p. 123)

Grid Selection

Decisions regarding the use of a grid and grid ratio should be made by balancing image quality and patient protection. In order to keep patient exposure as low as possible, grids should be used only when appropriate, and the grid ratio should be the lowest that would provide sufficient contrast improvement. (See p. 132)

Grid Errors

A radiographic image that has suboptimal exposure can be the result of many factors, one of which is grid cutoff. Before assuming that an underexposed image is due to technique factors and then reexposing the patient, the radiographer should evaluate grid alignment. If misalignment is the cause of the underexposure, the patient can be protected from reexposure with a technique factor adjustment. (See p. 135)

Chapter 8: Exposure Technique Selection

Kilovoltage Selection

Using higher kVp with AEC decreases the exposure time and overall mAs needed to produce a diagnostic image, significantly reducing the patient's exposure. The kVp selected for an examination should produce the desired image contrast for the part examined and be as high as possible to minimize the patient's radiation exposure. (See p. 203)

Monitoring Backup Time

To minimize patient exposure, the backup time should be neither too long nor too short. Backup time that is too short results in the exposure being stopped prematurely, and the image may need to be repeated because of poor image quality. Backup time that is too long results in the patient receiving unnecessary radiation if a problem occurs and the exposure does not end until the backup time is reached. In addition, the image may have to be repeated because of poor image quality. (See p. 205)

Patient Variability

Factors related to the patient affect the time of exposure reaching the IR and ultimately image quality. Increases or decreases in patient thickness result in changes in the time of exposure if the AEC system is functioning properly. Pathology, contrast media, foreign object, and pockets of gas are patient variables that may affect the proper exposure to the IR and ultimately image quality. (See p. 209)

Anatomically Programmed Radiography and Patient Exposure

When using a preprogrammed set of exposure factors (APR), the radiographer must evaluate the appropriateness of the exposure technique factors selected. Adjustment of the preprogrammed exposure factors may be necessary for that patient or procedure. (See p. 213)

Exposure Technique Charts and Digital Imaging

Exposure technique charts are just as important, if not more so, when using digital IRs. Underexposure or overexposure of a film-screen IR can result in a radiograph with decreased or increased density. Because image brightness is controlled by computer processing, the visual cues for overexposure or underexposure are missing. Exposure technique charts are an effective tool in selecting appropriate exposure techniques for a quality digital image. (See p. 214)

Answer Key for Chapter 9: Image Evaluation

Activity 1

Image Quality
Digital

An optimal digital image of the hip was produced using the following exposure technique:

200 mA	12:1 grid ratio
50 ms	CR image receptor
70 kVp	8 × 12 collimation
40-inch SID	Patient thickness 10 cm
0.6 mm small focal spot	Minimal OID

Without compensation, the proposed changes are made one by one. On the following chart, indicate the effect, if any, each change has on the brightness, contrast, and spatial resolution of the radiographic image.
1. If the image brightness, contrast, or spatial resolution of the image is increased, mark a + in the space provided.
2. If the image brightness, contrast, or spatial resolution of the image is decreased, mark a – in the space provided.
3. If the image brightness, contrast, or spatial resolution of the image is unchanged, mark a 0 in the space provided.

Proposed Individual Change	Brightness	Contrast	Spatial Resolution
85 kVp	0	–	0
1.25 mm focal spot size	0	0	–
45" SID	0	0	+
50 mA @ 0.20 s	0	0	0
Patient thickness 6 cm	0	+	+
Remove grid	0	–	0
Increase OID 4"	0	+	–
14 × 17 collimation	0	–	0

Activity 2

Image Quality
Film

An optimal film radiograph of the pelvis was produced using the following exposure technique:

100 mA
0.5 s
70 kVp
40-inch SID
1.25 mm large focal spot
92° F development temperature
90-second processing time

12:1 grid ratio
400 speed F/S
14 × 17 collimation
Patient thickness 14 cm
Minimal OID

Without compensation, the proposed changes are made one by one. On the following chart, indicate the effect, if any, each change has on the density, contrast, and recorded detail of the radiographic image.
1. If the radiographic density, contrast, or recorded detail of the image is increased, mark a + in the space provided.
2. If the radiographic density, contrast, or recorded detail of the image is decreased, mark a – in the space provided.
3. If the radiographic density, contrast, or recorded detail of the image is unchanged, mark a 0 in the space provided.

Proposed Change	Density	Contrast	Recorded Detail
Increase SID to 48"	–	0	+
Use 200 mAs	+	–	0
Increase kVp to 80	+	–	0
Film/screen relative speed 200	–	0	+
Increase patient thickness to 18 cm	–	–	–
10 × 12 collimation	–	+	0
Change SID to 25"	+	0	–
Use 200 mA @ ¼ s	0	0	0
Development temperature decreased	–	–	0
Patient moves during exposure	0	0	–
17 × 17 collimation	+	–	0
Angle tube 20 degrees	–	0	–
Change to 8:1 grid ratio	+	–	0
Use 50 mA station	–	0	0
Use 0.6 mm focal spot size	0	0	+
Increase OID 3"	–	+	–

Activity 3

Image Quality Calculations

Solve for the missing variable or calculate the new exposure factor to maintain exposure to the image receptor as in the initial exposure technique. Show all calculations.

mAs

mA = 100
time = 0.25 s
mAs = *25*

mA = 500
time = 100 ms
mAs = 50

mA = 50
time = 0.3 s
mAs = 15

$100 \times 0.25 = 25\,\text{mAs}$

$50 \div 0.100 = 500\,\text{mA}$

$15 \div 50 = 0.3\,\text{s}$

15% rule

Initial kVp = 70
Initial mAs = 10
  New kVp = 70 + 15% = **80.5**
New mAs = 5
$70 \times 1.15 = 80.5\,\text{kVp}$
$10 \div 2 = 5\,\text{mAs}$

Initial kVp = 80
Initial mAs = 100
  New kVp = 80 − 15% = **68**
New mAs = **200**
$80 \times 0.85 = 68\,\text{kVp}$
$100 \times 2 = 200\,\text{mAs}$

Initial kVp = 75
Initial mAs = 35
  New kVp = 75 + 2(15%) = **99.19**
New mAs = **8.75**
$75 \times 1.15 = 86.25 \times 1.15 = 99.19\,\text{kVp}$
$35 \div 2 = 17.5 \div 2 = 8.75\,\text{mAs}$

mAs-Distance Conversions

Initial mA = 100
Initial SID = 40″
  New SID = 72″
New mAs = **324**

Initial time = 0.5 s
Initial SID = 60″
  New SID = 25″
New mAs = **0.0868**

Initial mAs = 125
Initial SID = 56″
  New SID = 40″
New mAs = **63.78**

$$\frac{100}{X} = \frac{40^2}{72^2}$$
$1600\,X = 518{,}400$
$X = 324\,\text{mAs}$

$$\frac{0.5}{X} = \frac{60^2}{25^2}$$
$3600X = 312.5$
$X = 0.0868\,\text{s}$

$$\frac{125}{X} = \frac{56^2}{40^2}$$
$3136\,X = 200{,}000$
$X = 63.78\,\text{mAs}$

Grid Conversions

No grid, initial mAs = 10
Add 8:1 grid, new mAs = **40**

12:1 grid, initial mAs = 50
6:1 grid, new mAs = **30**

5:1 grid, initial time = 0.05 s
12:1 grid, new time = **0.125 s**

$$\frac{10}{X} = \frac{1}{4}$$
$X = 40\,\text{mAs}$

$$\frac{50}{X} = \frac{5}{3}$$
$5X = 150$
$X = 30\,\text{mAs}$

$$\frac{0.05}{X} = \frac{2}{5}$$
$2X = 0.25$
$X = 0.125\,\text{s}$

Film-screen Speed (F/s Spd.)

Initial mAs = 25
Initial F/s Spd. = 200
New F/s Spd. = 400
New mAs = **12.5**

$$\frac{25}{X} = \frac{400}{200}; \ 400X = 5,000$$

$$X = 12.5$$

Initial mAs = 10
Initial F/s Spd. = 600
New F/s Spd. = 300
New mAs = 20

$$\frac{10}{X} = \frac{300}{600}; \ 300X = 6,000$$

$$X = 20$$

Initial time = 0.25
Initial F/s Spd. = 100
New F/s Spd. = 50
New time = 0.4 s

$$\frac{0.2}{X} = \frac{50}{100}; \ 50X = 20$$

$$X = 0.4 \text{ s}$$

Activity 4

Image Quality Exposure Conversions

Calculate the new exposure factor to maintain a similar exposure to the image receptor as in the initial exposure technique. Show all calculations.

Initial Digital Exposure Technique
100 mAs
80 kVp
12:1 grid
56-inch SID

TO

New Digital Exposure Technique
40.82 mAs
58 kVp
No grid
40-inch SID

Calculations:

1. *The kVp is decreased by 15% twice and requires an increase in mAs by a factor of 2.*

$$100 \times 2 = 200 \, mAs$$
$$200 \times 2 = 400 \, mAs$$

2. *The grid is removed and requires a decrease in mAs.*

$$\frac{400}{X} = \frac{5}{1}$$
$$5X = 400$$
$$X = 80 \, mAs$$

3. *The SID is decreased and requires a decrease in mAs.*

$$\frac{80}{X} = \frac{56^2}{40^2}$$
$$3136X = 128,000$$
$$X = 40.82 \, mAs$$

Activity 5

Image Quality Exposure Conversions

Calculate the new exposure factor to maintain a similar exposure to the image receptor as in the initial exposure technique. Show all calculations.

Initial Film-Screen Exposure Technique		New Film-Screen Exposure Technique
200 mA		251.4 mA
0.05 s		⅕ s
65 kVp	TO	75 kVp
6:1 grid		8:1 grid
40-inch SID		56-inch SID
400 F/S speed		100 F/S speed

Calculations:

1. *The kVp is increased by 15% and requires a decrease in mAs by a factor of 2:*

$$\frac{10}{2} = 5 \ mAs$$

2. *The grid ratio is increased and requires an increase in mAs:*

$$\frac{5}{X} = \frac{3}{4}$$
$$3X = 20$$
$$X = 6.67 \ mAs$$

3. *The SID is increased and requires an increase in mAs:*

$$\frac{6.67}{X} = \frac{40^2}{56^2}$$
$$1600X = 20917.12$$
$$X = 13.07 \ mAs$$

4. *The film-screen speed is decreased and requires an increase in mAs:*

$$\frac{13.07}{X} = \frac{100}{400}$$
$$100X = 5228$$
$$X = 52.28 \ mAs$$

5. *The new mA needs to be calculated:*

$$\frac{52.28}{0.2} = 261.4 \ mA$$

Image Evaluation

The ability to recognize exposure technique errors and their resultant effect on the radiographic image is an important problem-solving skill. The following exercises provide you an opportunity to apply the knowledge gained from previous chapters in identifying causes of poor-quality images for both digital and film-screen image receptors.

Activity 6

Image Evaluation
Matching:

One of the four computed radiography (CR) images is good quality, whereas the others are results of errors. Match each image with its corresponding statement:

1. Good-quality lateral skull image   <u>D</u>

A.

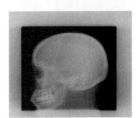

2. Imaging plate placed upside down   <u>A</u>

B.

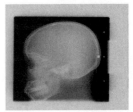

3. Grid placed upside down on imaging plate   <u>B</u>

C.

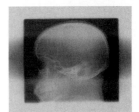

4. Grid removed with mAs adjustment   <u>C</u>

D.

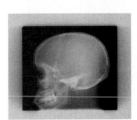

Activity 7

Image Evaluation
Multiple Choice:

Select the most likely exposure technique error responsible for the poor-quality image, and write your answer in the middle column:

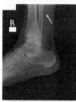

CR image

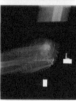

CR image

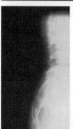

Film-screen AEC image

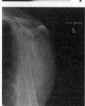

CR image

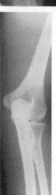

Film-screen image

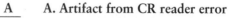

A   A. **Artifact from CR reader error**
B. Excessive fog
C. Insufficient quantity of radiation reaching image receptor
D. Upside-down imaging plate

C   A. Excessive quantity of radiation reaching image receptor
B. Upside-down grid
C. **Double exposure to image receptor**
D. Excessive quantum noise

A   A. **Off-centering using AEC**
B. Too high kVp
C. No grid
D. mA set too low

D   A. Excessive quantity of radiation exposure reaching image receptor
B. Motion unsharpness
C. Excessive collimation
D. **Insufficient quantity of radiation reaching image receptor**

B   A. Excessive fog
B. **Insufficient quantity of radiation reaching image receptor**
C. Too high kVp
D. Excessive quantum noise

Image Analysis

The ability to evaluate image quality and problem solve for improvement involves several skills. Knowledge of how exposure factors affect image quality individually and in combination is the first step to successful problem solving. In addition, the ability to calculate exposure factor changes accurately is necessary to improve image quality.

The following image quality exercises are opportunities to develop problem-solving skills by applying the knowledge learned from the previous chapters.

Activity 8

Image Analysis
Film Image Evaluation: Image Quality Analysis
Radiograph 1
kVp = 70
F/S speed = 400
mAs = 4
Grid ratio = 12:1
SID = 40 inches
Focal spot = small
Optical density = 1.04

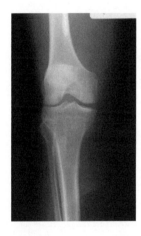

Radiograph 2
kVp = 60
F/S speed = 100
mAs = 6.3
Grid ratio = 6:1
SID = 34 inches
Focal spot = large
Optical density = 0.30

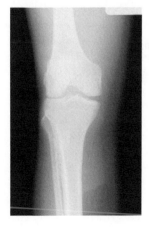

Evaluation:

➤ *Visually compare Radiograph 1 and Radiograph 2, and comment on the quality of the density, contrast, and sharpness of Radiograph 2. State whether Radiograph 2 needs to be repeated and explain why.*

➤ *Evaluate each change in exposure factor, and discuss its appropriateness and how it affected the density, contrast, or sharpness (even if not apparent) of the image and patient exposure.*

➤ *Calculate the appropriate mAs value for each of the cumulative changes to determine why Radiograph 2 displays its level of density, contrast, and sharpness.*

➤ *Identify the correct mAs value that should have been used for each of the exposure factor changes to maintain density as in Radiograph 1. Last, compare the actual mAs used in Radiograph 2 with the calculated mAs value that was needed to maintain density and contrast. In addition, make other exposure factor recommendations to improve the quality of the image.*

Calculate and Respond:

➤ *The kVp decreased by 15% in image 2 and requires an increase in mAs by a factor of 2:*

$$4 \text{ mAs} \times 2 = 8 \text{ mAs}$$

➤ *The SID was decreased from 40 inches to 34 inches, and the mAs would need to decrease:*

$$\frac{8}{X} = \frac{(40)^2}{(34)^2}$$
$$1600X = 9248$$
$$X = 5.78 \text{ mAs}$$

➤ *The film-screen speed was decreased from 400 to 100 and requires an increase in mAs:*

$$\frac{5.78}{X} = \frac{100}{400}$$
$$100X = 2312$$
$$X = 23.12 \text{ mAs}$$

➤ *The grid ratio was changed from a 12:1 to a 6:1, and the mAs would need to decrease:*

$$\frac{23.12}{X} = \frac{5}{3}$$
$$5X = 69.36$$
$$X = 13.87 \text{ mAs}$$

➤ *In comparing Radiograph 2 with Radiograph 1, there is decreased density on Radiograph 2. In the area of interest, Radiograph 2 had an OD of 0.30, which is below the diagnostic range. This image would be considered unacceptable and needs to be repeated because visibility of the area of interest is too low for diagnostic interpretation.*

➤ *Radiograph 2 has a decrease in kVp of 15% (70 to 60), which would decrease the density and increase contrast; an increase in mAs by a factor of 2 would be needed to compensate. The mAs would need to be 8 instead of 4. A kVp of 60 for the knee is lower than needed, which requires more mAs and results in increased patient exposure.*

➤ *The SID was decreased from 40 inches to 34 inches, which would increase the radiation intensity reaching the anatomic part and increase density. The mAs would need to be decreased from 8 to 5.78. Decreasing the SID would also increase magnification and decrease recorded detail in the image.*

➤ *The film-screen speed was decreased from 400 to 100, which would require an increase in mAs from 5.78 to 23.12. Decreasing the film-screen speed would not only increase the recorded detail in the image but also increase patient exposure.*

➤ *The grid was changed to a lower grid ratio from 12:1 to 6:1, which would decrease contrast because more scatter radiation reached the film and density would be increased. Radiographic contrast would be decreased because of the excessive scatter reaching the film. The mAs would need to be decreased to compensate and should have been 13.87 instead of 23.12. Using a lower grid ratio for the knee would decrease patient exposure.*

➤ *Last, a large focal spot was used instead of a small focal spot, and this would decrease recorded detail in the image.*

➤ *After all the changes in exposure factors, Radiograph 2 is too light because 6.3 mAs was used instead of 13.87 mAs. The SID should be 40 inches to improve the sharpness in addition to using a small focal spot. The film-screen speed should be faster to reduce patient exposure.*

Activity 9

Image Analysis
Computed Radiography Image Evaluation (Recommended S number Between 100 and 300)
Radiograph 1
kVp = 81
mAs = 5
Focal spot = small
Grid ratio = 12:1
SID = 40 inches
Central ray perpendicular
S number = 156

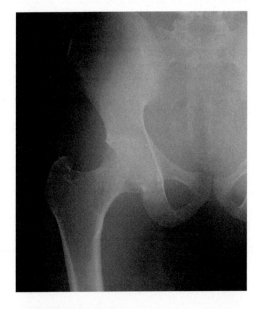

Radiograph 2
kVp = 59
mAs = 1.1
Focal spot = large
Tabletop = no grid
Grid ratio = 6:1
SID = 30 inches
Central ray angled 20 degrees caudad
S number = 620

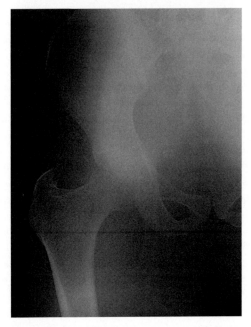

Evaluation:

➤ *Visually compare Radiograph 1 and Radiograph 2, and comment on the quality of the contrast and spatial resolution of Radiograph 2. State whether Radiograph 2 should be repeated and explain why.*

➤ *Evaluate each change in exposure factor, and discuss its appropriateness and how it affected the exposure to the IR, contrast, or spatial resolution (even if not apparent) of the image and patient exposure.*

➤ *Calculate the appropriate mAs value for each of the cumulative changes to determine why Radiograph 2 displays its level of contrast, spatial resolution, and S number.*

➤ *Identify the correct mAs value that should have been used for each of the exposure factor changes to maintain the quality as in Radiograph 1. Last, compare the actual mAs used in Radiograph 2 with the calculated mAs value that was needed to maintain sufficient exposure to the IR. In addition, make other exposure factor recommendations to improve the quality of the image.*

Calculate and Respond:

➤ *The kVp decreased by 15% twice in image 2 and would require an increase in mAs by a factor of 4:*

$$5 \text{ mAs} \times 4 = 20 \text{ mAs}$$

➤ *The SID was decreased from 40 inches to 30 inches, and the mAs would need to decrease:*

$$\frac{20}{X} = \frac{(40)^2}{(30)^2}$$
$$1600X = 18,000$$
$$X = 11.25 \text{ mAs}$$

➤ *The grid ratio was removed, and the mAs would need to decrease:*

$$\frac{11.25}{X} = \frac{5}{1}$$
$$5X = 11.25$$
$$X = 2.25 \text{ mAs}$$

➤ *In comparing Radiograph 2 with Radiograph 1, the densities are similar; however, the contrast is decreased, and there is an increase in quantum noise visible. This image would be considered unacceptable and needs to be repeated because visibility of the area of interest is too low for diagnostic interpretation.*

➤ *Radiograph 2 has a decrease in kVp of 15% twice (81 to 59), which would decrease the exposure to the image receptor and increase contrast; an increase in mAs by a factor of 4 would be needed to compensate. The mAs would need to be 20 instead of 5. A kVp of 59 for the hip is lower than needed, which requires more mAs and results in increased patient exposure.*

➤ *The SID was decreased from 40 inches to 30 inches, which would increase the radiation intensity reaching the anatomic part and image receptor. The mAs would need to be decreased from 20 to 11.25. Decreasing the SID would also increase magnification and decrease spatial resolution in the image.*

➤ *The grid was removed, which would decrease contrast because more scatter radiation reached the image receptor. Radiographic contrast would be decreased because of the excessive scatter reaching the image receptor, adding fog to the image. The mAs would need to be decreased to compensate and should be 2.25 instead of 11.25. A grid should be used with the hip because of the amount of scatter radiation reaching the image receptor. However, removing the grid requires a decrease in mAs, and this would reduce patient exposure.*

➤ *A large focal spot was used instead of a small focal spot, and this would decrease spatial resolution in the image.*

➤ *The central ray was angled 20 degrees caudad, which causes increased shape distortion and decreases the spatial resolution in the image.*

➤ *In comparing the S number between the two images, the S number is increased from 156 in Radiograph 1 to 620 in Radiograph 2. This indicates a low exposure to the image receptor and is outside the recommended range for the hip.*

➤ *After all the changes in the exposure factors, the mAs should have been 2.25 mAs instead of the 1.1 mAs actually used in Radiograph 2. The insufficient exposure to the image receptor is indicated by the high S number. The density was maintained in Radiograph 2 as a result of automatic rescaling during computer processing. The SID should be 40 inches to improve the spatial resolution in addition to using a small focal spot and remove the 20-degree central ray angulation.*

CHAPTER 1: RADIATION AND ITS DISCOVERY

1. B	3. D	5. D	7. B	9. A
2. C	4. A	6. C	8. D	10. C

CHAPTER 2: THE X-RAY BEAM

1. B	4. A	7. D	10. D	13. D
2. D	5. C	8. A	11. C	14. D
3. B	6. A	9. C	12. B	15. A

CHAPTER 3: IMAGE FORMATION AND RADIOGRAPHIC QUALITY

1. D	4. B	7. A	10. C	13. B
2. D	5. D	8. A	11. B	14. D
3. C	6. B	9. C	12. D	15. D

CHAPTER 4: EXPOSURE TECHNIQUE FACTORS

1. D	4. B	7. C	10. B
2. C	5. A	8. D	11. B
3. A	6. C	9. A	12. C

CHAPTER 5: SCATTER CONTROL

1. C	5. B	9. B	13. C	17. C
2. B	6. A	10. A	14. C	18. D
3. D	7. D	11. D	15. A	
4. B	8. D	12. A	16. B	

CHAPTER 6: IMAGE RECEPTORS AND IMAGE ACQUISITION

1. C	4. D	7. A	10. B
2. A	5. C	8. B	11. A
3. D	6. D	9. D	12. D

CHAPTER 7: IMAGE PROCESSING AND DISPLAY

1. C	**4.** D	**7.** D	**10.** B	**13.** A
2. A	**5.** B	**8.** A	**11.** A	**14.** D
3. C	**6.** A	**9.** D	**12.** D	**15.** B

CHAPTER 8: EXPOSURE TECHNIQUE SELECTION

1. B	**4.** D	**7.** B	**10.** B	**13.** B
2. C	**5.** D	**8.** A	**11.** D	**14.** C
3. D	**6.** D	**9.** C	**12.** C	**15.** A

CHAPTER 9: IMAGE EVALUATION

1. C	**3.** A	**5.** C	**7.** A	**9.** A
2. D	**4.** B	**6.** B	**8.** C	**10.** D

CHAPTER 10: DYNAMIC IMAGING: FLUOROSCOPY

1. A	**4.** B	**7.** B	**10.** B	**13.** D
2. D	**5.** D	**8.** B	**11.** B	**14.** B
3. C	**6.** C	**9.** B	**12.** C	**15.** D

CHAPTER 1

Figures 1-1 and 1-3, From *Glasser O: Wilhelm Conrad Roentgen and the early history of the roentgen rays, 1933.*

Figure 1-7, A, Courtesy *Siemens Healthcare, Malvern, Pennsylvania.* B, From *Bontrager K, Lampignano J: Textbook of Radiographic Positioning and Related Anatomy, 7e, St. Louis, 2009, Mosby.*

CHAPTER 2

Figures 2-9, 2-12, 2-14, 2-15, and 2-20, From *Johnston JN, Fauber TL: Essentials of Radiographic Physics and Imaging, St. Louis, 2012, Mosby.*

Figure 2-23, Courtesy *Varian Medical Systems, North Charleston, South Carolina.*

CHAPTER 3

Figures 3-4, 3-27, and 3-28, From *Johnston JN, Fauber TL: Essentials of Radiographic Physics and Imaging, St. Louis, 2012, Mosby.*

Figures 3-9 and 3-18, From *Mosby's Instructional Radiographic Series: Radiographic Imaging, St. Louis, 1998, Mosby.*

Figure 3-19, Modified from *Sprawls P: Physical Principles of Medical Imaging Online, 2e, http://www.sprawls.org/ppmi2/.*

Figure 3-23, From *Frank E, Long B, Smith B: Merrill's Atlas of Radiographic Positioning and Procedures, 12e, St. Louis, 2012, Mosby.*

CHAPTER 4

Figure 4-6 *(left)* and 4-7 *(left)*, From *Johnston JN, Fauber TL: Essentials of Radiographic Physics and Imaging, St. Louis, 2012, Mosby.*

Figures 4-17 and 4-18, From *Frank E, Long B, Smith B: Merrill's Atlas of Radiographic Positioning and Procedures, 12e, St. Louis, 2012, Mosby.*

CHAPTER 5

Figures 5-6 and 5-8, From *Mosby's Radiographic Instructional Series: Radiographic Imaging, St. Louis, 1998, Mosby.*

Figures 5-20, From *Johnston JN, Fauber TL: Essentials of Radiographic Physics and Imaging, St. Louis, 2012, Mosby.*

Figure 5-26, From *Martensen KM: Radiographic Image Analysis, 3e, St.Louis, 2011, Saunders.*

CHAPTER 6

Figure 6-3, From *Bushong SC: Radiologic Science for Technologists, 9e, St.Louis, 2009, Mosby.*

Figures 6-4 and 6-5, Courtesy *Fujifilm Medical Systems, USA, Inc., Stamford, Connecticut.*

Figures 6-10, From *Johnston JN, Fauber TL: Essentials of Radiographic Physics and Imaging, St. Louis, 2012, Mosby.*

Figures 6-12 and 6-13, © 2002 The American Registry of Radiologic Technologists®
The ARRT does not review, evaluate, or endorse publications. Permission to reproduce copyrighted materials within this publication should not be constructed as an endorsement of the publication by the ARRT.

CHAPTER 7

Figures 7-1, 7-2, 7-3, 7-4, 7-5, 7-6, 7-7, 7-13, and 7-14, Modified from *Sprawls P: Physical Principles of Medical Imaging Online, 2e, http://www.sprawls.org/ppmi2/.*

Figure 7-8, Photo courtesy and copyright *Barco.*

Figure 7-10, From *Bushberg J: The Essential Physics of Medical Imaging, 2e, Philadelphia, 2001, Lippincott Williams & Wilkins.*

Figures 7-11 and 7-12, From *Kuni C: Introduction to Computers and Digital Processing in Medical Imaging, Chicago, 1988, Year Book Medical Publishers.*

Figure 7-20, From *Johnston JN, Fauber TL: Essentials of Radiographic physics and imaging, St.Louis, 2012, Mosby.*

CHAPTER 8

Figures 8-1 and 8-7, From *Johnston JN, Fauber TL: Essentials of Radiographic Physics and Imaging, St. Louis, 2012, Mosby.*

Figure 8-6, Courtesy *Philips Healthcare, Andover, Massachusetts.*

CHAPTER 9

Figure 9-8, Activity 7: Figure 1 and Figure 2, Courtesy *Andrew Woodward.*

Activity 7: Figure 5, From *Bontrager K, Lampignano J: Textbook of Radiographic Positioning and Related Anatomy, 7e, St. Louis, 2009, Mosby.*

CHAPTER 10

Figure 10-1, B, From *Bushong SC: Radiologic Science for Technologists, 9e, St. Louis, 2009, Mosby.*

Figure 10-2, Courtesy *Siemens Healthcare, Malvern, Pennsylvania.*

Figures 10-3, 10-4, 10-8, and 10-9, From *Johnston JN, Fauber TL: Essentials of Radiographic Physics and Imaging, St. Louis, 2012, Mosby.*

Figure 10-5, From *Bontrager K, Lampignano J: Textbook of Radiographic Positioning and Related Anatomy, 7e, St. Louis, 2009, Mosby.*

Figure 10-6, A, Courtesy *Philips Healthcare, Andover, Massachusetts.* **B,** From *Curry T, Dowdey J, Murry R: Christensen's Physics of Diagnostic Radiology, 4e, Philadelphia, 1990, Lippincott Williams & Wilkins.*

Figure 10-7, A, Courtesy *Thales Group, Vélizy Villacoublay, France.* **B,** From *Bushberg J: The Essential Physics of Medical Imaging, 2e, Philadelphia, 2001, Lippincott Williams & Wilkins.*

Figure 10-10, From *Eastman Kodak Company, Dayton, Ohio.*

15% rule Rule stating that changing the kilovoltage peak by 15% has the same effect on image receptor exposure as doubling the mAs, or reducing the mAs by 50%.

absorption As the energy of the primary x-ray beam is deposited within the atoms comprising the tissue, some x-ray photons are completely absorbed. Complete absorption of the incoming x-ray photon occurs when it has enough energy to remove (eject) an inner-shell electron.

active layer The radiation-sensitive and light-sensitive layer of the film.

actual focal spot size The size of the area on the anode target that is exposed to electrons from the tube current. Actual focal spot size depends on the size of the filament producing the electron stream.

added filtration The filtration that is added to the port of the x-ray tube.

air gap technique Based on the simple concept that much of the scatter will miss the image receptor if there is increased distance between the patient and the image receptor (increased OID).

ambient lighting The level of light in the room while viewing images.

analog-to-digital converter (ADC) A device that takes the video (analog) signal and divides it into a number of bits (1s and 0s) that the computer "understands."

anatomic programming/anatomically programmed radiography (APR) A radiographic system that allows the radiographer to select a particular button on the control panel that represents an anatomic area; a preprogrammed set of exposure factors is displayed and selected for use.

anode A positively charged electrode within the x-ray tube composed of molybdenum, copper, tungsten, and graphite. It consists of a target and, in rotating anode tubes, a stator and rotor.

anode heel effect The x-ray beam has greater intensity (number of x-rays) on the cathode side of the tube, with the intensity diminishing toward the anode side. The heel effect occurs because of the angle of the target.

aperture diaphragm A flat piece of lead (diaphragm) that has a hole (aperture) in it used for beam restriction.

artifact Any unwanted image on a radiograph.

attenuation Reduction in the energy or number of the primary x-ray beam as it passes through anatomic tissue.

automatic brightness control (ABC) A function of the fluoroscopic unit that maintains the overall appearance of the fluoroscopic image (contrast and density) by automatically adjusting the kilovoltage peak (kVp) or milliamperage (mA) or both.

automatic collimator/positive beam-limiting device Automatically limits the size and shape of the primary beam to the size and shape of the image receptor.

automatic exposure control (AEC) A system used to control the amount of radiation reaching the image receptor consistently by terminating the length of exposure.

automatic film processing The method used to produce a visible permanent image.

automatic film processor A device that encompasses chemical tanks, a roller transport system, and a dryer system for the processing of radiographic film.

automatic rescaling Occurs during histogram analysis and is employed to maintain consistent image brightness despite overexposure or underexposure of the digital image receptor.

backup time The maximum length of time the x-ray exposure continues when using an AEC system.

beam restriction/collimation Interchangeably used terms that refer to a decrease in the size of the projected radiation field.

beam-restricting device Changes the shape and size of the primary beam, located just below the x-ray tube housing.

body habitus Refers to the general form or build of the body, including size. The four types of body habitus are *sthenic, hyposthenic, hypersthenic,* and *asthenic.*

bremsstrahlung interactions Occur when a projectile electron completely avoids the orbital electrons of the tungsten atom and travels very close to its nucleus. The very strong electrostatic force of the nucleus causes the electron suddenly to "slow down." As the electron loses energy, it suddenly changes its direction, and the energy loss reappears as an x-ray photon.

brightness The amount of luminance (light emission) of a display monitor.

brightness gain The product of both flux gain and minification gain; results in a brighter image on the output phosphor.

Bucky Located directly below the radiographic tabletop, the grid is found just above the tray that holds the image receptor. More accurately called the *Potter-Bucky diaphragm.*

Bucky factor/grid conversion factor Used to determine the adjustment in mAs needed when changing from using a grid to nongrid (or vice versa) or when changing to grids with different grid ratios.

caliper A device that measures part thickness.

cathode A negatively charged electrode (within the x-ray tube). It comprises a filament and a focusing cup.

characteristic interactions Produced when a projectile electron interacts with an electron from the inner (K) shell of the tungsten atom and ejects it. An outer-shell electron drops into vacancy and the energy difference is emitted as an x-ray photon.

charge-coupled device (CCD) A light-sensitive semiconducting device that generates an electrical charge when stimulated by light and stores this charge in a capacitor.

coherent scattering An interaction that occurs with low-energy x-rays, typically below the diagnostic range. The incoming photon interacts with the atom, causing it to become exited. The x-ray does not lose energy but changes direction.

collimator Two sets of adjustable lead shutters located 3 to 7 inches below the tube that consist of longitudinal and lateral leaves or blades, each with its own control; this makes the collimator adjustable in terms of its ability to produce projected fields of varying sizes.

comparative anatomy Concept that states different parts of the same size can be radiographed by use of the same exposure factors, provided that the minimum kVp value needed to penetrate the part is used in each case.

compensating filter Special filters added to the primary beam to alter its intensity. These types of filters are used to image anatomic areas that are nonuniform in makeup and assist in producing more consistent exposure to the image receptor.

Compton effect The loss of energy of the incoming photon when it ejects an outer-shell electron from the atom. The remaining lower-energy x-ray photon changes direction and may leave the anatomic part.

Compton electron/secondary electron The ejected electron resulting from the Compton effect interaction.

cone An aperture diaphragm that has an extended flange attached to it. The flange can vary in length and is shaped as a cone. The flange can also be made to telescope, increasing its total length.

contrast medium A substance instilled into the body by injection or ingestion that is used when imaging anatomic tissues that have low subject contrast. Also called *contrast agent.*

contrast resolution   The ability of the image receptor to distinguish between objects having similar subject contrast.

convergent line   If points were connected along the length of the grid, they would form an imaginary line.

convergent point   If imaginary lines were drawn from each of the lead lines in a linear focused grid, these lines would meet to form an imaginary point.

conversion factor   An expression of the luminance at the output phosphor divided by the input exposure rate; its unit of measure is the candela per square meter per milliroentgen per second.

crossed/cross-hatched grid   Grid that has lead lines that run at a right angle to one another. Crossed grids remove more scattered photons than linear grids because they contain more lead strips, oriented in two directions.

cylinder   An aperture diaphragm that has an extended flange attached to it. The flange can vary in length and is shaped as a cylinder.

densitometer   A device used to determine numerically the amount of blackness on the radiograph.

density   The amount of overall blackness of the processed image.

density controls   Controls that allow the radiographer to adjust the amount of preset radiation detection values. Each control changes the exposure time by some predetermined amount or increment.

detectors   The sensors, cells, chambers, or pick-ups within an AEC device that sense how much radiation has reached the imaging plate in order to terminate the exposure.

developing or reducing agents   Agents that reduce exposed silver halide to metallic silver and add electrons to exposed silver halide during film processing.

diagnostic densities   The appropriate range of optical densities.

differential absorption   A process whereby some of the x-ray beam is absorbed in the tissue, and some passes through (transmits) the anatomic part.

digital imaging   An image is constructed from numeric data.

digital imaging and communications in medicine (DICOM)   A communication standard for information sharing between PACS and imaging modalities.

distortion   Results from the radiographic misrepresentation of either the size (magnification) or the shape of the anatomic part.

dosimeter   A device that measures x-ray exposure.

double-emulsion film   Has an emulsion coating on both sides of the base.

dynamic range   Refers to the range of exposure intensities an image receptor can accurately detect.

effective focal spot size   Focal spot size as measured directly under the anode target.

electromagnetic radiation   Radiation that has both electrical and magnetic properties. All radiations that are electromagnetic make up a spectrum.

electronic collimation   Also known as *masking* or *shuttering*. A post-processing function that can remove regions of the digital image.

electrostatic focusing lenses   Focuses and accelerates the electrons through the image intensifier toward the anode.

elongation   Refers to images of objects that appear longer than the true objects.

emulsion   The radiation-sensitive and light-sensitive layer of the film.

exit radiation   When the attenuated x-ray beam leaves the patient, the remaining x-ray beam is composed of both transmitted and scattered radiation.

exposure indicator   A numeric value that is displayed on the processed image to indicate the level of x-ray exposure received to the digital image receptor.

exposure intensity   The amount and energy of the x-rays reaching an area of the image receptor.

exposure technique charts Preestablished guidelines used by the radiographer to select standardized manual or AEC exposure factors for each type of radiographic examination.

exposure time Determines the length of time that the x-ray tube produces x-rays. Exposure time is set by the radiographer and can be expressed in seconds or milliseconds, as either a fraction or a decimal.

extrapolated Mathematically estimated; the mathematical process used to create technique charts.

feed tray A flat metal surface with an edge on either side that permits the film to enter the processor easily and correctly aligned.

filament A coiled tungsten wire that is the source of electrons during x-ray production.

filament current Heats the tungsten filament. This heating of the filament causes thermionic emission to occur.

film speed The degree to which the emulsion is sensitive to x-rays or light. The greater the speed of a film, the more sensitive it is.

fixed kVp/variable mAs technique chart A type of exposure technique chart that is based on the concept of selecting an optimal kVp value that is required for the radiographic examination and adjusting the mAs for variations in part thickness.

fixing agent Clears undeveloped silver halide from the film during processing.

flat panel detectors (FPD) Solid-state image receptors using a large-area active matrix array of electronic components ranging in sizes from 43 × 35 cm to 43 × 43 cm.

fluorescence The ability of phosphors to emit visible light only while exposed to x-rays (with little or no afterglow).

fluoroscopy Allows imaging of the movement of internal structures. It differs from film-screen imaging by its use of a continuous beam of x-rays to create images of moving internal structures that can be viewed on a television monitor.

focal distance The distance between the grid and the convergent line or point; sometimes referred to as *grid radius*.

focal range The recommended range of SIDs that can be used with a focused grid. The convergent line or point always falls within the focal range.

focused grid Grid that has lead lines that are angled, or canted, to match approximately the angle of divergence of the primary beam.

focusing cup Made of nickel and nearly surrounds the filament. It is open at one end to allow electrons to flow freely across the tube from cathode to anode. It has a negative charge, which keeps the cloud of electrons emitted from the filament from spreading apart. Its purpose is to focus the stream of electrons.

fog Scatter exit radiation (Compton interactions) that reaches the image receptor and creates unwanted exposure on the radiographic image.

foreshortening Refers to images that appear shorter than the true objects.

frequency The number of waves passing a given point per given unit of time. Frequency is represented by a lowercase *f* or by the Greek letter *nu (v)*, and values are given in units of Hertz (Hz).

grayscale The number of different shades of gray that can be stored and displayed by a computer system.

grid A device that has very thin lead strips with radiolucent interspaces, intended to absorb scatter radiation emitted from the patient.

grid cap Contains a permanently mounted grid and allows the image receptor to slide in behind it.

grid cassette An image receptor that has a grid permanently mounted to its front surface.

grid cutoff A decrease in the number of transmitted photons that reach the image receptor because of some misalignment of the grid.

grid focus The orientation of the lead lines to one another. The two types of grid focus are parallel (nonfocused) and focused.

grid frequency Expresses the number of lead lines per unit length, in inches or centimeters or both. Grid frequencies can range from 25 to 45 lines/cm (60 to 110 lines/inch).

grid pattern The linear pattern of the lead lines of a grid. The two types of grid pattern are linear and crossed or cross-hatched.

grid ratio The ratio of the height of the lead strips to the distance between them.

half-value layer (HVL) The amount of filtration that reduces the intensity of the x-ray beam to one-half its original value is considered the best method for describing x-ray quality. The HVL also can be used as an indirect measure of the total filtration in the path of the x-ray beam. It is expressed in millimeters of aluminum (mm-Al).

health level seven standard (HL7) A communication standard for medical information.

heat unit (HU) The amount of heat produced from any given exposure.

high contrast A radiograph with few densities but great differences among them is said to have high contrast.

histogram Graphic display of the distribution of pixel values. Each image has its own histogram, and it is evaluated to determine the adequacy of the image receptor exposure to x-rays.

hydroquinone Slow reducer, producing black (higher) densities during film processing.

illuminator Device that provides light illumination so that the anatomy, displayed as various shades of optical densities, can be visualized. Also known as a *viewbox*.

image intensification The process whereby the exit radiation from the anatomic area of interest interacts with a light-emitting material (input phosphor) for conversion to visible light to create a brighter image.

image receptor (IR) A device that receives the radiation leaving the patient.

imaging plate (IP) Located in the CR image receptor, where the photon intensities are absorbed by the phosphor.

immersion heater A heating coil that is immersed in the bottom of the developer and fixer tank. It is thermostatically controlled to heat the developer solution to its proper temperature and maintain that temperature as long as the processor is turned on.

inherent filtration The filtration that is permanently in the path of the x-ray beam. Three components contribute to inherent filtration: (1) the glass envelope of the tube, (2) the oil that surrounds the tube, and (3) the window in the tube housing.

input/output phosphor Phosphors within the image intensifier. The input phosphor converts incoming radiation into visible light energy, and the output phosphor converts the electrons into a brighter image.

intensifying screen A device in radiographic cassettes that contains phosphors that convert x-ray energy into light, which exposes the radiographic film.

intensity of radiation exposure The amount and energy of the x-rays reaching an area of the image receptor.

interspace material Radiolucent strips between the lead lines of a grid; generally made of aluminum.

inverse square law The relationship between distance and x-ray beam intensity, which states that the intensity of the x-ray beam is inversely proportional to the square of the distance from the source.

ionization The ability to remove (eject) electrons; a property of x-rays.

ionization/ion chamber A hollow cell that contains air and is connected to the AEC timer circuit via an electrical wire.

kilovoltage (kVp) Set by the radiographer and applied across the x-ray tube at the time the exposure is initiated, kVp determines the speed at which the electrons in the tube current move.

latent image The invisible image that exists on film after the film has been exposed but before it has been processed.

latent image centers Several sensitivity specks with many silver ions attracted to them.

leakage radiation Any x-rays, other than the primary beam, that escape the tube housing.

line focus principle Describes the relationship between the actual and effective focal spots in the x-ray tube. A smaller target angle produces a smaller effective focal spot.

linear grid Has lead lines that run in only one direction.

long-dimension linear grid Has lead strips running parallel to the long axis of the grid.

long-scale/low contrast A radiograph with a large number of densities but little differences among them is said to have *long-scale or low contrast.*

lookup tables (LUT) Provides a method of altering the image to change the display of the digital image in a variety of ways.

luminescence The emission of light from the screen when stimulated by radiation.

magnification An increase in the image size of the object compared with its true or actual size. Also known as *size distortion.*

magnification factor (MF) Indicates how much size distortion or magnification is shown on a radiograph. MF = SID divided by SOD.

magnification mode Image intensifiers have a multifold function to increase the size of the area of interest displayed on the television monitor. Changing the voltage of the electrostatic focusing lenses tightens the diameter of the electron stream, giving the appearance of magnification.

manifest/visible image The visible image after processing.

mAs/distance compensation formula Formula that provides a mathematical calculation for adjusting the mAs when changing the SID.

mAs readout The actual amount of mAs used for the image is displayed immediately after the AEC exposure, sometimes for only a few seconds.

matrix A digital image is displayed as a combination of rows and columns (array) of small, usually square, "picture elements" called *pixels.*

milliamperage (mA) The unit used to measure the tube current.

minimum response time Refers to the shortest exposure time that the AEC system can produce.

Moiré effect An artifact that can occur when a stationary grid is used during computed radiography (CR) imaging if the grid frequency is similar to the scanning frequency. Also known as the *Zebra pattern.*

object-to-image receptor distance (OID) Distance created between the object radiographed and the image receptor.

off-focus radiation Occurs when projectile electrons are reflected and x-rays are produced from outside the focal spot.

optical density (OD) A numeric calculation that compares the intensity of light transmitted through an area on the film (I_t) to the amount of light originally striking (incident) the area (I_0).

optimal kVp The kVp value that is high enough to ensure penetration of the part but not too high to diminish radiographic contrast.

parallel/nonfocused grid A grid with lead lines that run parallel to one another.

phenidone A fast reducer chemical, producing gray (lower) densities during film processing.

phosphor layer Active layer that is the most important screen component because it contains the phosphor material that absorbs the transmitted x-rays and converts them to visible light.

phosphorescence Occurs when screen phosphors continue to emit light after the x-ray exposure has stopped.

photocathode Converts the visible light in the image intensifier into electrons.

photoelectric effect Complete absorption of the incoming x-ray photon occurs when it has enough energy to remove (eject) an inner-shell electron. The ionized atom has a vacancy, or electron hole, in its inner shell, and an electron from an outer shell drops down to fill the vacancy.

photoelectron The ejected electron resulting from ionization during the photoelectric effect.

photomultiplier (PM) tube An electronic device that converts visible light energy into electrical energy.

photon A small, discrete bundle of energy.

photostimulable luminescence (PSL) The emission of visible light from the photo-stimulable phosphor when stimulated by a high-intensity laser beam.

photostimulable phosphor (PSP) The phosphor layer of the image plate (IP) that is composed of barium fluorohalide crystals doped with europium.

phototimers Use a fluorescent (light-producing) screen and a device that converts the light to electricity in an AEC device.

picture archival and communication system (PACS) A computer system designed for digital imaging that can receive, store, distribute, and display digital images.

pixel The smallest component of the matrix. Also known as *picture elements*.

Pixel bit depth Number of bits that determines the amount of precision in digitizing the analog signal and the number of shades of gray that can be displayed in the image.

pixel density The number of pixels per unit area.

pixel pitch The pixel spacing or distance measured from the center of a pixel to an adjacent pixel.

quantum A small, discrete bundle of energy.

quantum noise Visible as brightness or density fluctuations on the image as a result of too few photons reaching the image receptor to form the image. *Quantum mottle* is the term typically used when referring to noise on a film image.

rare earth elements Chemical compounds of elements that are relatively difficult and expensive to extract from the earth and range in atomic number from 57 to 71 on the periodic table of the elements.

recirculation system Acts to circulate solution in a film processing tank by pumping the solution out of one portion of the tank and returning it to a different location within the same tank from which it was removed.

recorded detail The distinctness or sharpness of the structural lines that make up the recorded image. This is the term that is used in film-screen imaging.

reducing agents Developing agents that reduce exposed silver halide to metallic silver and add electrons to the exposed silver halide during film processing.

relative speed Results from comparing screen-film systems based on the amount of light produced for a given exposure.

remnant radiation When the attenuated x-ray beam leaves the patient, the remaining x-ray beam is composed of both transmitted and scattered radiation. Also known as *exit radiation*.

replenishment The replacement of fresh chemicals after the loss of chemicals during film processing, specifically, developer solution and fixer solution.

resolution   The ability of the imaging system to resolve or distinguish between two adjacent structures. Resolution can be expressed in the unit of line pairs per millimeter (Lp/mm).

rotor   A device in the x-ray tube that causes the target to rotate rapidly during x-ray production.

sampling frequency   How often the analog signal is reproduced in its discrete digitized form.

sampling pitch   The distance between the sampling points.

scale of contrast   The range of densities visible in a film image.

scattering   Some incoming photons are not absorbed but instead lose energy during interactions with atoms comprising tissue.

screen film   Radiographic film sensitive to light emitted by the intensifying screen.

screen speed   The capability of an intensifying screen to produce visible light. The greater the speed, the more sensitive it is.

secondary electron   The ejected electron resulting from the Compton effect interaction. Also known as a *Compton electron*.

short-dimension linear grid   Has lead strips running perpendicular to the long axis of the grid.

short-scale contrast   A film radiograph with few densities but great differences among them is said to have *high contrast*.

SID   The distance between the source of the radiation and the image receptor.

signal-to-noise ratio (SNR)   A method of describing the strength of the radiation exposure compared with the amount of noise apparent in a digital image.

silver halide   Material that is sensitive to radiation and light.

silver recovery   Refers to the removal of silver from used fixer solution.

size distortion/magnification   Refers to an increase in the image size of an object compared with its true, or actual, size.

source-to-object distance (SOD)   Refers to the distance from the x-ray source (focal spot) to the object being radiographed.

space charge   The electrons liberated from the filament during thermionic emission that form a cloud around the filament.

space charge effect   The tendency of the space charge not to allow more electrons to be boiled off of the filament.

spatial resolution   The smallest detail that can be detected in an image; the term typically used in digital imaging.

spectral emission   The color of light produced by a particular intensifying screen.

spectral matching   Correctly matching the color sensitivity of the film to the color emission of the intensifying screen.

spectral sensitivity   The color of light to which a particular film is most sensitive.

standby control   An electric circuit that shuts off power to the roller assemblies when the film processor is not being used.

stator   An electric motor that turns the rotor at very high speed during x-ray production.

subject contrast   A result of the absorption characteristics of the anatomic tissue radiographed along with the quality of the x-ray beam.

target   A metal that abruptly decelerates and stops electrons in the tube current, allowing the production of x-rays.

thermionic emission   The boiling off of electrons from the cathode filament.

tissue density   Matter per unit volume or the compactness of the anatomic particles comprising the anatomic part.

total filtration   The sum of the x-ray tube's added and inherent filtration.

transmission   The incoming x-ray photon passes through the anatomic part without any interaction with the atomic structures.

trough filter   A double-wedge compensating filter added to the primary beam to produce more consistent exposure to the image receptor.

tube current   The flow of electrons from cathode to anode, measured in milliamperage (mA).

values of interest (VOI)   Determines the range of the histogram data set included in the displayed image.

variable kVp/fixed mAs technique chart   A type of exposure technique chart that is based on the concept that kVp can be increased as the anatomic part size increases. The baseline kVp is increased by 2 for every 1-cm increase in part thickness, and the mAs is maintained.

voltage ripple   The amount of consistency in voltage waveforms during x-ray production.

wafer grid   A type of stationary grid placed on top of the image receptor.

wavelength   The distance between two successive crests or troughs.

wedge filter   The most common type of compensating filter. The thicker part of the wedge filter is lined up with the thinner portion of the anatomic part that is being imaged, allowing fewer x-ray photons to reach that end of the part.

window level   Sets the midpoint (center) of the range of brightness visible in the digital image.

window width   The range or number of shades of gray visible on the digital image.

x-ray emission spectrum   The range and intensity of x-rays emitted.

Page numbers followed by *f* indicate figures; *t,* tables; *b,* boxes.